# Sports
# Medicine

## FITNESS · TRAINING · INJURIES

Second Edition

# Sports Medicine

## FITNESS · TRAINING · INJURIES

Second Edition

Edited by
Otto Appenzeller, M.D., Ph.D.
and
Ruth Atkinson, M.D.

University of New Mexico
School of Medicine
Albuquerque

Urban & Schwarzenberg
Baltimore-Munich 1983

Urban & Schwarzenberg, Inc.
7 E. Redwood Street
Baltimore, Maryland 21202
USA

Urban & Schwarzenberg
Pettenkoferstrasse 18
D-800 München 2
West Germany

Printed in the United States of America

## NOTICES

The Editors (or Author(s)) and the Publisher of this work have made every effort to ensure that the drug dosage schedules herein are accurate and in accord with the standards accepted at the time of publication. The reader is strongly advised, however, to check the product information sheet included in the package of each drug he or she plans to administer to be certain that changes have not been made in the recommended dose or in the contraindications for administration.

The Publishers have made an extensive effort to trace original copyright holders for permission to use borrowed material. If any have been overlooked, it will be corrected at the first reprint.

**Library of Congress Cataloging in Publication Data**

Sports medicine.
  Includes index.
  1. Sports medicine. 2. Physical fitness. 3. Physical education and training. I. Appenzeller, Otto. II. Atkinson, Ruth R. [DNLM: 1. Athletic injuries. 2. Sport medicine. QT 260 S7648]
RC1210.S686 1983     617'.1027     83-3471
ISBN 0-8067-0132-3 (pbk.)

Compositor: Graphic Arts Composition
Printer: Port City Press
Manuscript editor: Molly Ruzicka
Indexer: Susan Lohmeyer
Production and design: John Cronin

ISBN 0-8067-0132-3 Baltimore

ISBN 3-541-70132-3 Munich

Dedicated
to the Memory of
Papa (1899-1980)
Who Inspired Us
by Example

# Contents

## Section 1
## The Nervous System
## and Sports

## Section 2
## Nutritional and
## Gastrointestinal Aspects
## and Sports

## Section 5
## Locomotion and Sports

# Contributors

**Bob Anderson**
P.O. Box 767
Palmer Lake, Colorado 80133

**Otto Appenzeller**, M.D., Ph.D.
Professor of Neurology and Medicine
University of New Mexico
    School of Medicine
Albuquerque, New Mexico 87131

**Ruth Atkinson**, M.D.
Associate Professor of Neurology
    and Pediatrics
University of New Mexico
    School of Medicine
Albuquerque, New Mexico 87131

**Robert L. Bergman**, M.D.
Harborview Community Mental Health Center
326 Ninth Avenue
Seattle, Washington 98104

**Maire T. Buckman**, M.D.
Associate Professor of Medicine/Endocrinology
University of New Mexico
    School of Medicine
Chief of Endocrinology
Veterans Administration
    Medical Center
Albuquerque, New Mexico 87108

**Karen A. Carlberg**, Ph.D.
Department of Physiology
University of Florida College of Medicine
Gainesville, Florida 32610

**Thomas J. Carlow**, M.D.
Clinical Associate Professor of
    Neurology/Neurophthalmology
University of New Mexico
    School of Medicine
7000 Cutler N.E., Suite E7
Albuquerque, New Mexico 87110

**Thomas W. Chick**, M.D.
Associate Professor of Internal Medicine
University of New Mexico
    School of Medicine
Chief, Pulmonary Function Lab
Veterans Administration
    Medical Center
Albuquerque, New Mexico 87108

**R. Philip Eaton**, M.D.
Professor of Medicine
Chief, Division of Endocrinology
    and Metabolism
University of New Mexico
    School of Medicine
Albuquerque, New Mexico 87131

**Dale G. Erickson**, M.D.
Renal Medicine Associates, Ltd.
201 Cedar Southeast, Suite 409
Albuquerque, New Mexico 87106

**Art Gardenswartz**
4410 Menaul Boulevard N.E.
Albuquerque, New Mexico 87110

**Jerry E. Goss**, M.D.
Director, Cardiovascular Laboratory
New Mexico Heart Institute
Presbyterian Hospital Center
Albuquerque, New Mexico 87106

**Vivian H. Heyward**, Ph.D.
Associate Professor of Physical Education
Department of Health, Physical Education,
   and Recreation
University of New Mexico
Albuquerque, New Mexico 87131

**Philip L. Hooper**, M.D.
Assistant Professor of Medicine
University of New Mexico
   School of Medicine and
   Veterans Administration Medical Center
Albuquerque, New Mexico 87108

**Ernst Jokl**, M.D.
Professor of Exercise Physiology Emeritus and
   Professor of Neurology
University of Kentucky
   Medical School
Lexington, Kentucky 40506

**Neil I. Kaminsky**, M.D., F.A.C.P.
Encino Medical Plaza, Suite 9
717 Encino Place N.E.
Albuquerque, New Mexico 87102

**Carol A. Kresge**, MsT.
New Mexico School of
   Natural Therapeutics
106 Girard S.E., Suite 107
Albuquerque, New Mexico 87106

**Ron Lawrence**, M.D., Ph.D.
President
American Medical Joggers Association
P.O. Box 4704
North Hollywood, California 91607

**Barry R. Maron,** M.D.
8324 Constitution Place, NE
Albuquerque, New Mexico 87110

**William J. O'Brien**, Ph.D.
Assistant Professor/Orthopaedics
Chief, Division of Physical Therapy
University of New Mexico
   School of Medicine
Albuquerque, New Mexico 87131

**Robert M. Parks**, D.P.M.
Albuquerque Associated Podiatrists
121 Sycamore Street N.E.
Albuquerque, New Mexico 87106

**Glenn T. Peake**, M.D.
Professor of Medicine
Director, Clinical Research Center
University of New Mexico
   School of Medicine
Albuquerque, New Mexico 87131

**Jonathan M. Samet**, M.D.
Associate Professor of Medicine
University of New Mexico
   School of Medicine
Albuquerque, New Mexico 87131

**David S. Schade**, M.D.
Associate Professor of Medicine
Division of Endocrinology and Metabolism
University of New Mexico
   School of Medicine
Albuquerque, New Mexico 87131

**William R. Schiller**, M.D.
Professor of Surgery
Director, Burn and Trauma Unit
University of New Mexico
   School of Medicine
Albuquerque, New Mexico 87131

**William Selezinka**, M.D., M.S., F.A.C.S.
7349 Via Paseo del Sur
Scottsdale, Arizona 85258

**Nicholas A. Volpicelli**, M.D.
Presbyterian Professional Building
201 Cedar S.E., Suite 409
Albuquerque, New Mexico 87106

**Stephen C. Wood**, Ph.D.
Associate Professor of Physiology
University of New Mexico
   School of Medicine
Albuquerque, New Mexico 87131

# Foreword

Interest in sports medicine has grown exponentially during the last decade. Traditionally, orthopaedic surgeons rendered aid to athletes. Now, however, physicians in various specialties are involved in athletic medicine. The multidisciplinary approach to treatment and health maintenance of athletes is an accepted fact. The editors of this book have provided a guide for interested physicians and medical students who have difficulty finding information "under one roof." As President of the American Medical Joggers Association and consultant to the United States Olympic Committee, I receive many letters requesting information on how to learn more about sports medicine. Until the appearance of this volume, it was difficult for me to direct these inquiries to a single source for information.

During the last decade, the evolution of new interest in sports medicine has been spectacular. Internists, cardiologists, family practitoners, pediatricians, and even dermatologists all may be involved with athletes. The large number of Americans who participate in sports is well known. The President's Council on Physical Fitness and the Department of Commerce estimate that there are twenty-five million Americans who are jogging or running. Similar figures are thought to apply to other sports.

In the past, orthopaedists treated mainly professional, high school or college athletes. The sports physician today, however, is called upon to treat large numbers of participants in activities ranging from racquet ball and tennis to baseball and soccer. Physical activity of some sort is now the rule for over one hundred million Americans. The medical management of athletes requires not only basic orthopaedics but an even greater understanding of general medical principles as applied to athletes. For example, the United States Olympic team physicians treat far more upper respiratory illness than orthopaedic injuries and an estimated eighty-five percent of athletes reporting for aid at an Olympic event do so for reasons other than musculoskeletal problems. The sports physician should, therefore, have a thorough grasp of many areas of medicine, including, of course, orthopaedics, all of which are touched upon in this book.

Norms accepted for the general population do not always apply to athletes. New standards of physical measures and laboratory values are being established. What might have been considered abnormal in an athlete several years ago is now understood to be physiologic. Athletics offers an area for challenging medical research where physiologic adaptations to physical and mental stress can be observed. Results of this research will ultimately be valuable to all individuals, be they healthy or sick.

Sports physicians are often called upon to give nutritional advice to athletes. An understanding of nutritional principles is, therefore, vital. Basic cardiology for competence in cardiac rehabilitation programs, and even ingenuity to unravel dermatologic problems in athletes, are all necessary for competence in sports medicine. Thousands of physicians treat athletes today in high schools, colleges, universities, and in their daily practice. Many are doing an excellent job, but most wish they had some formal background for this task. The sponsors of this series of lectures on sports medicine at the University of New Mexico School of Medicine have tried to give status to sports medicine within the medical curriculum commensurate with the importance of the discipline in health maintenance.

**Ronald M. Lawrence**

# Preface
## to the Second Edition

When King George III confronted the historian Gibbon, who had just completed another book, he remarked, "Scribble, scribble, scribble, eh, Mr. Gibbon? Another fat book, eh, Mr. Gibbon?" What are the justifications for continuously adding to the already gigantic piles of books in print? Is it possible that one is attempting to intrude into libraries without first asking permission to enter? But, publishers are not in the charitable business, and new editions appear because old ones have sold out or have become obsolete. Sports medicine is rapidly evolving, and interest in this country in providing training in this all-embracing discipline has quickened with the advent of participant rather than observational athletic activities. Justification for the Second Edition lies in the success of the first and in heeding the constructive criticism from many quarters which has been incorporated into the new version. The contributors to the new edition attest to the holistic nature of sports medicine and should make this volume more useful for students and practitioners who have little contact with other than the medical aspects of sports.

The importance and limitation of sports medicine must be reassessed in order to appreciate the value of this clinical branch of medicine in promoting a desirable lifestyle, in preventing disease, and in enhancement of ethical values, particularly as they pertain to the training of physicians and of athletes themselves. It is important to document the value of exercise and athletics not only for the young, as it was done in the past, but also its possible implication in maintenance of health in large segments of our aged, but otherwise healthy, population.

These as yet not widely recognized influences of sports medicine have led to the inclusion of new chapters into this volume in the hope that those for whom this book is intended will find it all-encompassing and a source of existing knowledge supported by adequate scientific investigation and of hypotheses which might stimulate further research in this important new field.

The editors share the enthusiastic interest of the contributors for the physiologic and clinical effects of athletic endeavors, but sports will also have an important impact on the quality of life to which physicians and others working in the field of health maintenance have contributed in the past and hopefully will continue to do so in the future.

Spring 1983                                                                    **Otto Appenzeller**
**Ruth Atkinson**

# Preface
## to the First Edition

Writings on sports medicine are not new and are best exemplified by Pindar who wrote poems in honor of Greek Olympic winners and to whom we are indebted for the maxim, "A happy state of mind is the best doctor." Unfortunately, since Pindar's time the literature on sports medicine has not kept pace with the growth of knowledge concerning athletic training and performance. Publications on the effects of sports on health of large populations heretofore not athletically inclined have been scarce. With resurgence of active participation in sports by huge numbers bent on improving their appearance and well-being and perhaps extending their life span, sports medicine has become a respectable subject for study, and knowledge of its scientific basis is necessary for the practice of medicine and of "primary care."

Formal courses on sports medicine are not standard in most medical schools in this country. Proponents of several specialties whose interests include a number of body systems have contributed to this book, thus emphasizing the holistic nature of sports medicine. This all-embracing specialty has a pervasive role in health maintenance, and its contribution to a happy and productive life, though not yet fully documented, is, nevertheless, alluded to by some contributors. The interest and enthusiasm of multitudes for unaccustomed physical activity has led to an increase in "injuries" attributable to overuse, which are no longer the exclusive province of the surgeon trained in orthopedics who is physician for a team involved in contact sports. Moreover, increasing recommendation of physical activity in treating and preventing certain diseases has made it necessary for primary care providers to learn how to use this valuable new tool.

Without formal teaching of sports medicine, most physicians are not able to assess the value of claims made for or against physical activity in the treatment and prevention of disease. This has led to proliferation of "health providers" who are not medically trained and who enthusiastically employ new physical methods and sports.

For these reasons the University of New Mexico School of Medicine has offered medical students a structured curriculum in sports medicine, for which this book is a text. We hope that the diversity of contribution and the review of knowledge accumulated about the effects of sports on the human body will help students and physicians acquire the knowledge necessary to deal with the newly created demand for expertise in this field.

Spring 1981

**Otto Appenzeller**
**Ruth Atkinson**

# Acknowledgments

Nature has implanted egomania in certain persons in order to "get things done" and perhaps prevent baboons from inheriting the earth. But, what is invariably forgotten is that doers never do things alone. Those egomaniacs who see their work eventually published depend largely on a number of "saints" who live their lives doing their duty without writing books or otherwise making much noise. We, like others of our kind, take advantage of these usually nameless people, but wish to mention them here in the hope that those who take the time to read this will share our indebtedness.

Katherine Miller has devoted herself to details and administrative tasks beyond the capacity of the editors, and, of course, the staff of Urban & Schwarzenberg, particularly Ms. Nan Curtis Tyler and John Cronin, have given more than is customarily required. Without their labors, readers would not see the Second Edition before it is outdated. With their help, we have managed to produce this volume while it is still relevant and useful.

# Chapter 1

# Introduction: Medicine, Science, and Sports

by Ernst Jokl

To understand the explosive development of the international sports movement, consideration must be given to a number of historically unique changes that occurred during the past century. Some of these changes are of a social nature; others were engendered by the revolutionary advancements of science and technology. The result is the establishment of standards of growth, health, and fitness that never before existed.

## Child Labor

Until the end of the last century, child labor was prevalent throughout Europe. It was a curse that originated with the invention of machinery. A horde of workless, starving vagrants flocked from the countryside into the towns. Children were driven by the poverty of their parents into factories and mines. Child-slaves, orphaned and friendless, were supplied in droves by the workhouses to employers. Children as young as even 3 years of age spent 12 hours at a time in the darkness of the mines.

Lord Shaftesbury was among the most active proponents of reforms. "Never," he said in a parliamentary debate on child labor in the House of Commons, "have I seen such a display of selfishness, frigidity to every human sentiment, such ready and happy self-delusion."

In 1859, children less than 10 years old and girls and women were excluded altogether from the mines, but it was not until 1875 that employment of boy chimney sweepers was prohibited. The 1870s saw compulsory free education established throughout Great Britain, and thus a barrier was interposed between children and the factories. In the same decade the first kindergartens were introduced. The Society for the Prevention of Cruelty to Children, founded in 1872, took the initiative in promulgating progressive social legislation. It goes without saying that children until then had been in poor health, neither willing nor able to engage in sport.

1

# Leisure

To understand why, during the past decades, sports have become one of the major leisure pursuits of human beings, it must be realized that the concepts of both leisure and sport have only recently assumed their present meaning. The idea that time for leisure would be available to the ordinary individual sounded revolutionary not so long ago, when the worker, unless he or she was working, rested to recuperate from and gather new strength for work. The boys and girls who slaved in coal mines and textile mills around the middle of the 19th century had neither the time nor the strength to play. Their situation, as well as that of their elders, was incomparably worse than the conditions prevailing during the preceding millennium, in the relatively stable, predominantly rural village environment throughout Western Europe.

# Health

That medicine would ever become a science was beyond imagination only a few centuries ago. For example, consider the gorgeous portrait of Louis XIV (1638–1715) by Hyacinthe Rigaud. It shows the grand monarch in his ermine-lined robes of state, scepter in hand, arm on hip, gazing out on the world with affable condescension and consummate poise. We see the epitome of majesty: grace, dignity, command. It is disillusioning to turn to the king's private life, as described by his doctors. A new and disconcertingly human figure emerges, a man plagued by chronic infirmities of all kinds, pestered by doctors and surgeons, subjected to incredible purges, enemas, and emetics. The health of even the humblest citizen today is infinitely better protected than was that of "The Sun King" 300 years ago. Throughout his reign Louis XIV was attended by three "premier médicins" who kept a *Journal de la Santé du Roi*. It describes the illnesses of the royal patient: "rheumatism, vapors, humors, fistula, insomnia, indigestion, fluxes, headaches, chronic fevers, anthrax, melancholy, urinary difficulties, night sweats, vertigo, erysipelas, colds, colic, bile, acid mouth, chronic toothaches," and inevitably, "a great deal of gout." It is not difficult to understand why, as his biographer Philippe Aries mentions, "Louis XIV showed a marked lack of enthusiasm for tennis."

# Military Recruits 1790–1819

To assess the extent to which physique, strength, and fitness of the present generation of youths in the United States and Europe have benefited from the advancements of science and technology, one must evaluate the status of young people two centuries ago. A book entitled *The Enlistings, Discharging and Pensioning of Soldiers During the Years 1790–1819*, published in 1839 by Henry Marshall, Deputy Inspector-General of British Army Hospitals, describes that the 100,000 men who during that period enlisted on a long service contract of 21 years were a miserable lot: For a regiment, recruited in 1797 at Cork for embarkation to Buenos Aires, minimum weight was 116 lb 9 oz (52 kg), minimum height 5 ft 5½ in (1.66 m). Every recruit who complied with these standards was accepted, irrespective of his age. In the French Army, minimum weight was 110 lb (50 kg), minimum height 5 ft 2 in (1.575 m). (In the United States today, many schoolchildren 12 years of age would thus have qualified for acceptance!) At that time, every conceivable disease—epilepsy, palsy, insanity, rheumatism, hernia, blindness, ulcerations, etc.—was either simulated or intentionally reproduced in attempts to avoid army service. Nor did lashes deter malingerers from their set purpose. Hernias were produced by incising the scrotum, inserting the stem of a clay pipe, and with the assistance of a pal, blowing until the skin was as tight as a drum. Men were quite prepared to lose the sight of one eye if it could get them their discharge. This was done by the application of a caustic, by scraping the surface of the cornea, or by piercing it with a sharp needle and scratching the lens to cause cataracts.

# Nutrition

The means to conquer hunger and malnutrition is but a recent triumph of science. The role of vitamins as essential elements of a good diet was unknown until the beginning of this century. In 1913 Sir John Boyd-Orr assessed the incidence of rickets in Glasgow, Scotland: 40% of the city's school population was afflicted. In a repeat survey in 1936, only 10% of the children in Glasgow had rickets. Vitamin D had been identified by Adolf Windaus of Goettingen who was awarded a Nobel Prize in 1928. The Glasgow study was repeated once more in 1965, when not a single case of rickets was found among children born in Glasgow. However, the incidence of rickets among Asian immigrants to England today is comparable to that found in Glasgow in 1913. Malnutrition is still widespread in Asia and Africa, whereas in affluent societies obesity has become a major health problem.

# Infectious Diseases

The greatest single contribution of medical research to society is that it has brought infectious diseases under control. In 1900, infectious diseases were responsible for most deaths in the United States. Throughout the preceding centuries no family was spared the sorrow of children dying from "fevers." In his Johann Sebastian Bach Memorial Lecture delivered at Hamburg in 1950, Paul Hindemith mentioned that Bach lost 11 children during his life. Today, few children die during infancy. The chief causes of death in the United States are no longer infectious diseases but cardiovascular afflictions, malignant tumors, accidents, and crime. The length of life has increased from 48 years in 1898 to 70 years today. Whooping cough, diphtheria, smallpox, and poliomyelitis were brought under control only after World War II.

# Acceleration of Growth

Against the background of such changes as the foregoing, the favorable status of children today must be assessed. Today's boys and girls are taller and stronger than their parents and grandparents. An average-sized high-school boy aged 17 does not fit into the armor of Elizabethan knights in the Tower of London. There has been a steady acceleration of growth and maturation over the centuries, with a noticeable spurt during the past decades. One manifestation of this spurt is the appearance today of children and adolescents in sports such as swimming, gymnastics, ice-skating, and other athletic disciplines. Children now run the 26-mile marathon, climb the highest mountains, and participate in long-distance ski races. In 1979, two 12-year-old boys swam the English Channel; at the Pan African Track and Field Games in Nairobi in July, 1979, a 12-year-old girl won the 1500-m final against adult competition.

The corresponding opposite to the acceleration of growth is a deceleration of aging, a phenomenon representing the physiologic basis for the participation of large numbers of senior men and women in a great variety of sporting events. At the Montreal Olympic Games in 1976, more than 400 athletes over 40 years of age entered the competitions, several of them with conspicuous success. At Moscow in 1980, the number of senior Olympians was even greater.

# Women in Sports

The athletic status of women reflects the far-reaching changes that have taken place in the Western world during this century. The unfolding of the "power potential of the Second Sex" is still in progress, even though the scientific evidence on women's physical performance capacities was available long before it was applied in practice.

"A horse sweats, a man perspires, but a lady only glows." This statement illustrates the general attitude toward exercise and athletics for girls during the Victorian age. Since then, social attitudes have changed profoundly. During the past 50 years, millions of women have indulged in sports, gymnastics and games; competed in swimming, track and field events, and in horseback riding; climbed many of the highest mountains; and swum through a thousand rivers and lakes. Participation in such activities has given women some of the most valuable experiences of their lives. All the evils of which they had been warned have been conspicuous by their absence. The women have not developed a masculine appearance; most of them marry and have children. None suffer physical damage or "over-strain," from muscular exertion; their hearts have not been "weakened through athletics;" and most of them attain a ripe old age.

That the present generation of women grows stronger, that their physical maturation is better balanced and their appearance more attractive, that the health of young mothers and their children today is superior, that physically active women no longer look old at the age of 30, and that many schoolgirls play on the same team as their mothers—all these facts are, at least in part, the result of the interest now taken in the physical education of girls.

Sports and games and athletics for women are significant elements of that which many consider best in contemporary culture.

The role of women in sport was discussed in antiquity. In Plato's *Republic,* Socrates raises the question whether "females should guard the flock and hunt with males and take a share in all they do, or be kept within doors as fit for no more than bearing and feeding their children while all the hard work is left to the males." Socrates' brother, Glaucon, agreed that "women are expected to take their full share, except that we must treat them as not quite so strong." The two disputants concurred that both men and women ought to receive the same upbringing and education. Such a system, Socrates remarked, would at first appear revolutionary, but he pointed out that "it is not so long since the Greeks thought it ridiculous as well as shameful for men to be seen naked in the gymnasium. When gymnastic exercises were first introduced in Crete and later in Sparta, the cynics had their chance to make fun of them." But, he observed, "a new attitude was soon accepted and it will be the same once women are given equal access to physical education."

However, Plato was concerned with the education of an elite, a selected group of leaders of proven excellence of character, mind, and body. Thus, he argued logically that once the principle of selection is recognized and the wide scope of individual differences among men and women accepted, a distinction between the educational systems for boys and girls is no longer justified.

The fact that well-trained women athletes are superior to untrained men in all branches of sport signifies a revolutionary change in society's attitude toward the female. Views held, until recently, that menstruation, pregnancy, childbearing, and menopause prohibit females from participation in sports were shown to be false.

In several athletic disciplines, women's performances at present are equal to those of men. In terms of aesthetic criteria, women athletes rank above men, e.g., in gymnastics and ice-skating. The magnitude of physical educability of women is much greater than was assumed until recently: A young woman became champion of the State of Washington in weight lifting in the flyweight class (52 kg), winning the event against male competitors. Few, if any, men could have beaten Olga Korbut and Nadja Comaneci on the uneven parallel bars and the balance beam in 1972 and 1976. The 400-m running world record of 48.6 sec established by Marita Koch in 1980 is remarkable. At several marathon races held in the United States, over 1,000 women started; 96% of them finished. The current women's world record of 2 h 27 min is about equal to, or faster than, most Olympic winning times by men prior to World War II. Most of the best women athletes in 1981 would have won the respective track and field events for men at Olympic games a few decades ago: Marita Koch (400-m, 48.6 sec); Tatyana Zelentsova (400-m hurdles, 54.89 sec); Evelin Jahl (discus, 70.72 m); Ruth Fuchs (javelin, 69.16 m); Sara Simeoni (high jump, 2.01 m) and Rosemarie Ackermann (2.00 m); Grazyna Rabsztyn (100-m hurdles, 12.48 sec) and Johanna Klier (12.62 sec).

# Athletic Records

The chief elements from which all physical performances are synthesized have been identified through scientific analyses of athletic records. The world's best performances in sport have been documented since the beginning of this century, some of them longer. It has thus been possible to construct growth curves of world records for all sports events, including those held at Olympic Games. From them, the magnitude of the performance explosion during the past decades in all branches of sport can be assessed. However, rates of performance growth differ for different athletic disciplines. In swimming, performance growth continues, whereas in the short- and middle-distance track, the steep ascent of record growth curves is about to come to an end. In a few events, terminal positions have already been reached: The probability is not great that Bob Beamon's long-jump record of 29 ft 2.5 in (8.9 m) established in Mexico City in 1968 will be improved by much. Altogether, it is not generally realized that "the expanding athletic universe" is bound to reach its limits.

# Unexplored Resources

As to the future of athletic records, it must be taken into account that the advancements of science and technology that, in many areas of the world, have eradicated hunger and controlled infectious diseases have not yet benefited more than a quarter of the human race. The medical status of most populations of Asia and Africa today is no better than it was in Europe during the Middle Ages. The extent to which infectious diseases affect the physical status of entire ethnic groups became evident during the past 20 years in East Africa when smallpox was eradicated through the introduction of vaccination. Only then did Hamitic athletes from Tanzania, Ethiopia, and Kenya appear on the international athletic scene. Their conspicuous successes at the 1972 Olympic Games established their countries as major track and field powers. Their status will continue to gain as further public health measures are effective. A worldwide upgrading of all sports performances is bound to occur when the results of preventive and curative measures that are currently being introduced by the World Health Organization throughout the Third World become effective. The issue has wide implications.

Generally held beliefs that medical science has conquered most of our great killer diseases are fallacious. In the *Listener* of August 9, 1979, Brian J. Ford pointed out:

> We cannot yet reliably cure any virus disease and know next to nothing of the cause or cure of a host of major scourges, from cancer and coronary heart attacks to schizophrenia, arthritis, strokes and the degenerative diseases, from cystic fibrosis to Huntington's chorea. The tropical diseases alone, from schistosomiasis and river blindness to an array of worm parasites and the trypanosomes which waste the body, afflict hundreds of millions of people.

During the next two decades, public health measures are likely to reduce the incidence of all diseases everywhere. A worldwide advancement in growth and development should thus occur and from it further improvements of all athletic records. Considering the achievements of medical research so far, such forecasts seem justified.

Technologic innovations will continue to play an important role in the athletic performance explosion of our century. The introduction of Tartan tracks, newly designed javelins and discuses, fiber glass poles, and foam rubber mats have noticeably altered the entire track and field scene. The temperature control of swimming pools, improved filtration systems, establishment of smooth water surfaces through vertical lane markers, have facilitated achievement of new swimming records. The availability of large indoor facilities, such as the air-conditioned Astrodome in Houston and the Louisiana Superdome in New Orleans, has opened vistas not yet fully explored, e.g., that of creating optimal temperatures and other advantageous environmental conditions for individual athletic events throughout the year.

Last but not least, the fact that numbers of participants in all sports are continually increasing throughout the world renders probable the appearance from time to time of "athletic geniuses" and thus the establishment of extraordinary records—the phenomenon of Bob Beamon is likely to recur, at some future date, in other athletic disciplines.

# The Fields Beyond

Once the limits of physical performance growth are reached, a chief objective of athletics will be to explore the aesthetic possibilities that are inherent in sports—possibilities derived from the inexhaustible choice of designs of expression and communication of human movements.

In a few decades from now, the athletic situation will be comparable to that of oil painting in the middle of the 17th century, of the ballet prior to World War I, and of piano music during the 1920s.

The development of oil painting extended over the better part of two centuries, starting in the 15th century with Jan van Eyck's search for a varnish that would dry without being put in the sun; his discovery was subsequently elaborated by Giovanni Bellini, from whom Albrecht Dürer learned the technique he applied in his masterpiece *The Four Apostles*. Oil painting reached its ultimate perfection with Diego Velazquez, Jan Breughel, and Peter Paul Rubens.

The technical possibilities of the ballet were explored during the early years of our century when Serge Diaghilev presented his Ballet Russe in Paris, with Michel Fokine as choreographer, Vaslav Nijinsky, Anna Pavlova, and Tamara Karsavina as dancers; and Picasso, Derain, and Benois as "decorators." From it emerged Émile Jaques-Dalcroze's *Musical Calisthenics,* Claude Achille Debussy's *Dance Plays,* Richard Strauss's *Joseph's Legende,*and, most recently, John Cranko's *Stuttgart Ballet.*

Piano technique as we know it started with Beethoven's use of the hammerklavier and its exploration through his pupil, Carl Czerny, who became the teacher of Franz Liszt. To Liszt's Weimar school belonged Eugen d'Albert and Ferruccio Busoni, under whose direction Egon Petri acquired the ultimate level of keyboard mastery equaled but not surpassed by today's great pianists, not even Vladimir Horowitz, Rudolf Serkin, Sviatoslav Richter, or Benedetti Michelangeli.

When the history of gymnastics is written, the names of Olga Korbut, Nadja Comaneci, Nelli Kim, and their teachers will rank in the chronology of the subject like those to whom the arts are indebted for the technical perfection of painting, dancing, and music.

Through the unprecedented differentiation of the motor system that physical performance in all its manifestations is able to accomplish, sport is destined to reveal its powers of experience and communication and thus create a new culture—the third culture, if one considers the humanities and the natural sciences first and second.

The number of those who will take full advantage of this "third culture" will remain limited, just as the number of those who realize the aesthetic and intellectual possibilities of the arts and sciences remains limited. The pursuit of excellence in all its forms has always been entrusted to an elite in the sense defined by Lord Kenneth Clark:

> If you don't have an elite in some sense of the word—and it does not mean a class elite—and some people of superior mind and character guiding the people then it all falls into barbarism. The general rough-and-tumble of uneducated people is not going to produce a civilization.

# Section 1
# The Nervous System and Sports

Chapter 2

# Temperature Regulation and Sports

## by Otto Appenzeller and Ruth Atkinson

The recent evolution in understanding of the thermoregulatory system has made it a recurrent subject of physiological investigation. Moreover, with heightened interest in sporting activities, disturbances in thermoregulation, induced by environmental heat or excessive heat loads due to physical activity, may cause serious and sometimes lasting disorders in well- or less well-trained individuals.

The term *homeothermy* implies the maintenance of body temperature within certain limits and normal functioning of the thermoregulatory systems, but the nature of the regulatory mechanism, or set point, and how it adjusts to external heat loads, internal heat production, or the way it responds to pyrogens is a matter of debate. Considerable evidence now shows that thermosensitive neurons in the anterior and preoptic hypothalamus respond to blood temperature changes, and that these same neurons are also activated by impulses from the periphery and cervical spinal cord. Various systems concerned with heat loss or preservation are brought into play. These include behavioral changes, which are important in conscious thermoregulation. Neurons participating in thermoregulation release a number of transmitters at their terminals. The thermoregulatory set point has been thought of in biochemical terms without much consideration of control theory. For example, a balanced release of neurotransmitters or a balance in calcium or sodium in the immediate neuronal environment probably maintains body temperature, but this does not explain how neurotransmitters are released or ionic balance comes about, thus addressing components of the system but not its operational principles.

The study of environmental and internal temperatures and their relationship to thermoregulation suggests that a simple neuronal connection exists between thermosensors and thermoeffectors. In humans, heat production, heat loss effectors, and their set point could be based entirely upon (neuronal) signals generated in the central nervous system (CNS). The injection of norepinephrine, 5-hydroxytryptamine, and the cholinomimetic substance, carbamylcholine, into the cerebral ventricles of a variety of animals shows that their thermoregulatory effects are the same as those obtained from disturbance-response analyses.

Increased heat storage from increased heat production or increased peripheral vasomotor tone with inhibition of heat loss from sweating occurs during fever and during heat stroke associated with physical exertion. Fever is caused by a pyrogen, which increases heat production and decreases heat loss. Such a pyrogen might act between cold sensors and the crossing inhibitory influences on evaporative heat loss, a hypothesis that has been tested in animals. Present evidence suggests that bacterial endotoxins or prostaglandin $E_1$, both pyrogens, act on cold sensors or pathways from them. This occurs prior to activation of inhibitory influences on heat loss processes. Numerous animal studies implicate aspartate, acetylcholine, carbamylcholine, dopamine, gamma amino butyric acid, histamine, 5-hydroxytryptamine, indoleamine, prostaglandin $E_1$, and taurine in normal temperature regulation. Marked species differences in response to intraventricular injection of these agents and to agonist or antagonist drugs have been noted. It is uncertain how many and in what capacity these substances are involved in human temperature regulation (Bligh [1]).

# Temperature Regulation and Exercise

During physical activity, several organs share the demand for increased blood supply. The heart must supply adequate blood to its own contracting muscle and to the skin for transfer of the excessive heat produced from muscular contraction.

## Cardiac Output

In thermally neutral conditions during exercise, cardiac output increases in proportion to the rate of oxygen uptake. Increased cardiac output is associated with increased muscular blood flow.

It is not clear, however, whether a simple relationship exists between cardiac output and oxygen uptake when skin perfusion demand is high. Cutaneous blood flow is determined largely by body temperature, but reflex vasoconstriction of skin vessels occurs during hypotension. Nevertheless, at the onset of exercise, metabolic heat increases at a rate directly proportional to exercise intensity and is far in excess of heat dissipation.

Because of this imbalance, body temperature rises until heat loss through the skin by increased blood flow and sweating equals heat production. When this is achieved, a new set point at a higher steady internal body temperature or homeothermy occurs and is maintained until further heat loads either change the set point upward or decreased work load lowers body temperature again. The combined circulatory demands of muscles and skin are determined not only by body temperature, but also in part by average skin temperature, which is, in turn, closely related to environmental temperature. Therefore, when exercise intensity is great and ambient temperature high, the circulatory demands are considerably increased. The heart must then provide sufficient blood flow to both muscles and skin or compromise delivery of blood to one or the other.

If heavy exercise occurs in very hot environments, contracting muscles demand a disproportionately large segment of the cardiac output, which is shifted away from the skin; this, in turn, limits heat dissipation from the body core to the skin. Core temperature increases and ultimately leads to progressive hyperthermia, which eventually limits exercise. If, on the other hand, adequate blood flow to the skin is maintained at the expense of contracting muscles, anaerobic work occurs and adenosine triphosphate (ATP) synthesis is decreased along with the ability to maintain continuing muscle contraction.

**Compromised Blood Flow**    To prevent compromised blood flow to muscles, skin, or any other tissue during exercise, particularly in the heat, cardiac output must increase continuously. Recent experiments on treadmills in neutral and hot environments suggest that splanchnic blood flow is progressively reduced with increasing exercise intensity and is further reduced during exercise in heat, compared to the same work performed in cooler conditions. This might, in part, compensate for additional demands of the skin, but in extreme conditions of both exercise and heat, the body is prevented from maintaining both skin and muscle circulatory homeothermy.

**Skin and Muscle Competition for Blood**    The competition between skin and muscle blood flow during exercise in maintenance of homeothermy is further complicated by increased cutaneous venous volume during elevated body temperature. This increase is thought to be due, in part, to vasodilation of the skin veins because of their high compliance and reduced tone, which may result from an increased thermoregulatory drive. Increased venous blood in the skin permits additional heat transfer because of decreased velocity of flow and increased time for heat exchange between the blood and skin. However, increased peripheral blood volume reduces central volumes and it, in turn, reduces the cardiac filling, thus potentially compromising cardiac stroke volume. If reduction in stroke volume occurs, compensatory increase in heart rate is necessary to maintain cardiac output. A further complicating factor that decreases the central blood volume during exercise is the loss of plasma water to the extravascular compartment. Many investigators report significant fluid losses from the intravascular compartment during relatively short or prolonged exercise. The cause of the movement from the intravascular to the extravascular compartment is thought to be the relative tissue hyperosmolality that occurs in active muscles. This transcapillary movement of fluid, however, could also result from increased filtration pressure in active muscles. The absolute fluid loss for the intravascular compartment during exercise seems most closely related to the intensity of exercise rather than to the ambient temperature.

**Body Fluid Loss**    Another factor leading to central volume depletion and, therefore, fall in cardiac filling, is body fluid loss through sweating, which is directly related to ambient temperature and intensity of exercise. The sweat rate may exceed 1–1.5 L/h during prolonged exertion in a hot environment. Eventually, progressive reduction in central blood volume causes decreased cardiac filling, reduced stroke volume and failure of appropriate perfusion for a given level of physical activity. As the systemic pressure drops, maintenance of cardiac output becomes more dependent upon increased heart rate brought about by activation of baroreceptor reflexes. These same reflexes also increase the force of ventricular contraction and the ejection fraction, but in healthy individuals this is not adequate to maintain cardiac output, particularly during high heart rates and short cardiac filling times.

# Cutaneous Vasoconstriction

When near-maximal heart rates are attained and the cardiac output is falling as a result of reduced filling pressure, cutaneous vasoconstriction occurs in spite of the firmly established vasodilator drive. This, in turn, decreases an already marginal heat transfer from the core to the surface, resulting in heat storage, but helps maintain arterial blood pressure, cardiac filling, and thus, indirectly, muscle perfusion. Vasoconstriction during falling systemic blood pressure is activated by baroreflexes, which override thermoregulatory activity. It is not clear, however, whether cutaneous vasoconstriction is initiated by critical decrease in blood volume, increased internal body temperature, a specific level of peripheral flood flow, or, perhaps, critical reduction in the cardiac output (Nadel et al. [2]). During cycle ergometer exercise for 20–25 min at 40%–70% of maximal aerobic power at different ambient temperatures, fit, non-endurance-trained subjects were able to maintain constant thermal and circulatory levels in all but heavy exertion in the heat. Thermal regulation was impaired during exercise in the heat (36°C). The esophageal temperature (an approximation of central temperature) at the termination of heavy exercise averaged almost 38.1°C during performance in comfortable ambient temperatures, but at an ambient temperature of 36°C the esophageal temperature reached almost 39°C. The cardiac output in the steady state exercise was appropriate to the oxygen uptake, but was significantly higher during exercise in the heat, and this was entirely due to increased heart rate. Thus, under varying increased ambient temperatures with moderate exercise, the cardiac output can be elevated above that found under cool conditions, in order to deliver the appropriate amount of blood to both muscles and skin. During heavy exercise in the heat, however, it becomes more and more difficult to increase cardiac output because the heart rate is approaching maximum levels for a given individual, and stroke volume is, therefore, limited. Under those conditions, cardiac output is maintained as in cooler ambient temperature but is achieved only with a relative cutaneous vasoconstriction superimposed upon the heat-induced vasodilation.

**Stroke Volume and Plasma Volume**   Cutaneous vasoconstriction occurred when stroke volume and plasma volumes began to decrease. Skin vasoconstriction, therefore, presumably prevented further reduction in stroke volume and stabilized central circulation. The price of stabilization by skin vasoconstriction is, of course, decreased heat transfer from the core to the surface, and central body temperature rises after 20 min of exercise. Therefore, in subjects who are not endurance-trained or heat-acclimated, circulatory regulation takes precedence over temperature homeostasis.

**Body Position**   There is some evidence that cutaneous vasoconstriction during exercise in heat is influenced by body position. Vasoconstriction is greater in the upright position than when the subject is semi-upright on a bicycle ergometer. Evidence that this vasoconstriction is produced by activation of cardiopulmonary baroreflexes has now been found (Roberts and Wenger [3]). The absence of this cutaneous constrictor response at a critical level of exercise in the heat may cause a precipitous fall in stroke volume and, therefore, of cardiac output, forcing termination of exercise and collapse of the athlete. Furthermore, if peripheral venous hydrostatic pressure due to upright posture is abolished by supine exercise, which increases venous return from the periphery to the heart, then the cutaneous vasoconstriction is abolished because, at least with moderate exercise duration, cardiac output is not impaired (Nadel [4]).

# Hydration, Exercise, and Thermoregulation

It has been known empirically for some time that dehydration profoundly affects body temperature and circulation during heating or prolonged submaximal exercise or both. Experimentally, core temperatures were higher in dehydrated subjects at a given intensity of work than when the same subjects were normally hydrated, and similar observations were made in dehydrated subjects at rest. Reduced sweating and forearm blood flow under conditions of dehydration have been attributed to higher internal body temperature and inadequate temperature regulation. The mechanism by which the thermoregulatory system is modified by hydration, however, is still controversial. It is not, for example, clear whether dehydration changes the thermoregulatory activity of central nervous system neurons or whether it decreases the activity of thermoregulatory effector systems in response to certain central signals.

## Blood Volume Effect

Some investigators have found that impaired cardiac output during exercise while one is dehydrated must result from dependence, at least to some extent, upon the initial blood volume. It seems, therefore, if one accepts this interpretation, that during exercise with a high initial blood volume, exercise-induced decrease in plasma volume is less likely to cause circulatory strain than if the same plasma volume were lost with a low initial blood volume. Therefore, in hypovolemia, circulatory adjustments must occur more quickly if physical activity is to continue. This, however, does not indicate whether peripheral circulation is impaired in order to maintain muscular perfusion during dehydration; nor does it examine how cutaneous blood flow is affected if the muscles are adequately perfused during dehydration-associated exercise.

Attempts to answer these questions were made in subjects who were exercised in a normally hydrated, dehydrated (approximately 5% of body weight loss), or overhydrated condition. Again, these subjects were fit but had not been trained for endurance. They exercised for a relatively short time in a semi-upright position on a cycle ergometer at 60%–70% of maximum oxygen uptake in the heat (36°C). During these experiments the thresholds for cutaneous vasodilation were considerably higher in dehydrated subjects, but once vasodilation occurred, the relationship between central temperature and blood flow were similar to that in normally hydrated subjects.

From this it may be concluded that heat transfer of the cutaneous circulatory bed is as responsive per unit of central temperature change in hypovolemic as in normovolemic individuals. Surprisingly, however, the vasoconstrictor influence was superimposed upon the heat-induced cutaneous vasodilatation at very much reduced blood flows during dehydration. The differences in blood flow between control and hyperhydrated subjects were not significant.

**Results of Dehydration or Hypovolemia**   The consequences of dehydration are that the increased central temperature threshold for vasodilation and the relative vasoconstriction at higher internal temperature in hypovolemic subjects cause much greater elevation in body temperature than in well-hydrated exercising individuals, even though total heat production is the same. The notion, therefore, that maintenance of adequate circulation takes precedence over temperature regulation in conditions of high demand upon multiple systems, suggests that the sparing of circulation varies between an initial hypovolemic state and progressive decrease in blood volume during heavy exercise.

During dehydration or initial hypovolemia, the vasodilator threshold shift to the right implies that the central nervous system is responsible for this phenomenon because a change in the gain of the thermal detector does not occur. When normal hydration prevails, however, the central nervous system increases the vasoconstrictor drive to the periphery during progressive fluid loss with exercise. Experiments on subjects with mild hyperosmolality have shown that central nervous osmoreceptors are also involved in the control of the peripheral circulation. They, however, seem to be subordinate to the "volume receptors" because the hypovolemic vasodilatory shift appears without an increase in plasma osmolality.

**Muscular Activity**   Muscular activity places a burden on both thermoregulatory and skin vasomotor systems by creating a thermal load proportional to exercise intensity and causes a reduction in central blood volume that is also related to the amount of work performed.

When extreme heat or dehydration prevails, compromises in cutaneous circulation and thermoregulation are made. Increased body temperature, attributed to increased metabolism of the exercising muscles, is perceived in the central nervous system. A central temperature threshold for vasodilatation in the cutaneous vascular bed exists, which allows increased blood flow proportional to the increased temperature.

When skin blood flow is high, venous return and cardiac filling are reduced. Egress of fluid from the vasculature during exercise also decreases plasma volume. At that point, cutaneous vasoconstriction occurs, and this redirects some of the blood to the heart. In turn, heat transfer is reduced from the core to the surface. If, under these circumstances, cardiac filling improves, as may occur with recumbent posture, cutaneous vasoconstriction is immediately abolished and the core-to-skin transfer of heat is improved.

When relative dehydration is present at the beginning of exercise, the threshold for cutaneous vasodilatation shifts to higher central temperatures, suggesting the presence of centrally generated inhibition of the vasodilator drive. How this occurs is not clear. Nevertheless, answers to these questions and elucidation of the mechanisms of temperature regulation operative in endurance-trained and heat-acclimated subjects may give an insight into physical capabilities and ways of improving performance during heat stress in athletes.

## Effects of Heat

The effect of a desert environment (dry heat) on work and cardiac output during rest and during exercise has been examined in young and old subjects (Myhre et al. [5]). Surprisingly, during short-term exercise, cardiac output was unchanged, irrespective of whether activity was in a comfortable, cool environment or in the desert sun. During short-term exercise the metabolic rate is, apparently, the sole factor that determines cardiac output and not the environmental heat stress. Therefore, short-term exercise in dry heat can be sustained, provided the heart rate increases to compensate for the reduced stroke volume.

An increased heart rate, however, is not the case for endurance events in which maximum heart rate occurs during exercise requiring less than maximum oxygen consumption. One subject in this study, who had been examined 50 years earlier and again under similar conditions at age 85, showed no change in his ability to cope with the dry heat of the desert during short-term exercise. The changes in his performance were attributable to decreased muscle mass and strength and decreased respiratory and cardiovascular reserve. No changes were observed in the thermoregulatory system.

Comparisons of the work capacity of acclimatized and unacclimatized subjects and of acclimatized fit subjects in the desert environment heat have also been made (Wells et al. [6]). Prior observations showed that trained, unacclimatized runners are heat-tolerant to the extent that exercise hyperthermia with training at any environmental temperature may "pre-acclimatize" them to perform better in hot ambient temperatures. Intensive running may improve capacity for heat acclimatization so that a highly trained, unacclimatized person may not actually exist. It has been reported that training in humid heat improves heat tolerance during subsequent performance in moderate ambient temperatures. Moreover, anecdotal reports from the Honolulu marathon, staged in hot and humid conditions, suggest that Hawaiian runners perform better than those from the mainland.

## Significance of Physical Fitness

Subsequent studies on work performance of subjects of varying physical fitness in dry heat with significant solar exposure also show that acclimatization both of those who are fit and those who are average nonfit persons offers definite cardiovascular advantages for work in heat. In the acclimatized subjects, heart rates were lower during equal work, and rectal temperatures of acclimatized, fit subjects, performing higher work loads did not reflect any greater metabolic heat load than those of unacclimatized subjects in the heat. Moreover, the better cardiovascular function of endurance-trained members of the study during work in the heat also suggested larger stroke volumes.

In unacclimatized subjects, even though evaporative rates did not differ from those of acclimatized subjects, skin temperatures were very much higher, a result suggesting that unacclimatized persons must have greater cutaneous blood flow. This may constitute a disadvantage, since the higher peripheral flow lowers stroke volume and increases heart rate to maintain cardiac output. If one assumes that the central temperature is the main drive for an increasing cutaneous blood flow with work, then those who were acclimatized and particularly those who were endurance-trained had less cardiovascular strain during work in the heat.

Endurance training probably does not increase sweating, but endurance-trained subjects may sweat at lower central temperatures, and continuous aerobic activity may enhance sweating sensitivity. Because heat acclimatization in both fit and physically untrained subjects causes lower central temperatures for a given amount of work in hot ambient conditions, a smaller fraction of the cardiac output need go to the skin to maintain temperature homeostasis. This might result from increased sweating sensitivity after acclimatization.

One may conclude, therefore, that heat acclimatization decreases work strain in hot environments and that endurance training 1) offers an added advantage when continuously high metabolic heat loads, preferably with an additional éxternal heat load, are used; 2) further improves the performance; and 3) decreases cardiovascular and homeothermic regulatory stress. It is clear that heat- and exercise-acclimatized subjects dissipate thermal loads more efficiently, thus decreasing peripheral circulatory demands, with the result that cardiovascular performance is improved (Wells et al.[6]).

**Plasma Volume Expansion**    One aspect of natural or artifical acclimatization to heat is a 10%–25% expansion of plasma volume. In addition, isotonic expansion of the interstitial fluid also occurs. A close correlation has been observed between increased plasma volume and the thermoregulatory and cardiovascular adaptations to heat. Increased plasma volume presumably enhances heat tolerance and improves physical performance during high ambient temperatures by decreasing core body temperature and heart strain. In addition, endurance training also increases blood volume, mainly as a result of increased plasma volume.

Hypervolemia is associated with decreased heart rate, increased stroke volume during both rest and exercise, and a reduced hematocrit. All of these are associated with increased maximum oxygen uptake and cardiac output. There are, therefore, close similarities between thermoregulatory adaptive responses to a hot environment and those to exercise training—namely, an increased sweat rate, decreased heat storage, and decreased core temperature at certain work loads.

Plasma volume expansion during heat acclimatization is a thermoregulatory adaptive response, but most studies employed exercise in addition to heat exposure. Therefore, it is unclear whether the hypervolemia after exercise training is primarily the result of thermal stress or is induced by endurance training with its associated increased metabolic demands and internal heat loads. Nevertheless, a recent study suggested that exercise-induced hypervolemia is associated with 40% thermal factors and 60% nonthermal factors. The nonthermal exercise-induced factors were a twofold increase in plasma osmotic and vasopressor forces during exercise and a fivefold increase in resting plasma protein, all of which contribute to the hypervolemia. Two groups of subjects were exposed to either exercise training or heat, each of which raised rectal temperatures to the same levels. Plasma volume increased more during exercise training in a cool environment than during testing in a hot environment, a finding that supports the proposition that metabolic factors, in addition to external heat loads, are important in raising plasma volume during endurance training in either hot or cool ambient temperatures.

The hypothesis, therefore, that increased metabolism or other factors induced by exercise in the heat are necessary for maximal expansion of plasma volume and maximal performance under hot environmental temperature is further supported. The question has also been addressed as to how often thermoregulatory and metabolic systems need to be stressed in order to maintain the adaptive responses induced by heat and exercise training for expansion of plasma volume. Studies suggest that chronic intermittent exercise and heat exposure should be applied at least at 4-day intervals and that the adaptive plasma volume expansion diminishes significantly within a week when no further stresses are applied.

The studies of plasma proteins and their relations to hypervolemia during exercise and heat exposure suggest that exercise rather than environmental body heating was the main stimulus to hyperproteinemia. The cause of the increase in plasma proteins, however, with the associated hypervolemia, is not clear. Whether the additional protein is derived entirely from cutaneous interstitial spaces by means of a "flushing action" on the lymphatics, or the additional protein is the result of increased synthesis or decreased degradation has not been established.

The relationships of plasma electrolyte osmotic and endocrine responses to the hypervolemia in the experimental conditions of exercise alone or heat exposure without exercise are complex and not fully understood. Angiotensin and vasopressin increase more during exercise than during heat exposure alone, and this rise is accompanied by increased plasma osmolality. The hyperosmolality associated with prolonged exercise seems to be the dominant stimulus for the release of angiotensin and vasopressin. The hypervolemia also occurring during exercise is a secondary stimulus.

Surprisingly, the increase in vasopressin during exercise did not stimulate an appropriate increase in plasma renin. This result implies that plasma renin was at an optimal level to produce maximum sodium retention and protect against stress-induced plasma volume loss. It seems, then, that reduced plasma volume during exercise training, exposure to heat, and increased plasma renin were not primary factors accounting for the increased plasma volume.

The changes in the angiotensin-vasopressin system and the increased plasma osmolality during exercise training were closely related to the chronic hypervolemia. Therefore, during either heat acclimatization or endurance training, elevated plasma renin enhances sodium retention, which, in turn, increases plasma osmolality and vasopressin and thus promotes fluid retention. Whether sufficient stimuli are left after intermittent exposure to stress to account for the progressive chronic hypervolemia of either endurance training or heat acclimatization or of both, is not clear. However, the fluid balance seems to be restored after stress in direct proportion to the length of exposure and the level of dehydration that occurred. Exercise depletes intracellular water more than does rest in a hot environment. Therefore, it is possible that depletion of intracellular fluid is more important than depletion of extracellular fluid volume in the production of chronic hypervolemia of heat adaptation and endurance training (Convertino et al. [7]).

The sauna has been used by some for heat acclimatization, particularly if ambient conditions are not suitable for this. Exercise on bicycle ergometers in saunas has been used for this purpose. It is also not uncommon to take a sauna after strenuous exercise. The exposure to the high temperatures places stress on the homeothermy and cardiovascular adaptive mechanisms.

Peripheral vasodilatation, which occurs during heat load in the sauna, is evidenced by increased heart rates and great variability in systolic and diastolic blood pressures. Myocardial ischemia and associated electrocardiographic changes during sauna exposure have been reported (Taggart et al. [8]).

The response of the normal person to additional heat in the sauna after heavy exercise and its metabolic heat load is not known. A recent study compared aspects of exposure to a sauna environment during recovery from heavy exercise with recovery in a comfortable environment (Paolone et al. [9]). Electrical repolarization of the cardiac conducting system differed during recovery following heat exposure from that during recovery in comfortable conditions, specifically increased J-point displacement, prolongation of the QT interval, and loss of T-wave amplitude were noted.

These changes were associated with decreased diastolic blood pressure, elevated central body temperature, and greater myocardial oxygen demand. The J-point displacement seen during the final periods of exercise was attributed to the increased heart rate, and recovery in the hot environment was much delayed. The decrease in T-wave amplitudes in intense heat is well recognized and is probably due to the decreased stroke volume that accompanies heat exposure. The clinical significance of the prolonged QT interval in hot ambient conditions after exercise is not fully appreciated. It may be a secondary response to the discrepancy between oxygen supply and demand and perhaps signifies impending ischemic ST change.

From this study it was clear that the putative reduction in myocardial oxygen supply did not produce ischemic ST segment changes in normal subjects. This was interpreted to show that the low myocardial oxygen demands in the healthy person at rest, even in the sauna, does not lead to myocardial ischemia, despite increased heart rate. Although a number of electrocardiographic changes during sauna exposure after heavy physical exercise occurred in normal subjects, it seems that these do not pose an undue risk to those who are clinically normal and wish to engage in this post-exercise activity.

# Deconditioning and Temperature Regulation

Although we have some understanding of the basic mechanisms of adaptation to chronic intermittent exercise in normal subjects, the mechanism of deconditioning during bed rest is less understood. During the Apollo missions, following bed rest and after prolonged water immersion, decreased maximal oxygen intake, reduced plasma volume, and loss of cardiovascular tolerance to tilting were found. Exercise, either prior to or during exposure to weightlessness or to bed rest provided some protection from the deconditioning effects.

Deconditioning seems to result from, or at least seems to be associated with, reduced hydrostatic pressure on the cardiovascular system from recumbency and the elimination of longitudinal pressure on bones and muscles, together with reduced daily energy output as a result of decreased physical activity. The physiologic changes that occur during deconditioning include diuresis, reduced plasma volume, decreased red blood cell mass, and lower body weight. There is also decreased heart volume, impaired vasomotor tone, and changed carbohydrate metabolism, all of which may contribute to the decreased maximum oxygen uptake and changes in orthostatic and acceleration tolerances.

Moreover, the hypovolemia and impaired vasomotor tone could clearly affect thermoregulatory responses. The effect of bed rest deconditioning on temperature regulation is not well known. Most data on temperature before, during, and after bed rest were derived from non-exercising subjects who felt chilly, especially in the legs, at normally comfortable ambient temperatures and humidities after the second month of a 4-month bed-rest study. The time taken for the rectal temperature to return to control levels after elevation from arm immersion in hot water was increased during bed rest, but the time to onset of sweating in response to progressively increased ambient temperatures was significantly shortened and occurred at lower skin temperatures after 14 days of bed rest. After prolonged bed rest, auditory canal temperatures decreased in humans. In animals exercised to exhaustion after prolonged confinement, rectal temperatures rose more rapidly.

Therefore, the evidence, though still fragmentary, indicates that impairment of body temperature regulation exists after deconditioning.

The question of whether bed rest changes thermoregulatory responses during rest and exercise, and if so, whether this can be influenced by isometric exercise during bed rest, was studied. Rectal and mean skin temperatures and sweating responses were measured in 7 men during 70 min of submaximal supine exercise while ambulatory and after three 2-week bed-rest periods separated by 3 weeks of normal ambulation. During each of the three bed-rest periods, isometric or isotonic exercises for 1 hour per day, or no exercise, were carried out. The results of this study suggest that the excessive rise in rectal temperature during submaximal exercise after bed-rest deconditioning is influenced by changes in skin heat conductance and that there is also a relative inhibition of sweating, which may be a factor in the increased core temperature. The mechanism, however, for the hyperthermic response is not definitively established, although decreased plasma volume found during all three bed-rest periods could account for the excessive increases in rectal temperature.

In ambulatory subjects, such a decrease in plasma volume would be accounted for by inhibition of sweating. The impaired peripheral vascular function during prolonged bed rest could also account for the feeling of coldness in the extremities. The maximum oxygen uptake decreased after bed rest and, in the experiments reported here, the work load given in the exercise experiments did cause a constant absolute oxygen uptake; subjects were, therefore, working at a greater load after the rest period. It is not clear whether this greater load, evidenced by relatively submaximal heart rates, could also have played a role in the hyperthermic response to exercise after bed rest. Fragmentary evidence suggests that greater skin conductance of heat is associated with lower rectal temperature and vice versa, implying variable heat transfer from the core to the periphery. Evidence so far on this aspect of temperature control in relation to deconditioning is incomplete, but it does suggest that the excessively increased rectal temperatures during exercise after various periods of bed rest might be, at least in part, due to changes in skin conductance of heat and also to increased sweating sensitivity and evaporative heat loss (Greenleaf and Reese [10]).

The influence of heat acclimatization combined with exercise at 50% of maximum oxygen uptake on the deconditioning responses after 8 hours of water immersion was examined (Schvarz et al. [11]). The question addressed whether or not heat acclimatization prevents deconditioning after water immersion and is superior to exercise training in a cool environment. Heat acclimatization, together with exercise in a hot environment, results in improved exercise tolerance after water immersion. This is attributed to increased stroke and plasma volumes, known to occur during heat acclimatization. In the acclimated group, the changes in maximum oxygen-carrying capacity, maximal heart rate, and decreased exercise tolerance were distinctly minor compared to the changes in the control group, whose members were not heat acclimatized before water immersion. The acclimated group started water-immersion periods with higher plasma volumes than those of the controls, but water immersion, known to result in decreased plasma volume, was in fact associated with an excessive loss in the experimental group so that the post-immersion plasma volumes in the control and heat-acclimated subjects were equal.

It is interesting that the increased stroke volume, evidenced by decreased resting heart rate after acclimatization, was maintained after water immersion, but this increase in stroke volume did not occur in the control group. This might partly explain the better exercise tolerance with heat acclimatization after deconditioning. One effect of water immersion is diuresis, but this was equal in the two groups. The diuresis may reflect sodium levels during water immersion and decreases in norepinephrine excretion. The latter may have been more marked in the control group than in those acclimated to heat, because acclimatization can cause sodium conservation. Impaired sympathetic nervous system activity may have unfavorably affected the exercise tolerance in controls.

It is clear, of course, that strenuous training in cool ambient conditions is superior to heat acclimatization without exercise in improving maximum oxygen-carrying capacity, cardiac output, and oxygen delivery to the working muscles. Nevertheless, heat-acclimated subjects tested in temperate environments do have better thermoregulation than those who are trained without heat exposure. Heat acclimation may prevent the adverse effects of water-immersion deconditioning on exercise capabilities to some extent. Whether exercise capacity can be maintained by heat acclimation alone during prolonged periods of bed rest or water immersion deconditioning has not been determined (Schvarz et al. [11]).

# Periodic Thermoregulation

Athletes are well aware of fluctuations in their performance that occur at different times of the day or night. This variation in physical capacity is often attributed to nonspecific causes such as diet, environmental conditions, winds, temperature, or just not feeling right. Body temperature also fluctuates over time and has been extensively studied, and the current views are summarized by Feldberg [12] and Benzinger [13]. Numerous endogenous biologic rhythms with periodicities that approximate 24 hours (circadian) or longer (infradian), or shorter than 24 hours (ultradian) occur in animals and man. Ultradian rhythms may occur either every few milliseconds or be recurrent every 90 min or so.

Rhythmic fluctuations in temperature have also been noted for many years, and the autonomic effectors of human skin have ultradian cycles with periods of several minutes. Variations in normal temperature control in homeothermic animals often are linked to periodicities of critical temperature fluctuations controlled by the thermostat, but the extent of variations in the periodicity of normal rather than critical temperature has not been extensively investigated.

An influence of biologic clocks upon perceptual phenomena has been found. For example, experiments on human subjects with visual perception measured by critical flicker fusion thresholds show a spontaneous endogenous rhythm of ultradian periodicity. Similar results have been found in subjects performing maximal speed tapping; again, an ultradian periodicity in performance has been found. These two perceptual tasks show the same ultradian periodicities and this, of course, suggests consistencies in quantitative aspects of perceptions. Therefore, any change in perceptual acuity might act as a *Zeitgeber* (time signal) in the regulation of perceptual clocks. An obvious *Zeitgeber* is, of course, the onset of sleep, at which time a change in body temperature occurs. Sleep onset is also, perhaps, accompanied by slowing of perceptual clocks. In a large number of healthy subjects, skin temperature was recorded every 60 sec, in both the awake or sleeping state. The rhythms were significantly longer during sleep than waking, in a subsequent study using autocorrelation analysis of the results. The ultradian periodicities of temperature were similar on the hand, in the axilla, and on the tympanic membrane. It is, therefore, suggested that hypothalamic temperature oscillations of ultradian periodicity may be the source of these temperature rhythms (Lovett–Doust [14]).

Blood flow in small capillaries of the skin is fluctuant rather than random. Periodic capillary flow may be necessary to ensure adequate oxygenation of small capillaries, particularly those with diameters smaller than red blood cells. Furthermore, it has been suggested that an animal's body weight, rather than its surface area, governs rhythmic fluctuations of temperature, blood flow, oxygen consumption, and heart rate (Iberall [15]). From the extensive studies of the ultradian perceptual clock, it is known that its properties include endogenous rhythm, and dependency upon neural integrity; it can be entrained by damage to the nervous system; it is capable of phase shifts by single perturbations; it has a small variance; and moreover, it seems to be independent of environmental and relatively free from chemical or hormonal influences. This perceptual clock maintains the foregoing characteristics independently of intercurrent events or reactive feeling states in humans. Skin temperatures in ordinary subjects at rest in a pleasant ambient environment are controlled by mechanisms that emit ultradian pulsations. The periodicity of these mechanisms is related to the subject's state of alertness and is much longer during sleep. It may be that body temperature and ultradian variation in alertness are responsible for the differential performance of individuals at different times of the 24-hour cycle. Whether endurance training with its profound effect upon homeothermic mechanisms influences the ultradian periodicity of temperature has not been established. In some highly abnormal states, as in schizophrenia during abnormal perception, the ultradian temperature fluctuations are prolonged, a finding that suggests that at least in humans, a change in the periodicities of temperature and perhaps ultradian rhythms in perception occurs in certain pathologic conditions (Lovett–Doust [16]).

# Temperature Regulation and the Marathon

Some regulatory responses during long-duration sporting events have been measured. The performance of athletes in such events depends to a great extent upon their capacity to lose the excess metabolic heat produced during long exertion. The transfer of heat from the core to the surface and dissipation through convection, radiation, and sweating become important in these circumstances. Anything that reduces blood flow to the skin or sweat evaporation markedly decreases efficiency of temperature regulation and increases the risk of overheating and cardiovascular collapse. Core temperatures in marathoners may reach 40°C or higher, even in cool weather.

During long-term athletic performances, such as marathon races, body temperature depends upon metabolic rate, and this, in turn, is affected by work load and body weight. Therefore, heavier athletes have higher rectal temperatures than do lighter competitors, even when performing at the same pace. In order to maintain body temperature, large evaporative sweat losses occur during prolonged competition. Those with unsuitable hydration prior to competition may, therefore, be at a disadvantage and have inordinate increases in body temperature, thus seriously limiting performance and increasing the risk of hyperthermia.

Animals that run at very high speeds can increase heat production to 60 times above resting values but will refuse to continue running, unlike human beings, if their central temperature reaches a certain level. The distance, therefore, over which they are conditioned to pursue prey is limited only by the rise of body temperature. Human beings, on the other hand, continue physical work in spite of high body temperatures until collapse or other serious consequences occur.

# Heat Illness

There are four varieties of heat illness: 1) heat stroke, or high body temperature in a setting of impaired consciousness, delirium, and convulsions; 2) heat hyperpyrexia, a condition in which none of the clinical features of heat stroke occurs, except for body temperature greater than 41°C associated with excessive heat load or abnormalities in thermoregulation; 3) anhidrotic heat exhaustion, the absence of sweating because of sweat gland abnormalities and hot environment, causing abnormally high body temperatures; and 4) acute anhidrotic heat exhaustion, associated with mild infections in hot and humid climates.

In the fourth condition, the first symptom of infection may be failure of sweating in hot ambient temperatures rather than the usual chill, rigor, and fever. Such patients may also notice sudden cessation of sweating during exertion, associated with headache, anorexia, confusion, and mild ataxia. In this condition, the skin is hot and dry but otherwise normal, and normal thermoregulation, including sweating, will return within a day or two with recovery, if cooling is accomplished and exertion is temporarily curtailed.

## Heat Stroke

When rectal temperatures reach 41°C to 43°C and are associated with disturbed consciousness, mortality ranges from 50% to 70%. This situation can occur during excessive heat storage generated by working muscle during a marathon run, particularly in adverse conditions that make heat dissipation difficult or impossible. An understanding of the pathogenesis of heat stroke makes it preventable and should reduce mortality during heat waves, which claim 4,000 lives per year in cities around the United States.

Preventive measures include education of those exposed to heat and humidity because of ambient conditions, and in particular, education of athletes to avoid excessive heat loads by limiting physical work. Close attention to hydration and adequate, but not excessive, salt intake during physical work may also help prevent heat stroke, a condition that is not confined to the healthy and young athlete or military recruit in training in hot and humid climates, but also occurs in the elderly during heat waves.

In the elderly, heat stroke is often associated with preexisting disease, such as atherosclerotic heart disease, diabetes mellitus, or alcoholism. The use of phenothiazines, anticholinergic drugs, sedatives, or diuretics predisposes to heat stroke by action upon the thermoregulatory effector system.

Deaths from all causes during the July 1980 heatwave in St. Louis and Kansas City, Missouri, increased by 57% in St. Louis and 64% in Kansas City. While deaths in the predominantly rural areas of Missouri increased by only 10%, one of every 1,000 residents in the two cities was hospitalized for or died from heat-related illness during the heatwave. The incidence rates of documented hyperthermia were 26.5% in St. Louis and 17.6% in Kansas City, and those for persons over 65 years of age were 12 times higher than for younger individuals (Jones, Liang et al. [17]).

Assessment of risk factors for heat stroke in the same heatwave indicated that, apart from air conditioning and shaded residences, those who were able to care for themselves and engaged in vigorous physical activity, but reduced their activity during the heatwave and took extra fluids, were less at risk for heat stroke than those who were less able or normally less inclined to physical effort (Kilbourne, Choi et al. [18]).

**Symptoms**   Heat stroke is a medical emergency, and delay in diagnosis and treatment may lead to death or irreversible damage. It should be suspected in any person whose behavior or mental status changes during heat stress.

The criteria for diagnosis include high environmental temperatures and humidity, high rectal temperature, sometimes (though not always) hot, dry skin, and cardiovascular and central nervous system disturbances leading to clouded consciousness and collapse.

In exercise-associated heat stroke, the hemodynamic changes are those that occur normally during adaptation to heat with exercise; that is, increased heart rate and cardiac output, and decreased systemic vascular resistance and appropriate responses of effector organs that increase heat dissipation. These hemodynamic changes occur in impending heat stroke in young or older individuals in whom exercise results in excessive circulatory loads.

In contrast, elderly patients suffering from heat stroke unassociated with exertion have decreased cardiac output and increased peripheral resistance. The exact mechanism of this response in the elderly is not fully understood, but may be related to their inability to counter ambient heat loads with tachycardia and cutaneous vasodilatation during increasing body temperature.

Hypovolemia is present in exercise-associated heat stroke in the young or in disease-associated heat stroke in the elderly, and correction of this with large amounts of intravenous fluids does not seem to result in pulmonary edema, perhaps because of the inappropriately low cardiac output.

A hyperventilatory response to extreme heat occurs, but patients with heat stroke continue to hyperventilate and develop respiratory alkalosis. In addition, because of the hypovolemia and hypotension, the increased metabolic demands cannot be met and lactic acidosis often is also present, so that combined respiratory alkalosis and metabolic acidosis coexist.

Temperature correction of arterial blood gas measurements is necessary for accurate assessment of the metabolic respiratory changes in patients with heat stroke. Though the heat stroke patient may appear to have respiratory alkalosis and hypoxemia, correction for the increased temperature may show metabolic acidosis without hypoxemia. Therapeutic decisions based on the metabolic status of patients should be made only after temperature conversion of the blood gas results.

Hypokalemia, hypocalcemia, and hypophosphatemia are common, and rhabdomyolysis may occur in exertion-induced heat stroke, but the latter is rarely seen in those who did not exercise prior to the hyperthermia. In addition, hypoglycemia is a feature of exertion-induced heat stroke, whereas hyperglycemia is the rule in other patients.

Heat stroke is the second cause of death among athletes in this country, despite the fact that it is preventable, and, in addition, it affects a significant proportion of people over the age of 50. It is important to avoid heat stroke, whenever possible, by heat acclimatization, adequate hydration, and endurance training, which, as mentioned earlier, improves the capacity of the homeothermic system to dissipate heat.

Abnormalities of nervous system function in heat stroke include loss of consciousness or a sense of impending doom, headache, dizziness, confusion, and weakness. On occasion, euphoria may precede coma. Agitated delirium can appear, once the patient is stuporous, and extensor plantar responses, abnormalities in pupillary reactions to light, and seizures have also been observed. Occasionally, in severe cases, hemiplegia, incontinence, and decorticate posturing occur.

With cooling, consciousness returns promptly if the hyperpyrexia has not persisted for too long. If unconsciousness persists for 24 hours or longer and seizures are present, recovery is rarely full, and neurologic deficits of varying degree may be found some time after clinical improvement. In such patients, cerebellar function is particularly affected and the cerebellar deficits may be permanent.

On examination of the circulatory system of patients with heat stroke, the rapid pulse and wide pulse pressures are striking, and ST segment depression and T-wave changes, often with supraventricular tachycardias, may be seen. Although the cardiac output falls eventually, survival depends upon an increased cardiac output to meet the excessive circulatory demands. In addition, blood flow is high in skin and muscles, particularly in heat stroke associated with exercise, a result of a decreased vascular resistance, but splanchnic blood flow is reduced. Even when body temperature is restored to normal, the cardiac output remains high and the peripheral resistance low for hours, a condition not dissimilar to that seen after trauma or during severe infection.

Myocardial injury and sometimes increased pulmonary vascular resistance are the causes of heart failure in heat stroke. In addition, the petechiae and often large hemorrhages that occur, together with consumptive coagulopathy, have been attributed to heat-induced vascular endothelial damage, which has been identified by electron microscopy. Dehydration and electrolyte imbalances are seen most often and are most severe in cases associated with sports, particularly marathon running. Acute tubular necrosis occurs in 10%–35% of heat stroke patients and is related to direct injury to the tubules by heat, circulating blood pigments, and reduced renal blood flow.

In some patients, histologic evidence of liver damage includes central lobular necrosis and extensive cholestasis, findings particularly prominent in liver biopsies from gold miners after heat stroke. In these subjects, heat exposure, exertion and dehydration must have been present. Occasionally in marathon runners with severe heat stroke, transient malabsorption syndromes have occurred, but these abnormalities did not persist for longer than 3 months. Perhaps heat damage to the ileal mucosa with subsequent regeneration accounts for the clinical course of this disorder.

**Treatment of Heat Stroke**    There are two principles of treatment of heat stroke. First, the body should be cooled, and second, vital systems should be supported. Clothing should be removed and the patient placed in an ice-cold bath or cooling blanket if available. Naturally, in the field, substitution of these cooling methods by wet clothing and increased air circulation, together with shading, may be the only modalities available. Massage of the extremities promotes cooling because it counteracts the cutaneous circulatory stasis.

Once the body temperature falls, the patient should be removed from the cold environment. Reflex shivering, which tends to raise body temperature, sometimes occurs concurrently with a precipitous drop in core temperature, together with a cold stimulus on the skin. Phenothiazines may be used during the continued cooling to avoid this occurrence.

Support of the cardiovascular system to ensure continuous high cardiac output by correction of dehydration, hypovolemia, and acid-base disturbances should be prominent on the list, particularly for heat stroke associated with exertion, such as marathon runs. Intravenous fluid (1400 ml) is usually recommended in the first hour of treatment, but more, of course, needs to be given to those patients in whom heat stroke occurred after prolonged exertion.

Urine output must be carefully monitored at hourly intervals through a catheter, and if necessary, mannitol should be given to promote diuresis. Digitalis for heart failure, when it appears, can improve myocardial contractility, but because of the occasional respiratory alkalosis, digitalis toxicity may occur. Sometimes beta-adrenergic stimulation by isoproterenol can increase cardiac output to its necessary level, but alpha-adrenergic drugs should not be used, because they decrease skin perfusion and, therefore, impede heat exchange. If oxygen tension falls, oxygen may be given, though hypoxemia and shunting of blood through the lungs is not common in heat stroke. The therapy of disseminated intravascular coagulation with heparin in a dose of 7500 units every 4 hours is also useful. If coma persists in spite of normal body temperatures and normal kidney function, diuretics and urea or other dehydrating agents to reduce brain edema are necessary. For seizures, anticonvulsants are used in the usual manner. Most patients recover in a few hours if cooling, maintenance of the circulation, and hydration are prompt.

# Heat Stroke During Marathon Running

The explosive growth of interest in long-distance running has led to serious problems in many endurance events during climatic conditions favoring heat stroke when sufficient precautions are not taken. The well-trained, heat-acclimated athlete may compete under conditions that would ordinarily cause heat stroke in the poorly trained or those trained in cold environments.

There are several climatic and situational factors that may lead to heat stroke, even in relatively cool ambient conditions, under continuous and high endogenous heat production such as that seen during marathon or ultramarathon competition. These factors are as follows:

1. At the beginning of a race, running speed is usually fast and large amounts of blood are shunted from the skin and other organs to active muscles.

2. Increased body temperature normally accompanies strenuous muscular activity and leads to sweating.
3. If the environment is hot or, particularly, humid and windless, decreased evaporative heat loss from sweating by convection and radiation from the skin occurs. Moreover, the decreased blood flow through the skin at a time when cardiac output must be maintained to sustain continuous muscular activity contributes to decreased convection and radiation and, therefore, considerable reduction in heat transfer from the body core to the surface.
4. The normally high sweat rates contribute to dehydration.
5. Once dehydration appears, the high cardiac output cannot be maintained, and skin blood flow is further reduced because of decreased intravascular volume and the overriding need to supply adequate blood to active muscles.

This is the vicious cycle that leads to heat stroke. Once this cycle occurs, sudden decrease in sweating heralds impending heat stroke and should be the signal for competitors to abandon further exertion. The decreased sweat rate is due to progressive dehydration and once this appears, body temperature increases rapidly and collapse ensues. Warning signs need to be heeded.

Impending heat stroke is associated with decreased capacity for continuous physical performance, clouding of consciousness, ataxia, and decreased sweat rate in spite of continuous muscular activity. It is imperative that preventive and restorative measures be taken at this stage rather than after collapse, when restoration of homeothermy may be difficult and the high body temperature is dangerous to a variety of organs.

# Hypothermia

The popularity of physical activity in relatively cold environments where participants might be scantily clad is increasing. Moreover, sudden worsening in the weather, increasing winds, and wet clothing make the risk of hypothermia unpredictable and often lead to fatal outcomes. It should be stressed that clinical hypothermia may occur in persons exposed to relatively mild temperatures if prolonged exertion, dehydration, and relative lack of food, with consequent hypoglycemia, are also present. Deterioration in the judgment and strength of the exposed person with impending hypothermia is often an early sign that needs to be recognized. Hypothermia can occur with great rapidity, leading to death if preventive measures are not instituted.

When the rectal temperature falls below 30.2°C, clouding of consciousness and soon restless stupor occur. Slurring of speech, ataxia, and occasionally involuntary movements develop. Pallor, cyanosis, sometimes edema of the face, slow cerebration, and a croaky voice may suggest the presence of hypothyroidism. The body is characteristically cold; the cold is not confined to the extremities but extends to covered portions, particularly the axillae and groins. The pupils may be abnormally dilated or pinpoint and react sluggishly to light. Muscle tone is increased and the patient may have generalized rigidity and neck stiffness.

At this stage, shivering is absent. When shivering occurs, particularly in those who have completed prolonged endurance events, it is a sign of impending hypothermia, and rewarming measures should be instituted by bystanders because the subject is unusually incapable of correct judgment. During hypothermia, deep tendon reflexes are decreased, and delayed relaxation of the ankle jerk, as in myxedema, may be seen. The plantar responses are often extensor but revert to normal with rewarming. Hypotension, compensatory tachycardia, slow atrial fibrillation, or sinus bradycardia are commonly present. The occasional occurrence of gangrene of the toes has been attributed to intense vasoconstriction. Slow, sighing respirations are characteristic, but occasionally Cheyne-Stokes respirations occur. With respiratory depression, hypoxia and acidosis are seen.

Occasionally, pancreatitis has been documented by elevated serum amylase and also at necropsy. The abdomen may be distended as a result of decreased peristalsis, bowel sounds are commonly absent, and sometimes gastric dilatation with vomiting occur. Massive hepatic necrosis has been reported, but it is uncommon. Decreased renal blood flow reduces creatinine clearance, and in spite of diminished glomerular filtration, diuresis usually occurs because of decreased secretion and responsiveness of tubular cells to antidiuretic hormones. Eventually, dehydration and continued fall in renal blood flow produce oliguria. Renal failure from acute tubular necrosis may occur.

## Hypothermia in the Elderly Person

Accidental hypothermia is not confined to healthy athletes exposed to adverse climatic conditions, but also occurs in elderly persons in whom the clinical picture may be slightly different. Though elderly people may have low body temperatures, and symptoms or complaints of cold, those with accidental hypothermia do show decreasing alertness with the decrease in body temperature. The patient, therefore, may not detect the problem. The incidence of accidental hypothermia in those involved in outdoor activities is increasing because of larger numbers of participants. Accidental hypothermia in the elderly seems also to be a large problem, but exact estimates of its incidence are not available. Most studies have been done in Great Britain. Hypothermia does not leave diagnostic postmortem findings, so that in the elderly, death from this condition is often erroneously attributed to concomitant disease.

Accidental hypothermia out of doors and also in the elderly is often complicated by the ingestion of drugs that interfere with thermoregulatory mechanisms or accelerate heat loss during inclement weather. Alcohol, particularly, has been implicated as a cause, and yet is often used in the treatment of accidental hypothermia. A number of controlled investigations, however, involving cold water immersion, showed no difference in heat loss in those taking alcohol as compared to controls. (Ledingham and Mone [19]). Furthermore, one report indicated decreased heat loss after alcohol ingestion, and it was concluded that alcohol intake could be beneficial because it reduced the discomfort and anxiety of cold exposure.

# Alcohol-Induced Hypothermia

Alcohol-induced hypothermia causes hypoglycemia, and the reduced core temperature may interfere with hepatic detoxification of alcohol. Moreover, alcohol may inhibit hepatic gluconeogenesis independently. Thus, hypoglycemia, apart from occurring in those who exercise for prolonged periods, may be additionally aggravated by alcohol ingestion. In a study of water immersion that examined the rate of cooling before, and for 24 min at room temperature after removal of the subject from the water, a rapid decline in core temperature continued after standing without drying for 24 min. When alcohol was given prior to immersion, central body temperature declined faster, and recovery of normal temperature after removal from the water was delayed. Shivering under those conditions was considerably decreased.

In spite of the lower core temperature and decreased shivering, the subjects ingesting alcohol perceived less cold and judged the environment warmer than did those who did not ingest the alcohol. Thus, exposure to cold (water immersion) plus alcohol ingestion may seriously reduce central body temperature. Alcohol intake during or after sporting events in cold weather is dangerous and may accelerate the fall in central body temperature, causing serious complications. In addition, alcohol potentiates exercise-induced cutaneous vasodilatation, with consequent increased heat loss from the extremities. Barbiturates and other psychotherapeutic drugs in question have also been associated with accidental hypothermia. In such persons, the prognosis is related to the disorder for which the drugs were taken and to the degree of the hypothermia.

# Preexisting Diseases

Hypothermia may mask preexisting disease. Severe infections may be concealed by depressed consciousness, hypertension, variable leukocyte counts, and the absence of fever. Neurologic lesions might escape clinical detection because of the generalized nervous system depression during hypothermia. Elevated enzymes from hypothermia or pressure necrosis of muscles related to unconsciousness, plus the electrocardiographic abnormalities that occur in both hypothermia and myocardial infarction, make the diagnosis of myocardial infarction difficult.

The usual criteria for brain death are not applicable in hypothermic patients. Patients may be deeply comatose, without reflexes, and with fixed dilated pupils and slow, deep, sighing respirations, marked bradycardia, and severe hypotension, and yet make complete recovery. Whether or not this is the result of decreased oxygen requirements during hypothermia is not known. Disorders resulting from hypothermia are potentially fully recoverable even though clinical examination suggests the contrary.

# Accidental Hypothermia

Accidental hypothermia from water immersion after shipwreck is uncommon. The main cause of low body temperatures in such subjects with normal thermoregulation is exposure to cold water. In spite of theoretic considerations and popular belief, exercise during cold water immersion accelerates heat loss irrespective of clothing, initial temperature, or amount of adipose tissue. The survival time, however, rarely longer than 7 hours in 15°C water, varies with the amount of body fat. Thick subcutaneous fat reduces heat loss. Moreover, long-distance swimmers, particularly those who brave the English Channel, are about the only athletes whose performances are improved by increased body fat.

# Diagnosis of Hypothermia

The diagnosis of hypothermia depends upon accurate measurement of body temperature. In normal subjects, variations in temperature exist among different body parts. Skin temperature of the extremities, for example, varies considerably with changes in the surrounding temperatures. In accidental hypothermia, extremity temperature may be much lower, as a result of vasoconstriction, than temperature in other parts of the body.

Because hypothermia poses a threat only if core temperatures are low, it is necessary to obtain a reasonable estimate of the central temperature for accurate diagnosis. Mouth or rectal temperature does not adequately measure the rapid changes in hypothalamic temperature that are closely related to thermoregulation in both animals and man. Rectal temperature reflects central temperature changes but sometimes is fallacious. For example, if warm saline is infused intravenously or one limb is immersed in warm water, little change in rectal temperature occurs, but oral temperature rises strikingly. Oral temperature measurement reflects arterial blood temperature changes better than rectal measurement and does not merely indicate changes in oral or pharyngeal blood flow.

Central temperature recorded from the external auditory meatus is satisfactory for experimental and clinical situations. In fever, when slow temperature changes occur, and perhaps also in accidental hypothermia, rectal temperature measurement is adequate and is not liable to many technical errors. Because thermometers are geared to measure fever rather than hypothermia, they are rarely shaken down below 37°C. It must, therefore, be remembered that this instrument measures temperatures only above the level to which it is shaken down. When central temperatures are low, a thermometer that registers appropriately should be used. Hypothermia is present if the central body temperature is below 35°C. Between 35°C and 32.2°C, shivering and behavioral thermoregulation prevent further hypothermia, provided consciousness is not impaired and other physical disabilities do not exist. If the central temperature falls below 32.2°C, depression of tissue metabolism with progressive clouding of consciousness occurs, and below 24°C death from ventricular fibrillation is usual. Mechanisms that prevent core-temperature drop, such as vasoconstriction and shivering, usually fail at these low temperatures. The body then loses heat like an inanimate object.

# Treatment of Hypothermia

Hypothermia is treated by rewarming, and the method used should be individualized. Active rewarming may be dangerous in older people because it leads to vasodilation in the skin, which is usually several degrees colder than the central temperature; thus further cooling of the blood occurs and ventricular fibrillation and relapse into coma may result. If the initial temperature is around 32°C or if the afflicted person is otherwise healthy, active rewarming in hot water has been advocated. In the field, however, a successful approach is rewarming with a jacket containing plastic tubing through which hot water is circulated to heat only the chest and upper abdomen, and covering the extremities with blankets. Sometimes surrounding the victim with warm, nonhypothermic bodies in a sleeping bag is effective. In a hospital setting, a warm water bath is useful.

Complications should be treated as they occur. Blood gases, routine blood, urine, and liver function studies should be performed in those in whom rewarming does result in rapid recovery.

Rewarming through inhalation of warm humidified air or oxygen can be performed with sophisticated equipment in the field, but is obviously more suited for hospital use. Heat uptake via the lungs is greater if inspired air is saturated with water vapor. The heat is transferred to the thoracic blood and then to the heart and brain and the respiratory and vasomotor centers respond in a way that conserves heat for the organism.

Comparisons show that rectal temperature and brain temperature rise more slowly during a warm bath than during warm air inhalation. The after-drop that occurs with hot water rewarming is not a feature of hot air inhalation, and thus the danger, during rewarming, of collapse due to further drop in central temperature does not exist. If assisted ventilation is used in addition to inhalation of warm and fully humidified air or oxygen, the core temperature rises even more rapidly. This method, obviously suitable for hospital use, is not practical in the field; chest rewarming with a jacket is probably the safest method that can be used out-of-doors (Low and Goethe [20]).

# References

1. Bligh, J. 1980. Central neurology of homeothermy and fever. In: Lipton J.M., (ed): Fever. Raven Press, New York, pp 81–89.
2. Nadel, E.R. et al. 1979. Circulatory regulation during exercise in different ambient temperatures. J Appl Physiol 46:430–437.
3. Roberts, M.F., Wenger, B.C. 1980. Control of skin blood flow during exercise by thermal reflexes and baroreflexes. J Appl Physiol 48:717–723.
4. Nadel, E.R. 1980. Circulatory and thermal regulations during exercise. Fed Proc 39:1491–1497.
5. Myhre, L.G. et al. 1979. Cardiac output during rest and exercise in desert heat. Med Sci Sports 11:234–238.
6. Wells, C.L. et al. 1980. Training and acclimatization: Effects on responses to exercise in a desert environment. Aviat Space Environ Med 51:105–112.
7. Convertino, V.A. et al. 1980. Role of thermal and exercise factors in the mechanism of hypervolemia. J Appl Physiol 48:657–664.
8. Taggart, P. et al. 1972. Cardiac responses to thermal and emotional stress. Br Med J 3:71–76.
9. Paolone, A.M. et al. 1980. Effects of postexercise sauna both on ECG pattern and other physiologic variables. Aviat Space Environ Med 51:224–229.
10. Greenleaf, J.E., Reese, R.D. 1980. Exercise thermoregulation after 14 days of bed rest. J Appl Physiol 48:72–78.
11. Schvarz, E. et al. 1979. Deconditioning-induced exercise responses as influenced by heat acclimation. Aviat Space Environ Med 50:893–897.
12. Feldberg, W. 1974. Body temperature and fever: changes in our views during the last decade. The Ferrier Lecture. Proc R Soc London [Biol] 191:199–229.
13. Benzinger, T.H. 1977. Temperature. I. Arts and Concepts. II. Thermal Homeostasis. Dowden, Hutchinson and Ross, Inc. Stroudsburg, Pennsylvania.
14. Lovett-Doust, J.W. 1979. An ultradian periodic servo-system of thermoregulation in man. J Interdiscipl Cycle Res 10:95–103.
15. Iberall, A.S. 1972. Blood flow and oxygen uptake in mammals. Ann Biomed Eng 1:1–8.
16. Lovett-Doust, J.W. 1962. Consciousness in schizophrenia as a function of the peripheral microcirculation. In: Roessler, W., Greenfield, D.A., (eds): Physiological Correlates of Psychological Disorder. Wisconsin Press, Madison, pp 61–69.
17. Jones, T.S., Liang, A.P., Kilbourne, E.M. et al. 1982. Morbidity and mortality associated with the July 1980 heatwave in St. Louis and Kansas City, Missouri. JAMA 247:3327–3331.
18. Kilbourne, E.M., Choi, K., Jones, T.S. et al. 1982. Risk factors for heat stroke. JAMA 247:3332–3336.
19. Ledingham, I. McA., and Mone, J.G. 1980. Treatment of accidental hypothermia: a prospective clinical study. Brit Med J 1:1102–1104.
20. Low, A., Goethe, H. 1980. Vergleich zwischen Wärmeabgabe und Wärmezufuhr über die Lunge und Körperoberfläche bei der Hypothermie bzw. bei deren Behandlung. Int Arch Occup Environ Health 45:231–249.

# Chapter 3

# Neurology of Endurance Training

## by Thomas J. Carlow and Otto Appenzeller

Limited scientific evidence documents the effects of endurance training on the nervous system. This chapter reviews this evidence by specific categories: electroencephalography (EEG), sensory-evoked responses, mental function, visual system, cerebellar control, peripheral nerve conduction, stretch reflexes, and treatment of neurologic disorders.

# Electroencephalography

Normally cortical alpha rhythm, 8–13 cps, is blocked by attention, eye opening, and mental activity. The percentage of time spent in alpha rhythm, the alpha index, can be enhanced by 25% after significant exercise (Pineda and Adkisson [1]) and the EEG tracing in general appears more regular. These changes are transitory, lasting for 5–10 min before reverting to the preexercise state. Fatigue and decreased sense of awareness are common after strenuous exercise and may be the primary sources of observed changes in the EEG.

Sleep can be divided by EEG tracings into a rapid-eye-movement (REM) and non-REM state. Non-REM sleep can be further subdivided into four stages. The later portion of non-REM sleep, the slow-wave stages, serves a restorative function for the body. Physical exercise increases the need for slow-wave sleep (Oswald [2]). The level of physical fitness determines the percentage of slow-wave sleep during the night following significant exercise. Slow-wave sleep increases in the fit person and does not appreciably change after unaccustomed exercise in the unfit or the person who has not had endurance training (Griffin and Trinder [3]). A possible explanation is that adrenocortical activity affecting sleep after exercise differs in fit and nonfit subjects (Buguet et al. [4]).

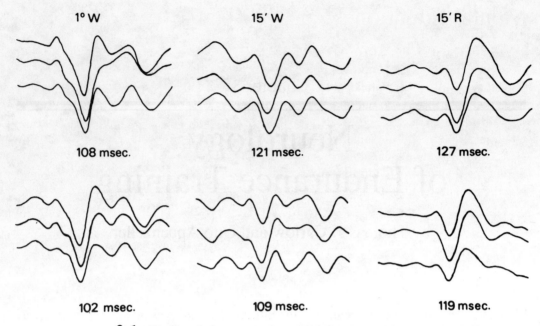

**3–1**  Visual-evoked responses from one endurance-trained individual (51-year-old male) at rest (*upper row*) and after the run (*lower
row*). 1°W, 1-degree white target; 15′ W, 15-min white target; 15′ R,
15-min red target. Latencies are measured from beginning of trace to
peak of first major positive wave in milliseconds.

# Sensory-evoked Potentials

Visual-evoked potentials (VEP) are electrical responses of the brain to visual stimuli,
reflecting central nervous system transmission from the retina to the occipital cortex. The
VEP have been monitored in highly trained marathon runners before and after endurance
efforts (Carlow and Appenzeller [5]; Carlow et al. [6]). Latencies in VEP "normally"
increase with age. Mean latencies to the major VEP peaks were shorter in the endurance-
trained compared to age-matched nontrained persons. After a 10–18 mile run, 75% of all
VEPs demonstrated a decreased latency when compared to baseline (Fig. 3–1). These
VEP changes could reflect an enhanced central nervous system (CNS) transmission in
endurance-trained subjects. Whether endurance training prevents age-related CNS deterioration observed in older persons is not clear, but it remains an intriguing and unresolved
question.

Brainstem auditory-evoked responses (BAER) are measures of electrical transmission
through the brain stem from the cochlear hair cells to the upper midbrain. Statistically
significant decreases in latencies to major BAER wave-shape peaks were observed in 10
long-distance runners after a 24.2-km run (Brenner and Appenzeller [7]).

Somatosensory-evoked responses measure conduction from a peripheral nerve to the
central nervous system, through the spinal cord. Shorter latency for spinal cord transmission in the endurance-trained person compared to the "normal" nonfit person have not
been reported but might, if found, pose intriguing theoretic possibilities concerning spinal
cord levels of response to athletic performance.

# Mental Function

Academic achievement improves with sustained endurance training (Barry et al. [8]; Powell [9]; Gutin [10]; Curetan [11]). The improvement might be the result of personality traits that contribute to initiation and maintenance of a conditioning program, rather than of a postulated effect of physical fitness on the mind. Endurance-trained persons are intelligent, sober, shy, imaginative, reserved and more self-sufficient (Hartung and Farge [12]). Many psychological aging processes are felt to be slowed if a high level of physical training is maintained. Unfortunately, cerebral blood flow, cerebral autoregulation, and blood chemistry before, during, or after an endurance effort have not been studied.

# Visual System

Intraocular pressure (IOP) decreased by 38% in normal subjects who ran on a treadmill until their pulse rates increased to 180 beats/min (Lenapert and Cooper [13]). The decreased IOP lasted for 3 h before reverting to pre-exercise levels. The decreased IOP in glaucoma patients after an endurance effort was independent of the initial IOP (Stewart et al. [14]). IOP decreased in marathon (42 km) runners but not to the same degree as in subjects who were not endurance-trained. On the other hand, IOP in 8 highly trained runners in the Himalayas showed an average increase of 37% at the end of 10 days when highest altitudes (17,700 ft) were reached (Fig. 3–2). At no time did IOP reach pathologic levels. The increased IOP was a comparison with normal values found in Katmandu. Changes in serum osmolarity, lactic acid, $pCO_2$, hyperoxia, hypocapnia, or hypercapnia during exercise and altitude exposure may all play a role in controlling IOP by either direct or indirect reflex mechanisms (Worthen [15]). Endurance training can decrease intraocular pressure at sea level and may be therapeutically important for glaucoma patients.

Impairment of night vision in the lower visual fields as a result of decreased adaptation to dark in the upper retina has been documented after a distance run. The investigators hypothesized that the abnormal adaptation to dark was due to low ophthalmic arteriolar pressure and a change in cerebral blood flow autoregulation, with a resultant decrease in blood supply to the upper retina (Jones and Wilcott [16]). Goldmann perimetry (a method for mapping visual fields), performed before and after an 18-mile run in two endurance-trained subjects, showed no abnormalities. Anecdotal reports suggest that runners have improved visual acuity immediately after a race (Graybiel et al. [17]). The ability to distinguish separate components of a flickering light, flicker fusion frequency, improves after exercise (Cureton [18]), a finding that supports the impression that visual acuity improves after an endurance effort.

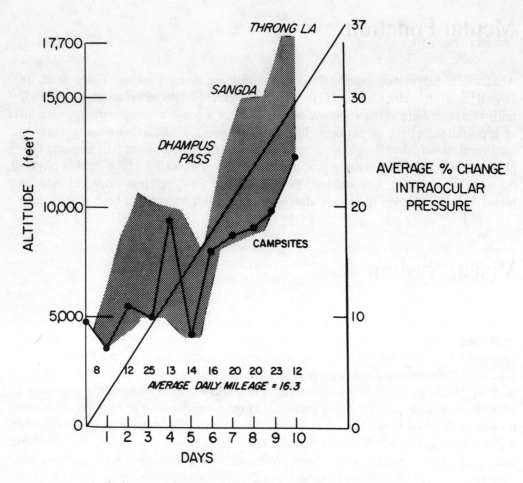

**3–2**   Average percentage change in intraocular pressure in 8 endurance-trained subjects. *Shaded area*, daily gains and losses in altitudes.
Overnight campsite altitudes and daily mileage are also indicated.

# Cerebellar Function

Cerebellar plasticity is the inherent capacity of the cerebellum to modify its function in
response to environmental change. Studies of monkeys (Floeter and Greenough [19]) and
mice (Pysh and Weiss [20]) raised with and without exercise show that animals reared
with sustained physical activity have larger Purkinje cells with more dendritic branching.
Structure of the cerebellum can, therefore, be modified with sustained and prolonged
physical effort.

Neuromuscular function, measured by dexterity, improves with training. The cerebellum integrates neuromuscular control and processes proprioception, vision, and hearing.
The effect of endurance training on cerebellar function has not been fully evaluated in
humans. Postural studies (posturography) performed before and after an endurance effort
have not documented the subjectively perceived ataxia after a marathon run (Appenzeller
and Seelinger [21]).

Is cerebellar plasticity responsible for the transfer of motor skills from one system to another? Numerous examples have been documented, e.g., a blind gymnast working on the parallel bars, substituting proprioception for vision (Jokl [22]). Can improvement in one system controlled by the cerebellum improve function in other systems? Is the observed visual reaction time of endurance-trained persons due to cerebellum-initiated change and its effect on improved neuromuscular control? These questions have yet to be answered.

# Peripheral Nerve Conduction

Warm-up activities prior to athletic efforts may not only increase muscle tone and blood flow but may speed up motor-nerve conduction velocity, facilitating subsequent muscular activity. Motor-nerve conduction velocities increase after only 5 min of exercise on a bicycle ergometer (Currier and Nelson [23]). An anecdotal report suggested that mean motor-nerve conduction velocity in long-distance runners is faster than that of age-matched controls. Running may improve motor-nerve conduction velocities and delay the age-related decline.

# Stretch Reflexes

The stretch or deep tendon reflex is initiated by a tendon tap, e.g., knee jerk, which stretches both muscle fibers and muscle spindles (Brodal [24]). The spindles have separate motor and sensory innervation, they monitor muscle length and control the contraction velocity of muscle fibers. This dual innervation is influenced by supraspinal structures acting upon anterior horn cells in the spinal cord. Increased spindle activity occurs in normal anxious subjects and in disease, e.g., decerebrate rigidity. Brisk deep-tendon reflexes are examples of suprasegmental influences on muscle spindles, and have been documented after athletic effort (Johnson et al. [25]). An elaborate study of 38 young men was performed to evaluate the Achilles tendon reflex. After a 1.1-mile run, significant shortening of the Achilles reflex responses was observed. The 19 fastest runners were compared to the 19 slowest runners before their run. The faster runners had brisker deep-tendon reflexes before the run. This suggests that better trained athletes may have shorter and brisker deep-tendon responses than do nontrained subjects (Johnson et al. [25]).

Contraction of a voluntary muscle and its motor units (alpha motoneuron and muscle fibers supplied by it) are typically independent of each other. Through training, motor units can become highly synchronized with resultant increased strength, e.g., those of weight lifters (Brown- Miller et al. [26]). Training influences supraspinal structures that are thought to modify spinal motoneuron firing rate and synchronization.

A Babinski sign or extensor response of the great toe to plantar stimulation is commonly accepted as "an upper motor neuron" sign. Fourteen percent of healthy officer-training candidates had an extensor toe response immediately after a 22-km march (Yakolevana and Farrell [27]). The response, which reverted to normal after 2 h, was attributed to disinhibition of supraspinal control or facilitation as a result of fatigue and variability in endurance. Could endurance training alter highly programmed spinal activity and allow even more complex motor acts to occur entirely at the spinal level?

Muscle fibers and spinal motor neurons change their enzymatic content in rats that have received increased physical training (Edgerton et al. [28]; Gerchman et al. [29]). Both muscle fibers and motoneurons in the anterior horn of the spinal cord adapt to chronic repetitive overload by increasing the percentage of specific mitochondrial enzymes. This is thought to be due to a suprasegmental influence on the spinal cord.

In animals and humans, type I (slow-twitch) muscle fibers can be transformed to type II (fast-twitch) muscle fibers by appropriate training. Four long-distance runners had muscle biopsies after aerobic and anaerobic training. Conversion of type I to type II muscle fibers occurred after anaerobic training, with a shift in the opposite direction after aerobic training (Jansson et al. [30]).

# Neurologic Disorders

Long-distance running decreases the frequency of attacks and the severity of migraine headaches (Atkinson and Appenzeller [31]). Effort migraine, on the other hand, appears frequently after near-maximal physical activity and has rarely resulted in focal neurologic deficits (Seelinger et al. [32]; Miller [33]).

# Summary

Endurance training affects the nervous system. The EEG shows an increased alpha index, the VEP and BAER latencies are shortened, and mental function improves with physical effort. Intraocular pressure decreases and visual acuity may improve. Even the structure of the cerebellum, the enzymatic content of the muscle fiber, and the histochemistry of the anterior horn cell are modified by exercise. Peripheral nerve conduction may improve and motor unit synchronization and deep tendon reflexes can be modified with training.

Running, swimming, and other forms of sustained effort may be useful therapeutic alternatives for highly motivated persons with migraine. The finding that endurance training shortens the latency of the VEP and BAER may be useful in monitoring or even preventing the expected decline with advancing age of CNS electrical transmission.

# References

1. Pineda, A., Adkisson, M.A. 1961. Electroencephalographic studies in physical fatigue. Tex Rep Biol Med 19:332–342.
2. Oswald, I. 1976. The function of sleep. Postgrad Med J 52:15–18.
3. Griffin, S.J., Trinder, J. 1978. Physical fitness, exercise and human sleep. Psychophysiol 15:447–450.
4. Buguet, A., Roussel, B., Angus, R., Sabistou, B., Radomski, M. 1980. Human sleep and adrenal individual reaction to exercise. Electroencephalogr Clin Neurophysiol 49:515–523.
5. Carlow, T.J., Appenzeller, O. 1978. Endurance training and the nervous system. In: Appenzeller, O., Atkinson, R., (eds): Health Aspects of Endurance Training, Vol. 12. Medicine and Sport, Karger, Basel, New York.
6. Carlow, T.J., Appenzeller, O., Rodriguez, M. 1978. Neurology of endurance training: Visual evoked potentials before and after a run. Neurology 28:390.
7. Brenner, R.P., Appenzeller, O. 1981. Neurology of endurance training. IV. Brainstem auditory evoked responses (BAERs). Electroencephalogr. Clin Neurophysiol 51:42 p.
8. Barry, A.J., Steinmetz, M.E., Page, H.F., Rodahl, K. 1966. The effects of physical conditioning on older individuals. II. Motor performance and cognitive function. J Gerontol 31:192–198.
9. Powell, R.R. 1975. Effects of exercise on mental functioning. J Sports Med Phys Fitness 15:125–131.
10. Gutin, B. 1965. Effect of increase in physical fitness on mental ability following physical and mental stress. Res Q Am Assoc Health Phys Educ 37:211–221.
11. Cureton, T.K. 1963. Improvement of psychological states by means of exercise-fitness programs. J Assoc Phys Ment Rehab 17:14–25.
12. Hartung, G.H., Farge, E.J. 1977. Personality and physiological traits in middle-aged runners and joggers. J Gerontol 32:541–548.
13. Lenapert, P., and Cooper, K. 1967. The effect of exercise on intraocular pressure. Am J Ophthalmol 63:1673–1676.
14. Stewart, R.H., LeBlanc, R., Becker, B. 1970. Effects of exercise on aqueous dynamics. Am J Ophthalmol 69:245–248.
15. Worthen, D.M. 1978. Effects of exercise on the visual system. Med Sport 12:38–46.
16. Jones, R.K., Wilcott, I.T. 1977. Topographic impairment of night vision related exercise. Am J Ophthalmol 84:868–871.
17. Graybiel, A., Jokl, E., Trapp, C. 1955. Russian studies of vision in relation to physical activity and sports. Res Q Am Assoc Health Phys Educ 26:480–485.
18. Cureton, T.K. 1957. Physical fitness work with normal aging adults. J Assoc Phys Ment Rehab 11:145–160.
19. Floeter, M.K., Greenough, W.T. 1979. Cerebellar plasticity: Modification of Purkinje cell structure by differential rearing in monkeys. Science 206:227–229.
20. Pysh, J.J., Weiss, G.M. 1979. Exercise during development induces an increase in Purkinje cell dendritic tree size. Science 206:230–232.
21. Appenzeller, O., Seelinger, D. 1980. Posturography after an endurance run. Personal communication.
22. Jokl, E. 1973. The physical structure of mind. In: Wartenweiler, J., Cerquiglinni, S., (eds): Medicine and Sport, Vol. 8. Karger, Basel, New York, pp 1–64.
23. Currier, D.P., Nelson, R.M. 1969. Changes in motor conduction velocity induced by exercise and diathermy. Phys Ther 49:146–152.
24. Brodal, A. 1969. Neurological Anatomy in Relation to Clinical Medicine. Oxford University Press, London.
25. Johnson, B.L., Jokl, E., Jokl, P. 1963. The effect of exercise upon the duration of the triceps surae stretch reflex. J Assoc Phys Ment Rehab 17:172–176.

26. Brown-Miller, H.S., Stein, R.B., Lee, R.H. 1975. Synchronization of human motor units: Possible roles of exercise and supraspinal reflexes. Electroencephalogr Clin Neurophysiol 38:245–254.

27. Yakolev, P.L., Farrell, M.J. 1941. Influence of locomotion on the plantar reflex in normal and in physically and mentally inferior persons. Arch Neurol Psychiat 49:322–323.

28. Edgerton, V.R., Gerchman, L., Carrow, R. 1969. Histochemical changes in rat skeletal muscle after exercise. Exp Neurol 24:110–123.

29. Gerchman, L.B., Edgerton, V.R., Carrow, R.E. 1975. Effects of physical training on the histochemistry and morphology of central motor neurons. Exp Neurol 49:790–801.

30. Jansson, E., Sjodin, B., Tesch, P. 1978. Changes in muscle fiber type distribution in man after physical training. Acta Physiol Scand 104:23–237.

31. Atkinson, R., Appenzeller, O. 1981. Headache in sports. Seminars in Neurology 1(4):334–344.

32. Seelinger, D.F., Coin, G.C., Carlow, T.J. 1975. Effort headache with cerebral infarction. Headache 15:142–145.

33. Miller, R.G. 1977. Transient focal cerebral ischemia after extreme exercise. Headache 17:196–197.

# Chapter 4

# Psychological and Behavioral Aspects of Sports Medicine

## by Robert L. Bergman

Consideration of the psychologic aspects of physical activity requires an artificial viewpoint, since it implies that mental and physical life are separate. Mental and physical experience, however, are as completely intermingled in sports and athletics as in any other human endeavor. Attitude and motivation are crucial in determining personal and competitive success, though they are perhaps overrated by persons unwilling to undergo the rigors of thorough training. Those who do exercise properly, however, can expect to enjoy the mental and emotional benefits of physical conditioning that have been recognized since antiquity.

In recent years, formerly sedentary persons of all ages and both sexes, and even disabled persons, have begun to train and compete, giving rise to imprecise, but impressive evidence that getting into shape physically is also good for you mentally. It has also become apparent that sports can exacerbate or cause certain emotional and interpersonal difficulties.

## Mental ''Gymnastics''

Physical improvement is a goal that many people despair of and try to ignore. By overemphasizing the distinction between body and mind and subscribing to the moralistic view that mind is more noble than body, they arrive at a somewhat comforting rationalization for their poor physical condition. They decide to stay overweight, weak, and clumsy for a variety of reasons that are only partially conscious. Most adults today believe that their physical condition and strength are unchangeable; long ago, they gave up the thought of serious athletics because of frustration and real or imagined ridicule whenever they were contrasted with physically able persons whom, they imagined received talents effortlessly. Even adults who competed in sports in youth, but who stopped competing at the end of school, or at middle age, fear embarrassment if they compare themselves with the envied men and women who are still competing. Until recently, the rare transformation of a fat weakling to an athlete was regarded as a miracle of determination or simply a miracle. Today, however, large numbers of formerly inactive people regularly swim, jog, bicycle, or weight train, for example. Many have learned to persist despite initial disappointment at their performance, and are exhilarated by having done that which they thought was impossible. In the process, they not only become more healthy and physically attractive, but their self-confidence improves. They soon recognize that appearance and physical ability are important parts of personality.

## Importance of Self-esteem

The self is fundamentally a body-self (Freud [1]). Our appreciation of ourselves is anchored in our earliest bodily pleasures and in the basic feelings generated by our mothers' and others' responses to us (Erikson [2, 3]; Kohut [4]). If we are well cared for, our pleasant sensations produce a sense of goodness that is the earliest perception of ourselves. Our family's pride and pleasure in us then confirms our basic self-esteem. In an optimum childhood, pride becomes based on real qualities and accomplishments. Parents who are empathically attentive to their child and neither overindulge nor over-demand provide healthy external support to self-esteem. Their reasonable expectations become the child's own, and from an approving parent, the child acquires the internal supports of self-esteem—the ability to value oneself and to be pleased by actual qualities and achievements.

Many things can go wrong with this process. Overindulgent parents for example, can create an exaggerated sense of self-importance in the child, regardless of the child's achievement. This attitude can promote conflict and bitterness when the child starts school or encounters those who are not as appreciative as parents. Both inattentive or over-demanding parents can fail to endow a child with a feeling of value and may cause the child to harbor an infantile, secret portion of his or her personality that is unrealistically ambitious, demanding, and full of rage. Variations on this theme include people who feel meaningless, insignificant, and empty because they do not acknowledge or benefit from love for themselves. They attach themselves to others whom they grossly overrate and expect to receive ultimate happiness from, only to suffer another disappointment. At the more normal end of the spectrum are people who plod along successfully enough, but who seldom allow themselves to have fun or feel special about what they do. Many of the recent happy converts to running or other sports come from this latter group.

## Self-image and Athletics

Children who do not evoke an adequately empathic response from their families may nevertheless feel good about themselves because of their pride in their parents. It is this type of feeling slightly transformed that makes professional sports so profitable. Children are often painfully aware of how much smaller, less knowledgeable, and skillful they are than the older people around them, but may console themselves by their close association with big impressive beings. Parents who are realistic about themselves and accepting of the child allow him or her this hero worship without undue encouragement or painful deflation of the overestimation of themselves. Eventually, in normal development, the need for hero identification is replaced by identification with cherished ideals. But pleasure in the success of heroes who occupy the place formerly occupied by idealized parents is still important to most people—and to all sports fans, for example. To sports fans, the beloved team becomes almost an extension of the self: "We're number one!" they shout when their team, with whom they have no real connection, wins the ultimate game.

For most people, however, the vicarious experience of the Super Bowl is not enough to maintain their spirits, not to mention the patency of their coronary arteries. Even the most devout fans long to participate. If something lures them onto the running track or to some other athletic activity that formerly seemed impossible, the rewards still include some of the old benefits of hero worship, but now in a more satisfying form intermingled with self-pride. The new athlete will probably join with other athletes to train, compete, or just to discuss the sport, and will benefit from a sense of belonging to a group that shares accomplishment, special knowledge, and sometimes pleasurable eccentricity.

# Psychology and Training

Converts to regular physical exercise find that they have decreased tension and an increased sense of well-being that comes partly from having satisfied ambitions that previously gave them pain. Training, however, should be initiated properly, increasing physical effort gradually.

## Danger of Overdoing It

Care should be taken to avoid over-exertion at the start of an exercise program, which can lead to injury and loss of motivation. Not uncommonly, an adult's childhood attempts to be special may have been rediculed or ignored, and the shame of those experiences causes the person to forget about being special in any way except in his or her secret dreams or fantasies that are kept alive by belief in the efficacy of really trying. An enthusiastic pep talk to people who are just beginning to get into shape can unleash a mania to do great things immediately, and the would-be athletes suddenly do an astonishing number of sit-ups or laps, only to injure themselves. The disappointment is proportional to the earlier hope and effort, and the individual may abandon the exercise program.

Bettelheim [5] has pointed out that children's stories of this century are less realistic than the old fairytales. The popular story of *The Little Engine That Could* tells of the hero, a small steam locomotive, that accomplishes the nearly impossible feat of pulling a heavy train across mountains by saying over and over, "I think I can, I think I can." Many people think that a marathon is run on magic, and in order to run 26 miles all they have to do is want to and think they can. When suddenly-released infantile grandiosity leads people to feel that they can do the impossible, the resulting injuries and feelings of defeat are likely to provide them additional strong reasons for never again allowing that side of themselves to emerge; the old defenses thus obliterate the wish to be good in sports.

## A Beneficial 'Addiction'?

To assist such persons, one needs to empathize with their pain and discouragement and help them to substitute persistence for belief in an overnight, magical transformation. Millions of people thus convinced have found that they become feverishly devoted to exercise they can do fairly easily every day, a devotion that is often called addiction. While many of these were formerly sedentary types who once defensively quoted Mark Twain to mask disappointment in themselves: "Whenever I feel the urge to exercise, I lie down until it passes over." Today, they are out doing their daily run, and talking about the "runner's high."

Once a person has persisted in endurance exercise long enough to increase capacity for oxygen utilization, frequent or daily runs or other workouts are accompanied by exhilaration. The activity itself is pleasurable and improves general mood; inability to exercise, on the other hand, can cause irritability and depression. Such phenomena have not been explained adequately. One rationale, however, is that doing something one enjoys is cheering and it makes one angry to be prevented from engaging in a pleasurable activity.

The suggestion that exercise is a beneficial addiction may be supported by the finding that runners have increased levels of beta-endorphin peripherally or changes in other central nervous system peptides that affect mood and pain perception (Appenzeller [6]; Carr, Bullen et al. [7]). If further studies confirm and expand on these findings, the "runner's high" may be explained from a physical point of view, but the psychological benefits will not be invalidated as a result. When we speak of emotional needs and their satisfaction, we refer to feelings mediated and perceived through the central nervous and other physical systems. The reason that people feel bad about themselves because they are overweight, ungainly, or weak, or that, on the other hand, they are glad to be attractive and strong, may be attributed, in part, to society's attitudes about such characteristics. Nevertheless, this author believes that such attitudes also reflect our biochemical state.

In those terms, the runner's high seems to confirm our self-esteem. Since the self is partly physical and most runners have altered their bodies, they have experienced changing themselves in visible and measurable ways. Exercise can also contribute a new dimension of satisfaction to peoples' lives—especially those, for example, whose jobs are repetitive or boring or who lack other opportunities for a major sense of accomplishment. The runner with watch in hand, knows for sure how far and how fast he or she has gone and can quickly compare this accomplishment to his or her own past or others' performances. Definite, achievable goals can thus be set.

Those in training can also recognize from their own experience the health benefits of exercise and can look forward to decreased chance of certain illnesses. Most important, they can see improvement in their bodies, and thus in themselves.

# Athletic High and Meditation

An athletic high may be similar psychologically to certain meditative states. Many cultures practice methods for the voluntary alteration of consciousness (Ornstein [8]). Some rely on psychoactive drugs. Others, who practice yoga or Zen Buddhism, use intellectual and institutional frameworks for teaching, learning, and practicing ways of attaining states associated with well-being and wisdom. Some of the methods, such as yoga, are also athletic. Whatever the mode of meditation, the mental states that are the goal of each are similar: a lessening of tension, detachment from petty issues, and an increased sense of meaningfulness. As a result, subjects are able to think more originally, freely, and creatively.

Though most of the published results of meditation are subjective, objective studies show unusual feats of autonomic control and of decreased awareness of pain. Skilled meditation can be correlated with measurable alterations of neurologic and physiologic states. The biographies of several creative geniuses such as Newton and Einstein suggest that though they were not students of a particular meditative technique, they were capable of highly personal, withdrawn mental states in which they achieved great insights by intuitive, nonverbal thought. Some mental phenomena of creative intellectual life may be responsible for the stereotype of the absent-minded professor (Nemerov [9]). Some people achieve meditative states naturally or learn to do it on their own, but, by whatever route, it appears that this kind of thinking is particularly characteristic of the nondominant cerebral hemisphere. Studies of patients whose cerebral hemispheres have been separated by interruption of the corpus callosum (Sperry [10]; Gazzaniga [11]), and other neuropsychological experiments indicate that the mental experience associated with right hemisphere activity is emotional, intuitive, and global rather than linear and logical. Meditation may result from alteration in the relationship between the two hemispheres, with increased access to right hemispheric functions.

Styles of meditative practice may be divided into two general types: in one, attention is greatly narrowed; in the other, it is greatly widened. Skillful meditators concentrating on a single object, mental image, or thought can be so oblivious to their surroundings that they show little or no response to sudden loud noises or other normally startling events. Others concentrate on nothing, but maintain attention on all stimuli and continue to be responsive to constant and monotonous stimuli such as the ticking of a clock. Either way, immediate goal-directed thought is lessened or abolished in favor of a mental and sometimes physical passivity that would usually be interpreted as boring. Perhaps, meditation might be described as highly refined boredom. The usual complaint about circumstances that produce boredom is that there is nothing to do, see, or hear. A person who has nothing to do that leads directly to a somewhat satisfying goal, and is not diverted by entertainment, must often resort to his or her own thoughts and often reluctantly. Meditators find the experience of becoming familiar with unknown parts of themselves hard at first, but ultimately rewarding.

Participants of bicycling, running, or swimming must also confront boredom. Some self-consciously train themselves to meditate and some learn to meditate without calling it that. In the process, they expose themselves fully to a new experience and like it. Repetitive solitary athletic activity for a few minutes or hours permits the athlete to discharge the tension of mental passivity and allows his or her attention to focus naturally or float freely without direct personal involvement. The physical activity can be attended to minutely, or can be allowed to continue automatically; either way, a good chance exists to turn down or tune out the incessant chatter of the verbal centers.

Often, the benefits are unexpected. Many people learn, for example, that when a direct, logical mental assault on a difficult problem is fruitless and wears them out, going outside to run, ride, perform some other exercise results in solution of the problem without their knowing they were thinking about it.

# Coaching the Beginner

The unexpectedness of some benefits of fitness and the difficulty of describing them make it hard to convince others to begin. One should remember, however, that even if a person expresses scorn for the idea, he or she is most likely really expressing insecurity at the idea of getting into shape, or even envy of the person who is in shape. Low-key reassurance allows the potential beginner to start with an activity that he or she can easily imagine himself doing, such as walking/running a short distance, and if repeated every day or so for a few weeks, easily results in the ability to do much more.

As mentioned previously, those who coach beginners should be aware of magical thinking and should tactfully discourage unrealistic notions that by super effort, great things can be accomplished all at once. Perhaps the most critical and difficult moment of encouragement comes when the neophyte runs a mile the first day or does 50 situps and awakens the following morning an invalid. At this point, one should help loosen the stiffness and then indicate that it is neither necessary nor desirable for training to be painful. This is the optimum time for a beginner to learn that athletic fitness is a matter of willpower and that continual training is important. Willpower should be applied to establishing regular training habits, rather than pushing oneself to the point of pain that may be dangerous. All advice and information given to the beginner should come from personal experience. Honest accounts of having gone through the same thing oneself from someone who is obviously physically fit are more likely to be effective than promises of how wonderful the beginner will later feel. For the beginner, a role model is important. It is more difficult for a person who is not training to talk someone else into starting. Especially when coaching young people in a competitive sport, a coach has a greater chance of inspiring his or her team to physical fitness if he or she is also physically fit. And the message may also thus be conveyed that fitness is not only for the young. A child or adolescent on a team should be starting a life of physical fitness. If such youngsters are not encouraged to maintain their conditioning year-round and beyond graduation, an opportunity is lost, and they will later be at risk for difficulties of retired athletes (a category that probably should not exist).

# Disadvantages of Training

## Changes in Lifestyle

There are also disadvantages to a life of regular training. Even if nothing goes wrong with the athlete himself, the way of life may cause conflicts with others. An hour or more every day devoted to training is a strain on many families, particularly if the training regimen is newly imposed. Many spouses resent their partner's suddenly getting up early or staying out in the evening for a daily workout and, in addition, they may be dismayed instead of pleased by his or her improved condition, thus feeling inferior in comparison. It may be hard for new athletes to realize that their spouses are not wholly pleased by their physical changes. Not wanting to acknowledge feelings of envy or fear, a spouse may instead complain bitterly about absences from home and other inconveniences of a training schedule. In trying to help people with these problems, one should keep in mind the possibility that behind the overt complaints is the fear of being scorned or abandoned. The athlete can be helped to see that the partner's objections are based on fear more than selfishness, and may also need to recognize the legitimacy of some of the complaints. Running 10 miles a day is usually at the expense of time at home and often at the expense of work around the house. The runner may also be sleepier immediately after going to bed than he used to be—thus, sexual habits may have to change. Many couples solve some of these problems by the nonathlete joining in sports, but this may create trouble with competitiveness, especially if there is a marked disparity in talent. In addition, with both partners training, less time between them is available for the housework, so that deciding who will do what requires considerable negotiation.

## Overreaction to Interruptions in Training

The sacrifices that athletic converts make indicate how much they value their sport and, therefore, help explain their fear and unhappiness if an injury or illness interferes with their pursuit of it. Even a brief interruption in an accustomed routine may result in an exaggerated reaction. A disabled runner may feel that all past accomplishments will disappear overnight and may further injure himself or herself by persistent ill-advised training because it is too painful to stop. These reactions are often based on magical thinking and unresolved conflict. Probably no one ever completely gives up secret dreams of having special power, and even an athlete who has learned that persistence in training works better than compulsive attempts may engage in self-delusion.

Popularization of results of limited studies or anecdotal reports in runners' magazines and medical journals has unfortunately led to an over rating of the benefits of various exercise regimes. Immunity from heart attack or to death from myocardial infarction, as well as reversal of aging are held out, for example, as rewards of exercise. It takes only a little wishful thinking to extend such ideas to covert belief in eternal youth and perhaps, even, eternal life. Such ideas, usually only partially recognized in oneself, combined with an intense, sublimated competitiveness produce the religious zeal often found in runners.

Such ideas alone do not explain, however, the over-reactions to temporary interruptions in training, because people who believe that they have found the secret key to eternal youth and health can fairly easily relax and wait to begin again.

The darker side of the conflict comes from anxiety and guilt. Commonly, a repressed or denied notion exists that it is wrong to try to be better than others and that punishment always hovers nearby. The conscious experience may sublimate a sneaky feeling that one is really a fake or that recognition and victories were somehow undeserved. An injury or illness sometimes tips the balance in favor of obsessive worry, and the disabled athlete has a vague sense of impending doom that can only be warded off by ever greater and foolish workouts. In the extreme case, exacerbation of an injury can result in a vicious cycle in which increased disability leads to increased panic and ever-more-intense and dangerous efforts.

The usual advice in such a case is to switch sports temporarily. If one has an Achilles tendon inflammation, swim instead of run. Sometimes panic is such that the less danger-ous activity is carried to harmful extremes or may take up inordinate time and energy. A physician or others in an advisory role should encourage the athlete to talk freely about his or her ideas and fears and help him or her to recognize the fantasies of super power and of punishment or shame. Gaining a more realistic view of the situation includes the under-standing that true athletic skills are not as wonderful as secretly wished or as likely to vanish as secretly feared.

## Anorexia and/or Bulimia

Almost all the common unrealistic beliefs about the benefits of physical activity are distortions of realistic benefits of such activity. Exaggeration of the value of endurance exercise to control obesity, for example, has lead to an increasing problem: the combina-tion of heavy training and anorexia and/or bulimia. Our society is increasingly preoccu-pied with sexual attractiveness, and the overall message is clear—fat is not sexually attractive. Yet, while sexual success for its own sake and as a form of competition has become important from childhood to senescence, at the same time, eating customs have not changed as rapidly as have caloric needs. Three hearty meals a day, at one time sensible for farm laborers, remains the habit of many sedentary bureaucrats. The result is the promotion of fat to the rank of popular preoccupation. The resulting insistence on weight loss—carried by some to the point of emaciation and dangerous illness, and sometimes combined with bouts of voracity during which one eats enormously, seemingly against the will and without enjoyment—has become a significant psychological problem.

While athletic training has helped many people lose weight, some have become overly reliant on it and believe in it as if it were omnipotent. Those who have lost weight despite eating as much or more than they ever did may believe that they can henceforth eat whatever they want without weight gain as long as they get in their daily exercise. As with the pursuit of any unrealistic but compelling belief, enormous efforts are spent in its defense. Individuals may spend greater amounts of time exercising to use up the extra calories that they are consuming. Suggestions that it is better to eat and exercise less are met with angry rationalizations about how much fun or how beneficial exercise is. The truth is that they believe that to cut back would be to abandon the magic that seems vital.

This situation is easy to deal with compared to that of a person for whom weight control has become a life or death struggle. Guilt, shame, and anger, experienced since early life, may intensify during the process of becoming independent and responsible, and in adolescence or young adulthood become focused on the problem of weight control in particular, and of autonomy in general. The unfortunate person feels ugly, fat, and helpless, and powerless to resist parents or others who encourage him to eat more. Bulimic episodes in which a person eats excessively, but loathes himself or herself for doing it, may alternate with periods of eating little or nothing. The patient's family and friends interpret the problem as a serious disturbance of eating habits; the person sees it as a desperate fight for thinness and self-respect. The patient believes that everyone completely misunderstands the situation because they do not recognize that obesity is about to overwhelm him or her.

Bitter interpersonal battles usually surround these people, not only about what the patient should eat, but, more recently, how much they should work out. Anorectic patients are noted for their ability to avoid food, to pretend to eat, and to falsify their weights. Today, many of them are also adept at endurance-exercising surreptitiously if others are trying to prevent it. One young woman who was severely malnourished and committed to a psychiatric hospital told her psychiatrist months later, after her condition had improved, that she did pushups for hours secretly in her room to rid herself of the unwanted nutritional energy that was forced on her.

Serious cases of this kind require expert treatment, but coaches, friends, or relatives of such athletes who are overly concerned about weight can help if they remember that empathy is more likely to be useful than advice. The magical beliefs and the unrealistic ambitions and fears that motivate the behavior may intensify in response to opposition. If the person has the chance to talk to an uncritical and intelligent audience about his beliefs, fears, and needs, he is likely to reappraise his own ideas and modify them gradually. Try saying, "It sounds as though losing another five pounds matters a lot to you," instead of, "You don't need to lose any more weight. You're a little too thin already."

## Psychologic Difficulty of Retiring from a Sport

Empathic medical help is now more available to athletes than formerly because many doctors are athletes themselves. It is important that an athlete find a physician who appreciates the physical and psychologic importance of sports. Despite increased awareness of sports, doctors who are not athletes themselves may not be knowledgeable about the psychologic aspects involved in advising a person to give up or reduce a sports program. Even if the patient's achievements are modest, they are almost certainly highly valued and the patient should not be asked to give up the sport except for a serious reason. Even then, the physician should help to find a substitute so that the patient can maintain his or her fitness. In any case, the doctor should expect to hear and accept the patient's grief about the painful loss that needs to be mourned.

The grief of professional athletes who are forced by age or injury to retire from their sport can be especially intense and they often have difficulty dealing with the loss of their abilities, their standard of living, and fame. This problem may be prevented to some extent if young athletes are taught to expect deterioration of their abilities with age but that athletics can be pursued throughout life. A former star should not experience the additional insult of being in poor physical condition; however, unless prepared in youth and encouraged in middle age, outstanding performers are likely to give up sports altogether and thus become physically unfit. Such people may be particularly demoralized, hypochondriacal and, indeed, have an abnormally high death rate, similar to that of intellectual geniuses whose extraordinary talents have deteriorated (Appenzeller [6]; Little [12]).

## Success Neurosis

Occasionally, star athletes mysteriously fall short of achievements that seem within their reach long before they are forced to retire. Some people in all pursuits are afflicted by success neurosis. Just as many graduate students fail to finish dissertations even though they seem quite capable intellectually, many sports competitors do not perform well at crucial times. Every sport has its own lore about this sort of failure. The common theme in such cases is unconscious guilt about unconscious fantasies of great personal triumph over adversaries that become confused with the potential real triumph over real rivals. One significant difference between the effects of this sort of neurosis in sports and in other life situations is that the potential for injury in sports can be great, and unconscious guilt may manifest itself not only in failure at a crucial time, but also in seemingly accidental injury. Most cases are highly treatable by skillful psychotherapy. The usual reason that an athlete continues to defeat or injure himself or herself is the failure to refer the patient for proper treatment, sometimes for fear of emotionally hurting or angering the patient. In most cases, however, referral for help is welcome.

# Psychiatric Patients and Athletics

It should be pointed out, as well, that increasingly, seriously disturbed psychiatric patients are being helped by involvement in sports. The improvements derived from physical fitness in emotionally healthy people may be even more beneficial to seriously demoralized patients, who may have given up hope of changing themselves for the better. Whether or not endurance exercise changes brain biochemistry in a way that overcomes depression is not established. Unquestionably, many depressed people who learn to do something that they admired, but thought was beyond them, experience long-lasting increased confidence in themselves, as well as pleasure from exercise.

# Conclusion

The lives of many people who were not thought to have athletic potential have been improved by serious participation in sports. The fact that women of all ages are increasingly becoming accomplished athletic competitors has probably been an important factor in overcoming ancient prejudices against woman's capacity for independence, autonomy, and full participation in life. Young girls are no longer told they will be spectators or, at best, cheerleaders and that sports heroes might be married, but never emulated.

Normal men and women of all ages and disabled persons of both sexes are now involved in sports, and the psychologic effects are probably at least as important as the physical. The continued and increasing participation of millions of Americans in sports, and their affirmation thereby of the rewards of athletic training have probably done more than any professional star to stress to society the importance of balancing mind and body.

# References

1. Freud, S. 1958. On narcissism. In: Complete Standard Edition of the Psychological Works of Sigmund Freud. Hagarth, London, pp 69–102.
2. Erikson, E. 1950. Childhood and Society. Norton, New York.
3. Erikson, E. 1968. Identity: Youth and Crisis. Norton, New York.
4. Kohut, H. 1966. Forms and transformations of narcissism. J Am Psychoanal Assoc 14(2):243–272.
5. Bettelheim, B. 1975. The Uses of Enchantment. Random House, New York.
6. Appenzeller, O. 1982. A symposium: mental health and illness. Exercise and mental health. In: Bernstein, E. Ed. 1983 Medical and Health Annual, Encyclopaedia Britannica, Inc. Chicago, pp. 134-141.
7. Carr, D.B., Bullen, B.A. et al. 1981. Physical conditioning facilitates the exercise-induced secretion of beta-endorphin and beta-lipotropin in women. N Engl J Med 305:560–563.
8. Ornstein, R. 1972. The Psychology of Consciousness. Freeman, San Francisco.
9. Nemerov, H. 1960. Absent Minded Professor, New and Selected Poems. University of Chicago Press, Chicago, p 56.
10. Sperry, R.W. 1964. The great cerebral commissure. Sci 1(64):142–152.
11. Gazzaniga, M.A. 1967. The split brain in man. Sci 8(67):24–29.
12. Little, J.C. 1979. Neurotic illness in fitness fanatics. Psychiatric Annals 9(3):49–56.

# Section 2
# Nutritional and Gastrointestinal Aspects of Sports

Chapter 5

# Nutrition for Physical Performance

## by Otto Appenzeller and Ruth Atkinson

Courses on nutrition are not usually taught in medical schools. This has led to criticism from a variety of activists who claim that physicians know nothing about nutrition, do not consider nutritional deficiencies in the diagnosis and treatment of disease, and rarely recommend nutritional remedies for the maintenance of health and personal well-being. Much of this criticism is unfounded.

Though food preparation is not taught in medical school, biochemistry and physiology are major courses in the first 2 years, and proteins, fats, carbohydrates, minerals, vitamins, and water are topics of primary importance.

Nutrition is especially important during periods of rapid prenatal and postnatal growth, following certain surgical procedures on the gastrointestinal tract, sometimes in cardiology, as part of preventive medicine, and in Third World countries.

Most textbook information on common sense about foods is based on studies of so-called normal people in the Western world. Comparisons between these populations and those in countries where food is sparse suggest that a large part of the world is starving. With the advent of physical activity as a legitimate part of one's daily life, a new view on nutrition is necessary because present opinions of adequate nutrition are based, in part at least, on evaluation of sedentary individuals. Certain principles of nutrition remain valid and need little modification. These include:

1. No single food can guarantee adequate nutrition. The corollary of this is that to be well-nourished, one must eat a variety of foods. This variety should include protein that supplies the essential amino acids in adequate amounts (meat, poultry, fish, eggs, or nuts, and vegetables), milk or milk products (cheese, ice cream, or yogurt), fruits and cereals, some of which should be lightly milled or whole grain.
2. Caloric intake must be balanced with output. The amount of physical activity is important in determining proper caloric intake.
3. Alcohol has a high caloric content; it may predispose to some forms of cancer, but in moderate amounts may retard atherosclerosis.

4. Calories are the same, irrespective of their source; it is important to ingest only as many as are expended, to maintain proper weight.

5. Consumption of one meal a day rather than several tends to increase the total number of calories over a 24-hour period. It is better, therefore, to have several small meals, rather than one large one.

6. Fluoride is essential for maintaining bones, and it retards or prevents tooth decay. Adequate fluoride is best provided, with few exceptions, by adding it to the water supply. Fluoridation is safe for any age or state of health.

7. Other nutritional supplements are not necessary for most people who consume a balanced diet. Exceptions are pregnancy, when iron and folic acid may be deficient, and certain disease states.

8. Increased blood cholesterol may be a risk factor for cardiovascular disease. Cholesterol levels are influenced not only by cholesterol intake or by the type of fat ingested but also by total caloric intake and expenditure. Cholesterol is made by the body in the absence of exogenous sources, and this is not appreciably influenced by dietary cholesterol. Although it is prudent to reduce dietary cholesterol, such as egg yolks, total fat intake can remain unchanged by partially replacing saturated with unsaturated fats from sunflower, corn, soy, or cottonseed oils, or by using soft margarines with minimum hydrogenation (necessary for solidification of the product made from these oils). Elevated blood cholesterol is only one of many factors favoring atherogenesis, and this subject is controversial. Genetics, hypertension, smoking, etc., also have a role.

9. Salt intake in the United States is much too high and may have something to do with the prevalence of hypertension. Minimizing dietary salt can be helpful in reducing hypertension in those afflicted. The salt used should be iodized.

Prospective studies on how healthy people cope with stress in later life and how they maintain mental and physical health indicate that nutrition, contrary to some beliefs, has little effect. The important factor is the means by which these people mastered their stresses.

# Myths and Facts About Nutrition

Nutritional nonsense is bantered about, and patients or athletes have a remarkable repertoire of unfounded beliefs. For example, the notion that healthful foods are found only in health food stores or appropriate health food sections of supermarkets is false. Many of these foods are claimed to have been produced without the use of pesticides and with manures or compost rather than chemical fertilizers.

Plants absorb only inorganic nutrients, and whether these are obtained from the bacterial action on soil, organic compounds in manure, or manufactured fertilizers makes no difference. All foods, if properly used, are healthful.

It is often claimed that processed foods are without nutrients and are inferior in quality to natural foods. Clearly, use of processed foods can contribute to a proper diet and can save time in preparation. If nutrients are missing from processed food, missing agents can be replaced. It is not necessary to know the caloric content of nutritional components, vitamins, and minerals in each food in order to achieve proper nutrition. People do not eat a single food at a meal, but eat groups of foods. The components must be considered in relation to the rest of the intake. An example is the avocado, which provides 260–280 cal, large quantities of vitamin A, and potassium. It also contains about 16% fat, but this is no reason to shun this excellent source of nutrition. Reducing-diets need only eliminate calories and not particular types of foods. Exercise is also helpful in body weight reduction.

Some proponents of health diets claim that sugar is a granular poison. Ordinary sugar makes up only about 15% of the total calories consumed by adults and perhaps up to 25% of those consumed by children. Most sugar is eaten as a constituent of other foods, as in ice cream or cakes. Sugar is completely utilized nutritionally. Carbohydrates in the diet, including honey, promote tooth decay when teeth are not cleaned after eating. It is the frequent consumption of sugar and the consistency of the sugar used, not its quantity, that cause tooth decay. Milk might be anticariogenic because of its phosphate content. If fluoridated water is consumed by children from birth or infancy, however, there will be, irrespective of the sugar consumption, a 70% reduction in tooth decay in comparison to those who do not drink fluoridated water.

Megavitamin therapy in excess of 10 times the recommended daily requirement is advocated by some for prevention of a variety of diseases. Large amounts of certain vitamins, particularly A and D, are toxic and cause, rather than prevent, disease. Moreover, there is no good evidence that megavitamin therapy can prevent cancer, cure colds, or achieve other similar claims.

It has been claimed by some that bananas and avocados have high cholesterol and fat content and should be avoided, particularly by those attempting weight reduction. This is false. Bananas, avocados, and other fruits and vegetables do not contain cholesterol, which is found only in animal products. Fat is present in trace amounts in bananas, which contain more carbohydrate than other fruits. Fat content in avocados is higher than in other fruits, but avocados are an excellent source of vitamins and minerals, and both bananas and avocados are good sources of potassium. Because of their high caloric content they should be used in moderation by people attempting to lose weight.

Physicians often err in assessing the nutritional status of their patients. Most patients suffer from problems related to excessive food intake or from the problems associated with food fads, leading to dietary deficiencies. Questions concerning eating between meals, what constitutes the usual breakfast, lunch, and dinner, how much alcohol is consumed, and how much salt is used are important in evaluating the nutritional status of patients and athletes. It should be emphasized that the help of professional dietitians and nutritionists should be sought, for they are an integral part of health care personnel. Certain athletes may require guidance to eat the right foods for a particular sport.

# Energy Expenditure

During optimal health, function of individual body parts depends upon total body function and vice versa. For this to continue, evolution has provided for a relatively constant cellular environment, and body fluid composition is kept constant. Muscle metabolism varies greatly from rest to maximal exercise. Muscles use about 100 times as much energy during peak activity as is used in rest, and they are similar to neurons during maximum metabolic activity. Nerve cells are always highly active metabolically, regardless of whether a person is asleep or is engaged in demanding mental gymnastics. The widely varying demands of muscles during rest and effort must be accommodated. The "machinery" must, from time to time, be turned on if the muscles and the mechanisms that service them are to be kept in proper working order. The only way to achieve this is by muscular work.

The resting metabolic rate for a 75-kg person is about 7 MJ (1700 kcal) per 24 hours, or equivalent to the energy expended in walking 35–40 km. Walking that distance, of course, requires an additional 7 MJ above that expended at rest. Carbohydrate and fat are the main substrates for muscle metabolism, but protein breakdown also occurs during extended or strenuous physical activity. Increasing work rates during certain athletic performances leads to greater carbohydrate utilization.

## Effects of Physical Training

A peculiar and important effect of physical training is the capacity of the body to oxidize fat for energy and decrease the use of glycogen for this purpose. The glycogen-conserving mechanism improves physical performance in many situations, but this is particularly seen in long-distance events. Training improves physical performances in several ways: The number and size of skeletal muscle mitochondria are increased, and mitochondrial enzymes are favorably modified. There is also increased capillary density per unit of muscle tissue, which reduces the distance nutrients have to travel between capillaries and muscle cells. With continuous and regular training, other benefits include increased tendon, muscle, and bone strength; better coordination; and perhaps delay in onset of fatigue.

Maintenance of constant body weight depends upon balanced energy intake and expenditure, even though energy expenditure may vary widely. If daily exercise is prolonged and intensive, calorie intake is often less than energy output, and reduction in body weight occurs (Tables 5–1, 5–2).

## Effects of Lack of Activity

On the other hand—and more commonly—if energy expenditure is less than calorie intake, and particularly if the energy expenditure is below a certain level, the surplus intake leads to obesity. In this condition, satiety is reached only after larger amounts of

**Table 5–1**    Weight Maintenance Based on Ordinary Activities 22 Hours/Day

| Activity | Length of Time* (h) | Energy Expenditure (MJ)† M | F |
|---|---|---|---|
| Sleeping (rest in bed) | 8 | 2.3 | 2 |
| Sitting | 6 | 2.3 | 1.75 |
| Standing | 6 | 3.75 | 2.25 |
| Walking | 2 | 1.5 | 1.25 |
| Maintenance energy intake (total) | | 9.85 (2364 kcal) | 7.25 (1740 kcal) |

*Suggested 2 h of exercise daily not included
†One MJ ≃ 240 kcal

**Table 5–2**    Energy Expenditure in Ordinary Activities and Some Sports*

| Type of Activity | Expended Energy (MJ†) | Type of Activity | Expended Energy (MJ†) |
|---|---|---|---|
| Housework | 10.5 | Waterskiing | 2 |
| Cycling 6 mph | 1 | Tennis singles | 2 |
| Tennis doubles | 1.5 | Paddleball | 2.3 |
| Cycling 8 mph | 1.5 | Cycling 12 mph | 2.3 |
| Volleyball | 1.5 | Alpine skiing | 2.3 |
| Badminton | 1.5 | Jogging 5 mph | 2.3 |
| Walking 4 mph | 1.7 | Swimming (continuous) | 2.75 |
| Cycling 10 mph | 1.7 | Running 8 mph | 2.75 |
| Cycling 11 mph | 2 | Cycling 13 mph | 2.75 |
| Walking 5 mph | 2 | | |

*For remaining 2 h or 24-h cycle (male and female)
†1 MJ ≃ 240 kcal

energy have been taken in than have been utilized. Much of the obesity widespread in the Western world is the result of too little physical activity in the face of excessive food intake, and the hypothalamic satiety center is set well above the energy expenditure. This state occurs in children who are reduced to little physical activity by modern conveniences and in adults who, because of the nature of their work, often lead a sedentary life.

It is important that the energy intake and satiety be regulated by the energy output, which can be achieved only if young people are encouraged to exercise regularly and if obese adults consciously regulate their diets to match energy output. If obesity occurs in infancy, the number of fat cells is increased and may predispose to obesity later in life. Treatment of obesity in such people is often difficult.

Appetite, which may have been a reliable guide to energy requirements and to the intake of appropriate nutrients in the past, is no longer a reliable indicator because it is manipulated by food manufacturers and the preparation of food. Therefore, under modern western conditions, food intake dictated by appetite even over short periods cannot be used to judge energy requirements. Two important changes that have occurred in modern society are social and cultural influences favoring large energy intake and reduction in the demand for physical work. The need for most nutrients, as opposed to the need for energy, is, to a large extent, independent of the individual activity level. Therefore, a subject who is less active runs the risk of nutritional inadequacies because the overall food intake is small if the subject is in energy balance (Wretlind [1]).

Thus, a linear relationship exists between the energy supply per 24 h and the supply of certain nutrients such as protein, calcium, thiamine, iron, and vitamin A. In general, a diet of about 12.5 MJ (3000 kcal) per day supplies the necessary nutrients to normal people, but it has been shown that the energy intake must exceed 10.5 MJ (2500 kcal) for an adequate supply of many nutrients. The western diet seems to be geared to an energy requirement of at least 10.5 MJ (2500–3000 kcal), an intake that is totally unsuitable for the majority of consumers. This, of course, accounts for obesity and malnutrition in areas where food is plentiful. The so-called "diseases of modern society," including iron deficiency, diabetes mellitus, and constipation, may at least in part be ascribed to chronic malnutrition or to inappropriate energy expenditure. One may speculate that low energy consumption and its associated malnutrition may be improved by providing more essential nutrients per unit of energy than are presently available; therefore, a change in dietary constituents is necessary for those who require only 6–8.6 MJ (1500–2000 kcal per day), or those people should become high energy consumers by participating in physical activity in different forms. By increasing energy output they can, without risking obesity, eat more and get adequate amounts of essential nutrients (Åstrand [2]).

# Body Weight

The ease of weighing a person and assessing nutritional state has obscured the complexity of the processes that underlie weight change. A number of athletes are anxious to decrease their weight, either to qualify for weight limits or to improve performance in long-distance events in which additional weight may be a disadvantage. Weight loss reflects a decrease in one or more body constituents sufficient to produce decreased body mass. Practically, the constituents usually contributing to weight loss over a short period are water, fat, protein, and glycogen. Over a longer term, deficits in mineral from bones and other areas may make a small contribution to weight loss.

## Components of Weight Loss

To assess the components of weight loss, one must remember that protein and glycogen are constituents of tissues and part of complex hydrated organic materials. Therefore, when glycogen or protein is lost, "obligatory water" that reflects the hydration ratio (grams of water per gram of body constituent) is also lost. The ratio for glycogen and protein is about 3–4:1 and for nitrogen alone is 19–25:1. These ratios are approximate because of individual variations; also, the range of hydration coefficients given in the literature is wide. Whether adipose tissue loses water in association with the mobilization of triglycerides is not known. In addition to the obligatory water losses with protein and glycogen, deficits, and sometimes retention of water during weight loss that are unexplained by hydration coefficients, occur. In these situations, the water seems to be drawn from the extracellular compartment or from a disproportionate loss of intracellular water, or a combination of both processes. During early weight loss, the composition of the loss is varied, depending on the diet and, what is more important for athletes, on the preexisting nutritional state of the subject. The variability of weight loss during the early stages is due to a varying water loss that, under some circumstances, may account for 100% of the weight reduction—for example during diuretic therapy or during excessive heat loads and physical activity.

With prolonged caloric restriction, however, water can be retained on occasion to the point that it may cause weight gain even though fat and protein losses continue. It is well known that on a weight-reducing regimen, all subjects tend to lose weight rapidly during the first week or two. Much of this rapid loss of weight is water, which reflects the natriuresis and reduction in renal-concentrating capacity that accompanies early starvation. The mechanism of the water and sodium losses in these situations are not fully understood. They may, perhaps, be related to increased glucagon secretion, and the increased anion load placed on the nephron by nutritional ketosis may explain the additional sodium excretion.

In addition, the obligatory water loss of 600–800 ml accompanies the depletion of body glycogen that occurs during fasting or carbohydrate deprivation. Attempts must be made to assess the meaning of weight loss, because it is essential to know the type of tissue that is being lost. One can estimate this from the energy value of the loss per unit weight. For example, the energy value is largest if a given kilogram of weight is entirely composed of body fat. On the other hand, if a given unit of weight loss is largely protein and water, less energy has been lost.

## Quality of Weight Loss

Empirically it has been found that the energy deficit or the quality of weight loss is likely to be highest when the rate of decrease in weight is slowest. To make an adequate judgment about the quality of the weight loss, however, the proportion of water per unit of weight lost needs to be assessed. Then, a better idea of the quality of weight loss can be based on the relative contribution made by fat and body protein to the energy deficit. It is customary to assume that an average weight loss of 0.45 kg (1 lb) corresponds to an energy deficit of approximately 14.5 MJ (3500 kcal). This, however, implies that 98% of the energy burned is derived from depot fat, the remainder being body protein. This very favorable composition of energy loss is, however, rarely achieved in weight control or reducing attempts. It is likely to occur only in obese subjects who fast for long periods, and the relative water loss is low. It is not likely to occur in nonobese subjects or athletes who are attempting to lose weight.

**Rate of Weight Loss**    Attempts to interpret the rate of weight loss with different diets can now be made by considering the differences between obese and nonobese subjects, both with respect to short- and long-term adherence to weight-reducing diets. Physically active adult male volunteers maintained for several weeks on approximately 5 MJ (1000 kcal) carbohydrate diets lost approximately 0.8 kg per day during the first 3 days, but the loss decreased to about 0.23 kg/day at the end of the second week. This difference was almost entirely due to increased water loss in the early phase of the diet and to some degree of water retention later on (Brozek et al. [3]).

Thirty-two male volunteers ate only salmon for 24 weeks. This diet supplied approximately 6.5 MJ (1570 kcal) per day, and was composed of 50 g protein, 30 g fat, and 275 g carbohydrates. The weight loss during the first 11 weeks was approximately 40% fat, 12% protein, and 48% water. During the remainder of the time, the mean composition of weight loss was 54% fat, 9% protein, and 37% water, and weight loss was only about 49 g/day during the second half of the experiment, compared to 150 g/day during the first half. The decreased weight loss was attributed to an adaptation of these nonobese subjects to the low-calorie diet. At the end of 24 weeks, the basal metabolic rate of the participants had dropped by an average of 31%, and their voluntary physical activity had decreased by 55%. Moreover, fat breakdown increased from a mean of 88% during the first half of the semi-starvation to a mean of 93% during the second half. In contrast to the energy equivalent of 14.5 MJ (3500 kcal) per 0.45 kg (1 lb) weight loss previously cited, the average energy equivalent in these nonobese subjects was only about 8 MJ/0.45 kg during the first 11 weeks of the experiment and about 10 MJ/0.45 kg during the second part of the experiment. This finding underscores the fact that in nonobese subjects during adaptation to undernutrition, the energy value of 0.45-kg weight loss is far below that usually cited.

In obese subjects, the rate of weight loss during the first 5 days of adherence to a diet comprised of 5 MJ (1200 kcal) was 0.45 kg (1lb) per day (Yang and Van Itallie [4]). There is, therefore, no difference in the rapidity of weight loss in the early phases of energy restriction in obese and nonobese subjects. In this situation, 66% of the weight loss was water, and the rest was very similar to that found in nonobese subjects.

**Ratio of Carbohydrates to Fat**    When the proportion of carbohydrates to fat was changed drastically and obese subjects were given a diet containing 90 g carbohydrate or a ketogenic diet containing only 10 g carbohydrate, but each yielding an energy of only 3.3 MJ (800 kcal), an absolute weight loss of 0.34 kg/day occurred, compared to 0.31 kg/day on the nonketogenic diet. The difference between the two rates of weight loss was due to increased water loss on the ketogenic diet.

**Starvation Diet**    In the same subjects studied during 10 days of complete starvation, the daily weight loss was 50% higher than the loss during the ketogenic diet, and the increase in loss was due to the greater energy deficit. Surprisingly, however, during the total fast, the energy lost was the same as that lost during the ketogenic diet, and the increased weight loss during complete starvation was entirely due to water loss.

During prolonged dietary restriction, obese subjects increase the energy contributed to maintaining metabolic activity by adding more of their fat stores to the fuel mixture. After 6 weeks on a very-low-energy diet, obese subjects oxidized a fuel mixture that was much higher in fat and lower in protein than that utilized by nonobese volunteers during similar stringent dietary restriction. Obese subjects, therefore, during prolonged severe intake curtailment, use their fuel reserves (fat) more efficiently than do lean persons. They also do not have the substantially decreased basal metabolic rate that occurs in nonobese volunteers, and they do not voluntarily decrease their physical activity, as occurs in their nonobese counterparts. Thus, obesity predisposes to a continued and better quality weight loss after prolonged periods of semi-starvation, whereas nonobese subjects, left to their own devices, decrease physical activity and, thus, energy expenditure, considerably.

From these studies, it is clear that the rate of body-fat loss correlates best with the energy deficit during food restriction. At a given energy deficit, the rate of loss in body weight depends upon the composition of the loss, and particularly on the proportion of water. During early calorie restriction, diuresis often occurs, and this can be increased and continued beyond its natural duration by a low-calorie ketogenic diet or by fasting. During prolonged restricted calorie intake, adaptation develops, and energy from fat stores is used to make up the deficit and conserve protein and water. Obese subjects adapt more successfully and can continue physical activities much longer than nonobese persons under similar dietary restriction (Van Itallie and Yang [5]). It cannot be determined from these studies, however, whether further adaptation occurs in athletes who continue physical activity during starvation. Athletes would undoubtedly hope that a continuous high-energy weight loss composed largely of fats with relative sparing of protein could occur.

# Food Selection

Selection of food is determined by a number of factors, the most important of which is the satisfaction of hunger. During famine, habits and preferences are forgotten, and sometimes products not normally regarded as fit for human consumption are eaten. Unfortunately, when ample food is available, the food choice is often largely influenced by habit. These habits are complicated and stem from a number of influences, especially the food available locally. For example, fish are a common part of the diet in coastal areas or near lakes or rivers. Where climate is appropriate, grain, complex carbohydrates, yams, tapioca, or similar plants are consumed.

In the Western world the wide variety of foods available makes the choice abundant and often leads the consumer astray. When common foods become scarce, as they did during World War II, they may be regarded as luxury items and eaten only rarely, together with those that are not considered appetizing. An example of this is the present shortage of herring in Europe, which a few years ago was a part of the daily diet of the poorer population but now is considered a delicacy because of its high price. The converse, of course, is also true when so-called luxury foods drop in price and become plentiful.

In addition to habits formed in early childhood, which are, of course, subject to familial traditions, religious and cultural influences play a large part in determining customary food intake. In many cultures, for example, the Indian culture, food is not only nourishment but is also an integral part of religious and other ceremonies. Of course, even today restrictions of certain foods, based on religious beliefs, are found in almost all countries.

Clearly, the dietary rules given in the Bible, the Koran, and the Talmud play an important part in the food selection of various ethnic groups. Moreover, the prescribed fasting during religious ceremonies and abstinence from certain foods play an important part in physical condition and food habits. Because of the very early adherence to a group of foods and habitual consumption of, or abstinence from, other foods, changes in dietary customs are hard for these people to accept and to follow.

However, in those who engage in various sports, food customs can easily be changed because of the athletes' desire for better performance and the promise often implied that consumption of certain foods will lead to improved athletic achievement. Nevertheless, in general, to achieve basic changes in food habits—whether to improve nutrition, prevent disease, or increase athletic achievement—requires strategies and technologies that, at least in the beginning, are integrated as much as possible with previous local habits and religious customs. Giving the impression that the products, timing, or changes proposed are in any way superior to those habitually used by the consumers must be strictly avoided.

# Starvation

Dietary manipulation to improve athletic performance includes starvation, carbohydrate restriction, protein ingestion, and excessive fat intake. The metabolic events of starvation need, therefore, to be delineated before such manipulations are recommended to athletes for improved physical performance. Human beings live for many months without food and maintain a nearly normal metabolic rate and physical activity (not athletic performance). Survival during starvation depends upon closely integrated adaptive changes.

Interest in starvation is an ancient one, but metabolic studies during starvation in normal people have been performed only recently. In a classic work entitled *A Study of Prolonged Fasting* (Benedict [6]), one subject was sealed in a calorimeter during the night, but was free to write his autobiography during the day. This subject, on the 31st day of fasting, claimed to be feeling very well, was "uplifted," and wished to prolong the fast further because he did not feel a trace of hunger or discomfort. He may of course, have had an easy time, being a professional.

Most other persons fasting for even shorter periods of time would not find it as uplifting. Nevertheless, the study showed that normal subjects can fast for a month without impairing either mental or usual physical capacity.

## Available Energy

The available energy during fasting comes mainly from fat (85%). The adipose tissue has little intracellular water and thus contains the most energy per unit of weight. Protein provides about 14% of the available energy, but because of its great importance in enzymatic, structural, and mechanical roles, it is usually preserved until very late, and the body engages in a number of stratagems to prevent the breakdown of protein.

**Carbohydrates**   The carbohydrate store is relatively small, providing only about 1% of available energy during fasting, but on the whole, the total energy available to the ordinary human body is enough to last for more than 80 days of total abstinence from food.

Even though carbohydrates are available in such short supply, they are essential for survival, and the clinical manifestations of hypoglycemia, particularly those due to central and peripheral nervous system dysfunction, suggest the importance of glucose. The central nervous system requires 115 g glucose in 24 h, and more is needed for muscle activity. Other tissues that require glucose for anaerobic glycolysis are, of course, bone marrow, the renal medulla, peripheral nerves, and erythrocytes (about 36 g/day). Total daily body utilization of glucose during fasting is about 150 g, and the small glycogen stores in the liver cannot supply enough for a 1-day fast.

Of the many adaptive changes that occur during fasting, an important one is gluconeogenesis, or production of glucose from proteins. Lactate, a product of glycolysis, can be resynthesized to glucose in the liver and kidney. This does not provide a net energy gain, since lactate was derived from glucose originally, i.e., the energy required for glucose resynthesis is offset by that derived from glycolysis. The advantage of this cycle (the Cori cycle) is twofold: 1) Energy for hepatic glucose synthesis comes from oxidation of fatty acids, which are available in large quantities; 2) The requirements for protein-derived glucose are minimized by the recycling of lactate, the glycolytic product.

**Fat**  Fat has a direct role as a source of glucose, in addition to providing the energy for glucose resynthesis in the Cori cycle. The glycerol skeleton of triglycerides is readily converted to glucose, yielding about 80 g/24 h at rest. When lipolysis increases during fasting, the released glycerol becomes an important, though minor, substrate for glucose synthesis.

**Amino Acids**  Finally, protein-derived amino acids can be used as a major source of glucose through gluconeogenesis, at great expense to the body, as illustrated by an old observation: When dogs are starved to the limit of survival, nitrogen excretion increases just before death, an indication that when all other stores are exhausted, the body turns to its protein. When this happens, death is near.

Fasting humans depend upon glucose production from many sources, but fat is the predominant substrate.

# The Kidney's Role

The kidney plays an important role in the metabolic adaptation to starvation. It not only contributes to the temporary diuresis at the beginning of starvation but also to gluconeogenesis, which increases to the point of providing almost half the total glucose production. The substrate for renal gluconeogenesis is glutamine, whereas the substrate for hepatic gluconeogenesis is alanine. The nitrogenous by-product of renal gluconeogenesis is ammonia, and the hepatic gluconeogenetic by-product is urea. The ammonia provides additional adaptive advantages because its excretion is in the cationic form, ammonium, which titrates the excess organic acid produced in fasting. Moreover, the ammonia may be resorbed, thus reducing the obligatory nitrogen loss that accompanies the hepatic urea formation. In addition, decreased urea excretion spares the major urinary solute and thus decreases the obligatory water loss and the need for water intake.

## Sequence of Events

During the early phase of starvation, blood glucose declines as a result of continuing glucose utilization, particularly by the central nervous system. The lowered blood glucose level signals insulin to fall and glucagon to rise, which in turn facilitate release of fatty acids and amino acids. Fatty acid oxidation, however, provides most of the body's energy requirements and gluconeogenesis supplies glucose to the central nervous system and glycolytic tissues. Insulin is the major regulator of peripheral lipolysis and proteolysis, and glucagon stimulates hepatic glycogen release and liver uptake of alanine for gluconeogenesis.

In early starvation, gluconeogenesis is achieved predominantly by rapid proteolysis. Death from starvation is not caused by hypoglycemia but occurs when one-third to one-half of body protein is lost. Therefore, survival in prolonged starvation necessitates reduction in the rate of protein catabolism. It was observed many years ago that nitrogen loss in starvation decreases with time. When fasting continues beyond 1 week, nitrogen loss measured as urea declines to 3–4 g/day after 4–6 weeks (Owen et al. [7]).

Blood glucose is unchanged after 3 days of starvation without additional physical activity. Therefore, the adaptation to prolonged fasting also includes reduced glucose utilization. Brain requirements for glucose (normally 100–125 g/day), in the face of a daily glucose production of only 80 g, are met by the use of ketone acids, which may provide up to 50%–60% of brain fuel needs. The increased use of ketones is, in part, due to a progressive hyperketonemia and, therefore, increased availability of ketones for the brain (Garber et al. [8]).

**Ketones**  Investigations of prolonged fasting suggest that ketones have a dual role, particularly in the late phase of starvation—that of energy substrate and a signal for change in the type of substrate consumed. The energy to the brain provided by ketones reduces the demand for glucose, and the ketonemia signals to the muscles to reduce protein catabolism and output (Saudek and Felig [9]). The decrease in alanine availability, in turn, causes a reduction in hepatic gluconeogenesis. Ketones coordinate the reduction of glucose utilization and production during prolonged fasts. Thus, metabolic adaptations during starvation maintain glucose homeostasis and conserve body protein. These adaptations are accomplished early by the release of alanine from muscles for hepatic gluconeogenesis. The signals for the initial responses are reduced plasma insulin and increased plasma glucagon. The negative nitrogen balance and depletion of protein stores threaten survival during prolonged fasts, and the organism's metabolism, therefore, shifts toward protein conservation. Hyperketonemia is then the main adaptive mechanism for the late phase.

A number of factors influence the normal human metabolic rate during fasting and refeeding. Normally, metabolic rate increases after a meal, and this increase is even greater when subjects exercise or when they have been overfeeding for several weeks. On the other hand, diminished metabolic rates after a meal were reported in underfed or starved subjects, in obese individuals, and in normal individuals at high altitude (Stock et al. [10]).

**Body Changes**    The efficiency of the human body changes in response to the nutritional status, and this may provide long-term control of energy balance over and above that provided by food intake. Acute changes in energy intake, such as those often practiced prior to competition by athletes, may also affect diet-induced thermogenesis, and, indeed, the magnitude of the thermic response to a meal during light exercise depends on the previous day's energy intake. Contradictory claims concerning this effect have been reported. More recent investigations of this important dietary manipulation (Stock [11]) showed that acute changes in energy intake do not affect the overall efficiency of the body's energy utilization, either at rest or during exercise. However, the normal changes in blood glucose and free fatty acids in response to food intake are considerably altered by the previous day's diet. The thermic effect of a meal during exercise is enhanced considerably by the subject's having overeaten on the previous day. Thus, carbohydrate loading or starvation prior to competition may profoundly affect the metabolic response to eating on the day of competition. Whether such dietary manipulation and thermic re-sponse alter performance have not been established.

# Diet and Life Span

In laboratory animals, dietary restrictions increase life span. A nutritionally adequate diet was fed every second or third day, intermittently with a nutritionally inadequate diet, or animals were fed *ad libitum* a diet with sufficient protein to support maximal growth. The increased life span in animals with dietary manipulation was thought to result from caloric restriction alone. Nutritional manipulation was imposed during early growth and the concept arose that senescence follows growth cessation and is delayed by caloric restriction during early growth.

More recent studies, however, have shown similar beneficial effects of dietary restrictions upon the life span of adult animals. This type of dietary manipulation has not been scrutinized scientifically in human beings. Nevertheless, the increase in life span with a restricted caloric intake has been found in a variety of species and may represent a basic biologic process that is also active in man. The mechanism for this is not known. Physiological and biochemical variables were examined in animals in which dietary manipulation delayed senescence and increased life span. The incidence of various diseases was also studied in these animals. For example, animals with an increased life span due to low protein feeding have lower rectal temperatures than controls.

Conversely, little is known about the effect of body temperature on life span in homeothermic animals. The life span of poikilothermic animals increases with decreased environmental temperature. This has been attributed to a lower metabolic rate resulting from a slowing of biochemical reactions by reduced temperature. However, low body temperatures of mice fed a low protein diet are, in fact, associated with increased oxygen consumption. Results are conflicting concerning the relationship of longevity to basal metabolic rate and increased oxygen consumption due to dietary restrictions, and at present the two factors cannot be definitively related.

Several diseases increase with age in animals and humans, but the relationship between the diseases and aging is not known. Dietary restriction and increased life span in mice and rats are associated with delayed onset of a number of diseases, but this is not a consistent occurrence, and the relationship between diet and disease is not clear. Mice fed two dietary regimens, either of which increased life span—namely, a low-protein diet and intermittent feeding—had small cells (judged from the DNA content of hepatic and renal cells) that increased in size with refeeding. The small cells contained less protein and had reduced activities of succinoxidase, cholinesterase, and malic dehydrogenase. No common biochemical alteration was found that could explain the increased life span due to dietary protein restriction or intermittent feeding, nor was there support for the hypothesis that dietary restriction increases life span by reducing protein synthesis and, consequently, reducing use of the genetic code.

Athletes manipulate their diets in many ways. This may include intermittent or continuous insufficient protein intake to sustain cellular activities. However, no studies have been able to relate dietary manipulations or athletic activities during caloric or specific nutrient restriction to longevity.

# Recommended Dietary Allowances

It is difficult to establish guidelines for nutrient and energy needs in humans. The standards are estimates based on judgments of expert committees. In the United States, the recommended dietary allowances (RDAs) are only aims to achieve. The RDAs are not minimum requirements but are amounts of nutrients and calories thought to nourish most people adequately in this country. There are no RDAs designed to provide adequate calories and nutrients for athletes in a variety of different sports, though human beings can maintain health within a wide range of nutrient and caloric intake. This includes short-term deficits in both caloric and dietary essentials. Most short-term deficits can be made up, but the effects of prolonged dietary inadequacies for those actively engaged in physical work have not been sufficiently studied. Nevertheless, for sedentary individuals, the most common nutritional deficit in this country is iron.

## Achieving a Suitable Balance

Excessive intake of nutrients and calories, on the other hand, is not always associated with deleterious effects. What is excess for a sedentary individual might not be excessive for an athlete. Moreover, the efficiency of liver and kidney function and the presence of compensatory and detoxification mechanisms are important in determining whether caloric and nutrient excess will be associated with symptoms. There are no recognized advantages to the ingestion of nutrients, and certainly not of calories, that are vastly greater than those needed for either correction of deficiency or replenishment caused by exaggerated requirements or by metabolic or absorptive diseases. Because of this, a widely varied diet makes the probability of excessive exposure to a noxious component, either natural or environmental, less likely. Moreover, it also assures that adequate essential nutrients are taken.

**Differences in Dietary Needs**    The balance of energy intake and output and of nutritional sufficiency is most acutely disturbed in the mature members of our society. The only-too-common weight gain is related to overeating and, even more importantly, to lack of exercise. Metabolic rate and energy expenditure usually decrease with age in our present society, but total caloric and nutrient intake does not. Therefore, in those who are not habitually physically active, caloric restriction is essential. Nutrient and caloric intake prone to restrictions, particularly in young people who are conscious of weight and figure control, may lead to disease or injury, and, during pregnancy, may compromise the offspring nutritionally.

Nutritional anemias common in women and older men in this country are related to inadequate dietary iron and folic acid. Osteoporosis, also common in elderly women and some men, is related not only to deficient dietary calcium but also to inactivity. Poor nutrition of the elderly in conjunction with their decreased physical activity is a growing public health problem.

**Dietary Trends**    Surveys of dietary trends in the United States indicate that protein-derived calories are about the same as in 1910. However, in the early part of this century, 50% of the protein came from grains and vegetables, and now 70% of the protein consumed is of animal origin. The increased dietary use of animal protein—meat, poultry, fish, and dairy products—is associated with decreased physical activity.

Carbohydrate consumption has declined, and the carbohydrates used are of different types. Starch consumption has dropped off much more rapidly than that of carbohydrate as a whole during the last six or seven decades, and refined sugar intake has increased, even though it was scarce during World War II. The use of flour and other grain products has also decreased considerably. The reduced use of complex carbohydrates in the diet, accompanied by decreased fiber intake, is a matter of concern for those engaged in dietary advice.

In this country, dietary fat has steadily increased, and has been accompanied by a shift in the type of fat used. Saturated fatty acid content in foods has changed little during the past decades. Polyunsaturated fatty acids have increased only modestly, but noticeably during the last 20 years, mainly as a result of the increased consumption of edible oils. Moreover, cholesterol intake at present is only 10% above that consumed a century ago. Over the past 20 years the consumption of eggs, lard, butter, and various dairy products has decreased while meat consumption has increased. These are all trends that are applauded by those advocating dietary manipulation to prevent certain diseases.

Vitamin and mineral intake has not changed much during this century, but calcium, vitamin D, and vitamin A are used slightly more than they were 65 years ago. Since the 1940s, iron, riboflavin, niacin, and thiamine have been added to flour, considerably increasing the per capita availability of these nutrients. The enrichment of certain cereals with the same nutrients has contributed to a slight increase in their consumption.

It should be reemphasized that since the early part of this century, dietary calories in this country have remained essentially the same, but there has also been a concomitant decrease in energy expenditure, related to transportation modes and changes in life-style. This trend has led to major health problems not usually evident in those who are physically active but predominant in the obese sedentary person. It has also contributed, though the mechanism is not understood, to increased vascular disease and other conditions that are probably related to dietary habits. In this setting, the reduced consumption of complex carbohydrates associated with decreased fiber intake has also been blamed for a number of degenerative diseases, but final proof that this aspect of dietary change is, in fact, influencing the occurrence of gastrointestinal disorders such as diverticulosis and certain types of cancer is not available.

## Dietary Protein

Dietary protein provides amino acids for growth and tissue maintenance, for enzyme production, and for gluconeogenesis. Amino acids that the body is unable to manufacture, or essential amino acids, are tryptophan, phenylalanine, methionine, lysine, threonine, leucine, isoleucine, valine, and histidine (mainly for infants and possibly for healthy adults). About another 15 amino acids can be made in quantities sufficient to provide the necessary building blocks for body tissues, provided enough nitrogen is available. The biologic value of protein is determined by the dietary composition of essential amino acids, the need for which is related to body requirements.

The need for protein and essential amino acids normally varies with age and is determined by their rate of turnover. In the average sedentary adult, this is about 2.5 g/kg/ day or about 175 g of protein. The obligatory losses of nitrogen are only about 30 g protein; there is therefore about an 80% reutilization. The essential amino acids form about 40% of the amino acid content of tissue protein. Essential amino acids need only provide half (20%) of dietary protein in the adult, so they must be even more highly conserved in total turnover of amino acid nitrogen. The essential amino acid requirement for new-tissue formation in growing children is increased to 43% of dietary protein. Standards proposed for a "safe level of protein intake" are 0.55 g/kg/day of excellent quality protein as an average value for adults, and 2 g/kg/day for infants from birth to 6 months of age.

The actual dietary intake of protein in the United States is much higher, and the possible deleterious effects of this on longevity have already been touched upon. Moreover, long-lived people in other parts of the world (Ecuador, Pakistan, and the Caucasus) subsist on low-energy and low-protein diets. These low-protein requirements may help eliminate much of the so-called world "protein gap" but, nevertheless, a number of activists clamor for closure of the protein gap and are reluctant to accept the practical implications of the latest thinking on protein requirements.

The human body is capable of infinite adaptive changes. When the energy intake falls below the requirement, the living organism burns its own tissue to help bridge the gap between intake and requirement. In the young this is sometimes evidenced by reduction or total cessation of growth. The adaptive changes to low-protein intake, known for years, include reduced urinary nitrogen excretion, especially in the form of urea. In prolonged or even short-lived protein restriction, the hepatic urea cycle is depressed, and amino acid synthesis is increased. The opposite occurs with protein feeding. In severe malnutrition (energy-protein reduction), the most significant deficit is caloric and not protein (McLaren [12]).

Glycogen and free fatty acids are the major energy sources for short-duration physical activity, and protein utilization probably occurs in exercise of long duration. For example, alanine output from skeletal muscle increases in proportion to work intensity (Felig [13]).

It may be that amino acids are transaminated in skeletal muscles, thus permitting *de novo* synthesis of alanine from glucose-derived pyruvate.

An intramuscular enzyme efflux after exercise is another explanation for increased protein involvement in exercise. The enzyme efflux, at least in isolated preparations, occurs only after the muscle work capacity is considerably reduced by fatigue, a finding suggesting that when the muscle's ability to synthesize ATP decreases as a result of glycogen depletion, the cell membrane breaks down and enzymes are released. The enzymes are then degraded into their component amino acids and are subsequently deaminated.

Another possibility is that protein involvement is directly related to the available substrate. Thus, serum urea increases linearly with exercise duration, beginning after about 70 min. At this time, liver glycogen is decreased and muscle glycogen is severely depleted. It is, therefore, possible that protein catabolism occurs with prolonged exercise, similar to that seen in short-term starvation (Saudek and Felig [9]). Therefore, the protein catabolism that occurs during or after prolonged exercise may be related to glycogen depletion and the consequent decreased ATP, and is not directly related to exercise.

The relationship between initial muscle glycogen content and protein catabolism has been examined (Lemon and Mullin [14]). When subjects exercised after carbohydrate depletion, serum and sweat levels of urea nitrogen were significantly higher than those seen with exercise after carbohydrate loading, and serum urea continued to be high into the recovery period. Protein breakdown during carbohydrate depletion was 13.7 g/h, and protein provided 10.4% of the caloric cost of the exercise. The possible mechanisms contributing to increased protein utilization with prolonged exercise have been discussed. In the studies of prolonged exercise in human subjects, the excretion of urea nitrogen in sweat was the most important mechanism in preventing an exercise-induced rise in serum urea nitrogen in both carbohydrate-loaded and -depleted subjects. The importance of urea nitrogen excretion in sweat was emphasized when the highest serum urea values were seen during the recovery period after sweating had ceased. Therefore, serum urea nitrogen probably is not a reliable index of protein catabolism but depends upon the exercising individual's capacity to sweat and on his or her thermoregulatory responses and heat acclimation (see Chapter 2, Temperature Regulation and Sports).

Changes in plasma and urinary amino acids were studied in participants in a 70-km cross-country ski race that lasted 4½–6 h and was associated with slight dehydration (Refsum et al. [15]). An average of 8 μmol/min/kg body weight of urea were produced during the race. This is more than twice the average urea production for normally active similar persons with ordinary protein intake. A marked change also occurred in plasma amino acids during the race, a finding supporting the suggestion that protein and amino acid metabolism is an integral part of the metabolic response to prolonged heavy exercise. The changes in the amino acid pattern were not influenced by the amino acid composition of serum albumin or muscle, materials probably metabolized during heavy exertion. The explanation was that heavy exercise causes muscle glycogen depletion, reduced pyruvate, and decreased alanine release. The amino acid changes in this study, as in previous studies, were similar to those found during prolonged starvation. Thus, it is clear from many well-conducted studies in humans that prolonged heavy exercise places demands on protein and amino acid stores that should be replenished by appropriate diet.

**Excessive Protein Intake**   Athletes engaged in heavy short-duration physical activity such as weightlifting, throwing, wrestling, and body building commonly eat excessive amounts of protein. This practice is based upon a tradition that goes back to the ancient Greek athletes who ate large quantities of meat to replace muscles spent during exercise, and is supported by the theory first propounded by J. Von Liebig in 1851 (Consolazio and Johnson [16]) that protein is the principal source of energy for muscle contraction. Though this is clearly not the case, recent reinvestigation of the theory has shed light upon the beneficial effects of increased protein intake, particularly in athletes engaged in muscle building. During such exercise, lean body mass and nitrogen retention increase, and this increase is augmented by higher protein intake. On the other hand, short-term exercise at both high-and low-caloric or nitrogen intake is usually accompanied by increased nitrogen excretion. Thus, athletes engaged in weightlifting, throwing, and other lean-body-mass building exercises over long periods of time and accompanied by increased muscle mass would benefit from increased protein intake on the order of 2.4 g/kg body weight per day. In endurance events, when excessive weight is undesirable, minimal protein intake, as recommended by the World Health Organization, is adequate to replace the muscle breakdown (Marable and Hickson [17]).

**Fad Diets**   Because increased physical activity is growing in popularity, the desire to lose excessive weight rapidly has tempted many to embark upon severe dietary restrictions and to use some diets that have been recommended for rapid weight loss. In 1976, a book entitled *The Last Chance Diet* was published (Linn and Stuart [18]). Within a short time, several liquid-protein-modified-fast diets became popular and were used for rapid weight reduction by large numbers of people. Though these dietary modifications were intended for the grotesquely obese and were to be the sole source of calories for those attempting this method of weight reduction, it soon became clear that a number of people who wanted to reach ideal weight rapidly to improve athletic performance were also using the diet.

By August, 1977, sudden death in several young diet users was reported, and between July 1977 and January 1978, 60 deaths occurred among avid users of the liquid-protein-modified-fast diet. Detailed clinical and necropsy information was available for 17 of these patients who had been healthy except for obesity before embarking on the diet. Electrocardiographic abnormalities, particularly prolongation of the QT interval, were ominous of and may have presaged sudden death in these patients. All those who died suddenly while on the liquid-protein diet were extremely obese, and it was unlikely that they had engaged in physical activity of any sort either before or during the diet. Nevertheless, the temptation to engage in extreme dietary manipulation of this or other types in order to, as it were, lighten the burden, particularly in endurance events, is often great enough that any method might seem minor if it leads to the desired effect. It should be emphasized that the use of various liquid-protein-modified-fast diets is dangerous. Their value in improving athletic performance is certainly questionable, and for those who are more than moderately obese, the chance of serious complications is great (Isner et al. [19]).

## Fear of Obesity

Obesity is seen as a serious threat to continued health because of its ill-defined relationships to morbidity and mortality from cardiovascular disease, and a number of other conditions, and those who are obese are often subject to derogatory assessments by themselves and their social contacts. It has been said that "whenever fat people have existed and whenever a literature has reflected aspects of the lives and values of the period, a record has been left of the low regard usually held for the obese by the thinner and clearly more virtuous observer" (Mayer [20]). Because, in this country at the moment, the obese are classed as immature, passive-dependent, and of low self-esteem, and are given the responsibility for their fatness, they not only face the hazards of their adiposity but also must contend with serious psychologic and social difficulties. It is, therefore, not surprising that some obese individuals embrace exercise and dietary manipulation of the type discussed in the foregoing sections as a panacea for their adiposity. Although both approaches are useful in weight reduction, one should be cognizant of the possible risks of exercise and dietary manipulation in those who are obese and not accustomed to energy expenditure. Moreover, physicians often have negative attitudes toward obese patients, and failure of weight reduction in many individuals may be due to feelings of shame, self-derogation, and the embarrassment that they experience when facing physicians (Maiman and Wang [21]).

# Lipid Metabolism

The main substrate for energy production in human skeletal muscle after prolonged exertion is lipid. Studies were performed, therefore, to assess the effects of training, particularly of the endurance variety, on lipid metabolism. After endurance training, muscle glycogen utilization is reduced and the carbon source of energy for muscular activity is shifted to lipids. This is a major advantage in delaying fatigue in events limited by muscle glycogen content (Gollnick [22]).

Subsequent studies confirmed these findings and showed that equally trained males and females with similar aerobic capacity and muscle fiber composition derive a comparable portion of their energy requirements from lipids. In such persons, however, *in vitro* measurement of a selected muscle mitochondrial enzyme suggests that female muscle adapts less well than male muscle under similar conditions of training. This finding was attributed to a lesser mitochondrial density in the trained female muscle than in the male muscle. However, even though these *in vitro* measurements suggest a difference in female muscle fibers, there was no functional effect on lipid utilization during prolonged exertion.

Although the capacity for muscles to metabolize fat is markedly enhanced by endurance training, the actual regulation of lipid use during prolonged physical activity is not limited by the ability of muscle fibers to oxidize fatty acids. Moreover, even untrained muscle can increase lipid oxidation markedly when plasma free fatty acids are increased (Costill and Coyle [23]), a finding that is theoretically explained by the known catecholamine increase with exercise and consequent release of free fatty acids from fat (Appenzeller and Schade [24]). It may be that changes in cyclic AMP are responsible for alpha- and beta-adrenergic stimulation. Catecholamine activity on beta receptors stimulates adenyl cyclase and increases intracellular cyclic AMP, which in turn changes cell function appropriately.

On the other hand, similar interactions with alpha receptors cause decreased cyclic AMP and opposite changes in cell activity. This hypothesis may not apply to all adrenergic responsive cells, but it has been tested in isolated human fat cells, and agrees closely with theoretic considerations (Robison et al. [25]. Epinephrine stimulated cyclic AMP in fat cells from obese subjects in the fed state, and glycerol was released into the incubation medium. Phentolamine (an alpha-adrenergic receptor blocker) enhanced this action and propranolol (a beta-receptor blocker) reduced it to below basal levels.

However, epinephrine suppressed cyclic AMP lipolysis when incubated with fat cells from fasted individuals. The reversal of epinephrine effect on fat cells by fasting appears to be due to decreased beta-receptor activity rather than increased alpha-receptor activity. This change in alpha- and beta-adrenergic receptor action occurred after 1 day of fasting and remained the same for an 8-day observation period.

These findings suggest that during fasting the sympathetic nervous system and circulating catecholamines act to conserve adipose tissue triglycerides (Burns et al. [26]). It should, at this point, be emphasized that some athletes fast prior to competition. If the competition extends beyond 60 min, then clearly the availability of free fatty acids for fuel is crucial to performance. The epinephrine effect of reversal upon lipolysis of human adipocytes from fasting subjects suggests that fasting is not indicated prior to endurance events but may, of course, be of some use during shorter athletic feats.

## Exercise Intensity

Under ordinary dietary conditions, the extent to which energy is supplied from carbohydrates or fat is determined by the relative exercise intensity. Increasingly more energy is derived from fat at exercise intensities of 65% maximum oxygen consumption ($\dot{V}_{O_2 \, max}$) during prolonged activity, but if the intensity rises to 75% $\dot{V}_{O_2 \, max}$, fat is not used and the muscle needs carbohydrate for fuel. Fat utilization during prolonged exercise is higher after a fat-rich diet than after a carbohydrate-rich or a normal diet.

Thus the implications are clear concerning dietary manipulation prior to sports that require prolonged activity of relatively low intensity, which would benefit, presumably, from a fat-rich rather than a carbohydrate-rich diet. This is not to say, however, that carbohydrate "loading" (to be discussed later) is not indicated for athletes who will engage in high-energy activities, even for 2 or more hours. Free fatty acid uptake from plasma into the muscle during exercise is related to plasma concentration of the free fatty acids, but the increased combustion of fat during prolonged exercise—clearly a useful adaptive mechanism—can only in part be explained by increased uptake of plasma free fatty acids. The plasma fatty acids might be supplied in part from hydrolysis of triglycerides by an enzyme (lipoprotein lipase) present at the endothelial surface of muscle capillaries. It is possible, therefore, that a training-induced increase in this enzyme might make more fatty acids available during muscular activity in trained individuals.

## Lipid Stores

Increased utilization of intramuscular triglyceride occurs in animals and man during prolonged activity, and has been attributed to an intracellular muscle enzyme called hormone-sensitive lipase. In recent studies of lipoprotein lipase activity and lipid stores in human skeletal muscles during prolonged exercise (Lithell et al. [27]), the enzyme increased in skeletal muscle during an 85-km cross-country ski race. Moreover, this increase was most striking in those athletes who had the best training and the fastest times in this competition. The training and $\dot{V}_{O_2\ max}$, as well as the finishing times, were closely correlated so that it is not possible to be certain which of these factors was, in fact, the determinant for the increased lipoprotein lipase activity. In the best-trained athletes, the largest triglyceride stores were in muscle biopsies taken before the race, and the largest decrease in triglyceride stores occurred during competition. The lipoprotein lipase activity increased only minimally in the best competitors. The least-trained participants in this study, on the other hand, had a sixfold increase in lipoprotein lipase during the race so that in these subjects there was greater capacity for free fatty-acid uptake from serum triglycerides in comparison to highly trained participants in the same race. Thus, these studies confirm numerous previous reports that muscular energy during prolonged heavy physical work is, in part, and probably most efficaciously, derived from intracellularly stored lipids, and in highly trained subjects the stores are both larger and more easily used than in less-well-trained competitors. It seems, therefore, advantageous to increase fat consumption during training in order to make free fatty acids more available and, perhaps, induce lipoprotein lipase formation in muscle capillary endothelium.

# Dietary Fiber

It has been suggested that the increasing prevalence of obesity in western countries may, in part, be due to increased refined carbohydrate and, therefore, reduced fiber in the diet. Several physiological activities of dietary fiber tend to reduce the chances of obesity. Fiber displaces nutrients from the diet and requires more chewing, thus reducing the rate of food ingestion. It also promotes secretion of saliva and gastric juice, which contributes to gastric distention and satiety, and decreases small bowel absorption of some foods, particularly fat and protein. Moreover, consumption of refined products such as white flour and sugar are more likely to cause excess calories because they can be eaten rapidly and absorbed efficiently.

In countries where obesity is rare, the population usually ingests a diet rich in complex carbohydrates with their high fiber complement. *Ad libitum* intake of high-fiber diets provides greater satiety than does that of low fiber diets of comparable energy content. This finding is attributed to a larger undigested residue in the intestine with corresponding increase in the feeling of bulk and distention.

The Egyptian sand rat, which normally eats a high-fiber diet, becomes obese on reduced fiber diets, and rats given snack foods become obese and then revert to normal weight when the ordinary rat-pellet diet is reinstituted. Snack foods are high in energy and sugar and are practically devoid of fiber. The overall role of food fiber in obesity is far from clear. It is, however, believed that consumption of fiber-rich food may help prevent obesity and promote weight loss in obese people if calories are simultaneously restricted.

## Vegetarian Diet

The dietary practices of athletes vary widely according to their sport. Many endurance athletes are vegetarians. Most, fortunately, are "lacto-ovo" vegetarians or are, at least, lactovegetarians. It is rare to find "pure" vegetarians or those who refuse eggs, dairy products, and all flesh foods. The true or pure vegetarian (vegan) whose philosophy prohibits exploitation or "cruelty" toward animals is at risk of serious malnutrition, particularly when engaging in high-energy output for a prolonged time.

Many athletes, and particularly vegetarians, also prefer organic or natural foods in the belief that vegetables grown with the addition of pesticides, herbicides, or inorganic fertilizers are, somehow, contaminated and have lost their nutritive values. This idea, of course, is not supported by scientific evidence, and belongs to the cultists espousing counter-culture philosophies, which have, until recently, also included the so-called Zen macrobiotic diet.

Athletes using vegetarian diets, however, have a large fiber intake, which affects gastrointestinal motility and nutrient absorption, both important considerations before competition. For example, if food energy content is reduced because of fiber, then adequate energy may not be available during competition, particularly in endurance events. The bulky residue and decreased speed of absorption of high-fiber foods may seriously affect performance by causing increased bowel motility and gastrointestinal discomfort.

The role of high-fiber foods in the maintenance of desired weight in some athletic disciplines is not clear. Nevertheless, vegetarianism is now widespread among certain athletes and merits consideration of its effect on performance during both competition and training (Calkins [28]). Claims have been made that increased dietary fiber prevents or treats diabetes, atherosclerosis, cancer of the large bowel, and many other disorders. Most of these claims are based on epidemiologic data comparing very different populations and important factors other than dietary fiber that may have been instrumental in changing the disease incidence.

Dietary fiber is the skeletal remnant of plant cells, which resists human gastrointestinal enzymatic digestion. Phytic acid (inositol hexaphosphate), closely associated with dietary fiber and an important component of bran and whole-grain flour, may combine with calcium, magnesium, iron, and zinc and cause deficiency of these ions when dietary sources are marginal or when the body requires larger amounts of them. Other constituents of the plant skeleton may have profound effects. These include silica and lipids found in fruit leaves and seeds, and nonmetabolizable sugars, such as raffinose, which may promote production of bowel gas in man. Whether these effects of dietary fibers are detrimental to athletic performance has not been determined.

## Effects of Fiber on Carbohydrates and Lipids

Well-documented clinical studies suggest that some types of food fiber have a beneficial effect on carbohydrate metabolism in diabetics. All studies agree on the glucose-lowering effect of guar and pectin often found in fruits. The glucose-lowering effects of dietary fibers, particularly cellulose, are less certain. In some diabetic patients, food fiber may significantly decrease or totally eliminate the need for insulin, an advantage that may be particularly valuable in those diabetics who are athletes.

Dietary fiber is also important in serum lipid regulation. For example, Seventh Day Adventists who are lacto-ovo vegetarians have a greatly reduced risk of coronary artery disease in comparison to others, but the specific dietary component responsible for the reduced risk in this group has not been identified. Neither cellulose nor bran has a definable effect upon serum cholesterol, whereas dietary guar and pectin lower it.

The role of high-fiber diets in the treatment of hypercholesterolemia is not established. Attempts have also been made to assess the value of dietary fiber in changing triglyceride levels in the management of atherosclerosis, but at present, information is insufficient to reach a conclusion. The value of athletic pursuits in the prevention or treatment of certain so-called degenerative diseases, including atherosclerosis, is also not clear because most athletes manipulate their diets, a factor that may affect the target disease in addition to increasing energy output.

Unquestionably, dietary fiber decreases transit time through the colon and also increases the average daily weight of stools. Small bowel transit time is relatively constant. A high-fiber diet also alters gastrointestinal bacterial flora. The lack of dietary fiber has been implicated on epidemiologic grounds as, perhaps, responsible for widespread diverticulosis in North America. Bran, which is not widely used by most people, shortens bowel transit time in normal subjects and in those with diverticular disease. Whether dietary fiber is at least partly responsible for bulky and frequent stools often occurring in endurance athletes is not clear.

Dietary fiber may also influence certain so-called degenerative diseases of western society. The typical "western diet," high in fat and protein and low in fiber, has been blamed for a number of ills, and the thrust is increasing for dietary modification to prevent disease, particularly among athletes. The effect of increasing dietary fiber upon athletic peformance, in preventing diabetes, atherosclerosis, diverticulitis, and perhaps colonic cancer is poorly understood, and one may not conclude, on the basis of present studies, that high dietary fiber benefits athletic performance or prevents disease (Levin and Horwitz [29]).

# Nutritional Supplements and Vitamins

Certain conditions must be met to evaluate claims for nutritional supplements and vitamins. These include answers to the following questions: Is the information based on personal observation, or can it stand the scrutiny of other scientists? Is it anecdote or science? Can the results be reproduced by those not involved in promoting the product, or does the recommended dietary change work just in the hands of its promoters, as suggested in a Harvard Medical School Health Letter [30]? Did control studies show that treatments are superior to placebos or "doing nothing"? What happens in the absence of supplementation or therapy? Are the results pure coincidence, the result of the natural history of the disorder, or the effect of other not-controlled-for conditions? Has the recommended manipulation, dietary or otherwise, been proven to be safe when compared with doing nothing or with other therapy? Is the risk of taking the supplement justified? In other words, what is the risk:benefit ratio? Lastly, the burden of proof that a certain dietary manipulation or therapy is effective is upon those who propose it, particularly if it involves methods or procedures that are not generally accepted medically.

## Megavitamins

Megavitamin therapy is the use of one or several vitamins in amounts that are 10 or more times greater than those recommended by the Committee on Dietary Allowances of Food and Nutrition, National Research Council of the United States. The recommended daily allowance (RDA) for each vitamin is substantially above the range that is commonly found in proper nutrition, to allow for a safety factor. Over the years, the RDA for most vitamins has decreased as knowledge about nutritional requirements has improved. Megavitamin therapy, as advocated by various cultists, is chemical and not nutrient therapy.

In general, vitamins function as coenzymes or hormones, or when combined with body protein to form holoenzymes, usually referred to as enzymes. A vitamin is useful only when combined with its apoenzyme, and the apoenzyme that is manufactured per unit of time is limited. Saturation of apoenzyme occurs at vitamin levels that are roughly those recommended in the dietary allowances, and excess vitamins become pharmacologic agents. Therefore, they are no longer nutrients, but are then medication.

A vitamin is an organic compound that the body cannot make in adequate amounts—that is, it is not protein, fat, or carbohydrate—and that is necessary for normal human metabolism. Vitamin deficiency produces a specific disease such as beriberi, rickets, or scurvy, which is corrected by administration of the deficient vitamin.

The 13 human vitamins need not be enumerated here. Four of them are fat soluble and nine are water soluble. The last vitamin to be discovered was $B_{12}$ in 1948, and further intensive research has not added new ones. Several growth factors, para-aminobenzoic acid, bioflavonoids, choline, inositol, lipoic acid, and ubiquinone, are necessary for other organisms such as bacteria. Some of these are also used by humans but can be produced in the body as needed.

Megavitamin therapy is rational and efficacious in certain genetic diseases associated with an inborn error of metabolism, in which the defect in vitamin utilization may be overcome by large doses of the vitamin. Occasionally, disorders occur that are associated with defective transport of vitamins across membranes. Megadose vitamins may be useful for treatment of toxic states produced by antivitamins—such as methotrexate, used in the treatment of malignancy; the antibacterial agent, trimethoprim, or the diuretic, triamterene. Megadoses of vitamin A have resulted in death, and death occurred in one person who had received 80 g of vitamin C intravenously (Herbert [31]).

There are no scientifically acceptable published data indicating that healthy, usually active individuals need vitamin supplementation, provided they eat a diet that includes grain, fruits, vegetables, meat, and milk products. It is not clear whether increased physical activity, including athletic performance, raises the demand for certain vitamins. Acceptable studies, for example, have not shown that vitamin C supplementation in excess of 200 mg/day is safe. In spite of these caveats, many athletes take megadoses of a variety of vitamins and, in particular, vitamin C. In this population, vitamin C ingestion of 15–20 g/day for many years has not, however, produced adverse effects, and the influence of such doses on athletic performance is purely anecdotal. Benefits from megadoses of vitamin E, also widely ingested by athletes, are anecdotally reported.

# Vitamin C Usage

The effects of large doses of ascorbic acid (vitamin C) on a variety of functions of human and animal cells have been assessed. Enhanced neutrophil motility to endotoxin-activated autologous serum, a chemotactic stimulus, occurred in normal adults after the ingestion of 2 and 3 g of ascorbate daily, whereas lower doses had no effect. Other functions of neutrophils were unaltered by vitamin C. Serum immunoglobulins and mitogen-induced protein synthesis were totally unaltered by ascorbic acid. Thus, vitamin C stimulates some cellular but not humoral immune function in humans. This effect should be considered when assessing the value of supplementary vitamin C in the protection from certain infections (Anderson et al. [32]).

Physical stress may require additional vitamin C. In studies of black mine workers in South Africa, subclinical vitamin C deficiency was common despite adequate daily intake from dietary sources. To prevent this, the addition of approximately 250 mg per person per day was recommended by the National Research Institute for Nutritional Diseases (Visagie et al. [33]).

Recent reports indicate that vitamin C stimulates prostaglandin $E_1$ formation in human platelets. This occurs at physiologic concentrations of vitamin C. Prostaglandin $E_1$ is important in lymphocyte function and, therefore, plays an important role in immune responses. Moreover, prostaglandin $E_1$ is also important in collagen and ground substance, in the metabolism of cholesterol, in the regulation of insulin, and in the responsiveness of the human body to insulin. It may be that defective prostaglandin $E_1$ formation accounts for many features of scurvy or partial vitamin C deficiency and additionally explains many of the reputed therapeutic effects of vitamin C. These hypotheses are unproven, but if correct, vitamin C is of value only if adequate dihomogammalinolenic acid, the precursor of prostaglandin $E_1$, is available. Adequate precursor in turn, depends upon the presence of enough essential fatty acids, pyridoxine and zinc (Horrobin, et al. [34]).

Because metals are involved in the function of various vitamins, studies were done to assess the bio-availability of dietary iron, copper, and zinc, and how this might be affected by vitamin C megadoses. It is known, for example, that such megadoses enhance absorption of iron and inhibit dietary copper absorption. Since zinc is particularly important in the reputed therapeutic effects of megadoses of vitamin C, its bio-availability after ascorbic acid supplementation was also examined in humans, and no effect was found over a dose range of up to 2 g ascorbic acid per day (Solomons et al. [35]). Because many athletes consume a relatively high fiber diet, it was also suggested that this might interfere with absorption of trace metals. Lacto-ovo-vegetarian nonathlete adolescents were compared to omnivores with regard to zinc in hair and dietary fiber. A significant positive correlation between zinc and fiber intake in the omnivores was noted. No significant correlation was found in the vegetarians, but a slight inverse relationship between zinc in hair and dietary fiber was present. This was attributed to the chelation effect by dietary fiber of, perhaps, phytic acid on zinc in the vegetarians (Treuherz [36]).

# Nutrition and Nervous System Function

Numerous studies have shown that inadequate nutrition during development can cause permanent structural and chemical changes in the nervous system, which correlate with long-term alterations in intellectual and sensorimotor activities. It is also agreed that the effect of such malnutrition is not as easily reversed when it occurs early in development as during later growth. In spite of the necessity still to prove that early malnutrition results in later behavioral alterations, overwhelming evidence exists for the great vulnerability of the nervous system to dietary manipulations or malnutrition during the time when glial cell hyperplasia and neuronal migration are most active. On the other hand, during adolescence and adulthood, the effects of malnutrition on nervous system function are easily reversed by improved nutrition.

More recent findings, however, suggest that brain composition, neurotransmitters, interneuronal communication, and therefore, nervous system function are sensitive to quantity and quality of food throughout the organism's life span, irrespective of whether growth is occurring. All central and peripheral neurotransmitters are dietary components or are relatively simple metabolites of dietary constituents. Minor changes in nutrient quality and quantity can, not surprisingly, produce changes in brain neurotransmitters and in the physiologic and behavioral responses of the organism, which depend, to a large extent, on the levels of these neurochemicals. In laboratory animals, for example, changes in the available tyrosine, tryptophan, or choline affect the synthesis of dopamine, norepinephrine, serotonin, and acetylcholine in the central nervous system (Wurtman et al. [37]).

It has not been established whether nutritional manipulation during maturity or senescence alters brain function by either structural alterations or change in neurotransmitter storage, release, or inactivation comparable to that in immature animals. Nevertheless, elderly people are particularly prone to nutritional deficiency as a result of social factors, advancing chronic disease, or mental dysfunction. Even in those who have access to complete diets, nutritional deficiencies may develop because of medical or dental dysfunction, gastrointestinal diseases, or other causes, thus limiting nutrients to the brain for appropriate neurotransmitter synthesis and maintenance of neurons and glia.

Whether morphologic abnormalities found in human and animal brains with advancing years are the result of insidious malnutrition has not been established. It is possible that the decreasing functional capacity of the aged nervous system might, in fact, be related to dietary abnormalities in some way still to be defined. The need exists to understand the relationships between aging, nutrition, nervous system structure, and the effect of physical activity on all three. Physical activity, however, has been shown to slow certain aging-associated processes of the human nervous system. Moreover, it is not known to what extent age-induced changes in brain structure, chemistry, and function directly alter nutritional status by influencing dietary habits and food utilization. Clearly, then, answers to these questions may provide understanding of the effects of nutrition on physical performance and, in turn, knowledge of how these interrelate with nervous-system aging and perhaps change its rate of progression. It should be remembered, however, that "no man can have a peaceful life who thinks too much about lengthening it" (Lucius Annaeus Seneca).

An accepted practice and one often suggested to those engaging in athletic activities is to indulge in the craving for certain foods if these develop. Recent evidence from animal studies suggests that such cravings may indicate nutritional requirements and may, in fact, result from changes in neuronal systems due to dietary-induced alterations in neurotransmitters.

Thus, although it has been recognized for years that extremes in dietary protein content and composition result in distortion of plasma amino acid patterns and depressed food consumption, it is now borne out in laboratory rats that shifts in plasma amino acids caused by normal food intake signal messages to the brain that control feeding behavior. These signals arise from amino acids that function as neurotransmitters or their precursors. Since it is known that at least two neuronal systems, one depending on 5-hydroxytryptamine and the other on catecholamines for neurotransmitters, are involved in the control of food intake, it is postulated that the neurotransmitters are influenced by the availability of their dietary amino acid precursors. The synthesis, for example, of 5-hydroxytryptamine and of the catecholamines is directly related to the level of precursors, tryptophan and tyrosine, respectively, in the brain. The brain uptake of these amino acids is exquisitely regulated by their plasma level. Therefore, changes in plasma amino acid patterns and availability influence serotonergic and catecholaminergic neurons to signal behavioral responses to food.

For example, if an animal selects among dietary options, it can change either the quantity or the quality of food consumed. Thus, evidence indicates that the quantity of food intake is influenced by shifts in plasma tyrosine in relation to other large neutral amino acids with a consequent alteration in brain tyrosine and catecholamine activity. On the other hand, changes in plasma tryptophan in relation to other large neutral amino acids alter brain tryptophan and 5-hydroxytryptamine, alter food preference, and regulate protein consumption. It is easy, therefore, to suggest (without scientific evidence) that the often reported cravings for certain foods during athletic activities or during changes in athletic performance and, perhaps, at other periods of life (pregnancy) are the result of changing levels of amino acids at least and possibly of other nutrients, and that they are best followed, in order to ensure adequate nutrition and energy balance for the task at hand (Anderson [38]).

Endogenous opiate-like substances have tentatively been linked with symptoms in some schizophrenic patients, and other anecdotal reports suggest that such patients may improve on gluten-free diet. Investigators at the National Institute of Mental Health looked at the possibility that peptic digestion of a variety of proteins, including wheat gluten, might produce opiate-like activity, and to their surprise, this was the case. These compounds are called exorphins, analogous to endorphins and the endogenously produced opiate-like materials. Isolation and sequencing of the peptides in hydrolysates of beta-casein (a constituent of milk) with opioid properties show them to be slightly different from the endogenously produced enkephalins, including beta-endorphin, and they have been called beta-casomorphins. These substances, like the endogenously produced beta-endorphin, produce a pain-free state (analgesia) after intracerebroventricular injections in animals, which is reversible by the opium antagonist, naloxone. It is not clear whether exorphins produce central nervous system effects after oral ingestion.

The instillation of digested gluten into the stomach of animals produces a rapid rise in postprandial peripheral insulin and glucagon, and simultaneous administration of naloxone intragastrically prevents increase in these blood hormones. This supports the view that the digested gluten test meal activates opiate receptors.

Other peptide-like substances have been isolated from foods. For example, a peptide with thyrotropin-releasing hormone (TRH) activity has been found in alfalfa; it differs from endogenous TRH, a prolactin releaser, by inhibiting prolactin release. TRH, distributed throughout the gastrointestinal tract, affects gastric acid and pancreatic secretions and gut mobility. Oat leaves contain a substance with activity similiar to luteinizing hormone-releasing hormone. The biologic significance of the neuropeptides has not been determined.

While some evidence exists that these food hormones are absorbed unaltered and produce systematic effects, the present feeling is that they have a significant role locally. Clearly, their local effects on gut motility, absorption of energy-producing foods, and other gastrointestinal functions also influence mood and performance (Morley [39]).

# Dietary Constituents and Disease

The eating habits of athletes include vegetarianism, and the effect of this on dietary lipids is of great interest, particularly in view of the reputed effects of exercise upon atherosclerosis (reviewed in another chapter). In acute clinical studies in human volunteers, it was shown that onion and garlic supplementation prevents alimentary hyperlipemia and increases fibrinolytic activity, effects that would presumably decrease lipid deposition in vessel walls and reduce atherosclerosis. Moreover, evidence also indicates that garlic and onion have hypocholesterolemic activity. In experimental animals, garlic inhibits atherogenesis.

In a recent study from India, the effects of the dietary use of onion and garlic upon serum cholesterol, triglycerides, lipoprotein, and phospholipids in members of the Jain community were investigated (Sainani and Desai [40]). These people, if strictly adhering to their religious tenets, abstain from garlic and onions. However, many members of Jain families consume either small or large quantities of onion and garlic and these, along with the abstainers, formed the three study groups whose serum lipid profiles were compared. All study participants were vegetarians and consumed fat and refined sugar approximately equally. It was clear, in this long-term epidemiologic review, that total abstention from garlic and onions throughout life was associated with significantly higher levels of serum cholesterol, triglycerides, beta-lipoprotein, and phospholipids. Small intake of these vegetables reduced these substances in the blood, and inclusion of large quantities of onion and garlic in the diet reduced serum lipids even more. These findings, combined with vegetarianism, complicate the assessment of the value of exercise in preventing atherosclerosis and its influence on morbidity and mortality due to vascular disease (Sainani and Desai [40]).

## Trace Elements

Dietary trace elements also probably influence cardiovascular disease. Geologic, geochemical, and soil maps were compared with epidemiologic maps to assess the influence of "geochemistry on the incidence of cardiovascular disease" (Masironi [41]). Changes in the content or in the availability of trace elements in rocks or water may contribute to certain chronic diseases including atherosclerosis.

The geographic distribution of cardiovascular disease is associated with geochemical differences, a trend particularly evident in the United States and Europe, where mortality from cardiovascular disease is high. High mortality rates from cardiovascular disease correlate well with areas where the underlying soil is poor in essential trace elements.

This finding has been further confirmed by observing a relationship between the incidence of cardiovascular disease and the degree of mineralization of water supplies. Thus, in parts of the world served by soft water, there is usually a high rate of cardiovascular death compared to parts of the world served by hard water. This negative association between mineralization of water and cardiovascular death is not confined to highly industrialized countries but is also present in the developing world.

Thus, evaluation of the reputed beneficial effects of exercise upon cardiovascular disease are further complicated by dietary factors such as the ingestion of hard water, clearly beyond control or manipulative capacity but nevertheless important and, speculatively, even more so to those who ingest large quantities of dietary fiber that may chelate trace elements otherwise available from the water.

## Environmental Effects

The environmental effects upon nutritional requirements are, of course, multiple and include the effects of altitude upon energy expenditure and intake. For example, it has been shown that body composition changes among sea-level residents when they are abruptly exposed to altitudes of 4000 meters or so. It has been suggested that the observed loss in body weight at altitude is due to decreased body fat and reduced blood and plasma volumes, changes, however, that were mostly due to the redistribution of body water.

Body composition does change with acute altitude exposure, and not only fat but protein, water, and minerals are lost. However, when the body fat of natives of high altitude, approximately 4000 meters, was compared with that of sea-level natives, no significant differences were observed. The effect of a 10-month sojourn at high altitude on body fat, measured by anthropometric techniques, showed that a significant decline occurred after exposure to 4000 meters, but there was increased lean body weight, and the total change in body weight was very much smaller than that observed after acute exposure to altitude. Moreover, fluctuations in body fat at high altitudes during a prolonged sojourn might be influenced by the seasons of the year as well (Bharadwaj [42]). During abrupt altitude exposure, increased energy is required to perform standard amounts of work when compared to sea-level requirements. Thus, increased energy is necessary during acute high altitude exposure of about 4000 meters, which might, perhaps, be due to the greater metabolic requirements for cardiac and respiratory function at altitude or perhaps to decreased efficiency of performance (Johnson et al. [43]).

Tissue hypoxia in exercising humans leads to increased free fatty-acid mobilization and utilization in spite of ongoing anaerobic metabolism. This has been tentatively ascribed to increased circulating catecholamines (Jones and Robertson [44]).

All these studies attributed the changes in body fat and metabolic alterations during exercise to altitude alone. However, in the field, altitude is almost always accompanied by cold, and the effects of cold have mostly been ignored in these studies. Moderately obese nonathletes fully clothed in arctic clothing exercised for 2½ h/day for a week in a climatic chamber where the ambient temperature was −40°C and the air was still. Their total daily energy expenditure was about 13 MJ. Only a small energy deficit occurred when energy expenditure was compared to daily caloric intake, but cold exposure led to a significant reduction in skin-fold thickness and increased body density, measured by underwater weighing. The body fat loss during that week was estimated to be from 0.8 kg to 2.3 kg, and lean body mass increased approximately 1.5 kg. These observations were attributed to protein synthesis under cold conditions, ketosis associated with exercise, and a small energy deficit (O'Hara et al. [45]).

Athletes have not been studied under comparable conditions. Their low body fat could affect work in the cold considerably and change the magnitude of body fat loss, energy intake, and lean body mass from that seen in moderately obese, middle-aged nonathletic males. High density lipoproteins reached 148 ± 29 mg/dl in whole blood in male mountaineers during a strenuous 8-week climb. This rise was attributed not only to the physical exertion and improvement in athletic fitness, but also to cold exposure, the hypoxia itself, and, perhaps to mental stress. Other factors that affect high-density lipoproteins such as body weight, alcohol consumption, or cigarette smoking did not change significantly during the climb, though dietary changes were significant in that the caloric intake increased considerably and consisted mainly of carbohydrates, which tend to decrease high-density lipoproteins. The rapidity with which high-density lipoproteins rose under these conditions is extraordinary. Similar studies should be undertaken to see what the actual rate of change might be. During high altitude exertion, changes in blood constituents of even greater magnitude have been observed within several hours (Nestel et al. [46]) (see Chapter 14, Oxygen Transport During Exercise at Sea Level and High Altitude).

# Dietary Principles

For optimum support of athletic performance, appropriate timing of food intake is essential. Clearly, large, infrequent meals cause discomfort during athletic performance and provide excessive calories. Meals before training or competition should be varied.

The training diet should be the standard one for a particular sport and should not precede physical effort too closely.

Ideally, 4–6 h should elapse between the last meal and the beginning of competition. A time lapse of several days exists between carbohydrate ingestion and muscle glycogen storage. The food mix is important. Free carbohydrates should be avoided before prolonged competition, since insulin release often leads to reactive hypoglycemia if physical activity is continued during the metabolism of sugar. The importance of fats in preparation for endurance competition has already been mentioned, and the value of vitamin supplements is not established. Most endurance athletes use megavitamin supplementation, but the effect upon their performance has not been documented.

The Oxford English Dictionary defines *brawn* as "pickled or potted boar's flesh." This is an apt description of the large, lean body mass that is attained by a diet that is predominantly proteins and fats and few carbohydrates.

Endurance events, on the other hand, require high caloric intake in the form of carbohydrates and fats and relatively little protein in proportion to the total calories consumed. The quantity of fiber in the diet is important when preparing for competition. For events lasting more than a few minutes, dietary fiber should not be taken, if possible, for a day or two to avoid gastrointestinal motility problems and defecation at inappropriate times.

# Carbohydrate Loading

Muscle glycogen supercompensation by athletes in endurance events is traceable to a report claiming that this improved marathon running significantly. Not all world-class endurance athletes find carbohydrate loading useful. Proper carbohydrate loading requires that the muscles be receptive to glycogen storage, which is the case only during the first 10 h after exhaustive exercise, and that muscles can sustain carbohydrate abstention, or total depletion of muscle glycogen. Moreover, the mean time to achieve maximum glycogen storage is approximately 3 days, with considerable individual variation.

The high carbohydrate intake, best ingested in the form of complex carbohydrates, must be preceded by an exhaustive workout, and followed by little or no exercise of the muscles to be used during competition. Moreover, the considerable changes in body weight—first the decrease associated with body water loss, and then the inordinate increase in body weight occasioned by water utilization in glycogen synthesis—make athletic performance sometimes difficult, particularly at the beginning of a long-distance race.

Investigations of substrate utilization during prolonged exercise preceded by the ingestion of glucose in glycogen-depleted and control subjects has shown that the principal substrate for energy in controls is carbohydrate, whereas in those who are glycogen depleted it is lipid (Ravussin et al. [47]). Clearly, therefore, for prolonged exertion, the glycogen depletion without repletion is preferable, since lipids are a better source of energy during long-distance races than carbohydrates. Moreover, in spite of glycogen depletion, these subjects did not utilize ingested glucose to a greater extent than did control subjects. This was probably due to their high free fatty-acid plasma levels, a factor that again suggests that the glucose intake during prolonged energy expenditure is not advantageous. Muscle glycogen use was not improved, and glucose ingestion may cause decreased water resorption from the gastrointestinal tract.

Thus, while it is well-established that during exercise the endogenous glycogen stores of muscles are an important source of energy, they are also the limiting factors in prolonged exertion. The alternate energy source from lipids is preferable if athletic performance is to continue beyond 1 h. The assumption that the exogenously administered glucose during exercise improves its utilization in those who are glycogen depleted has not been proved, and the experience of many suggests that such glucose intake may, in fact, lead to hypoglycemia during continued athletic performance and thus decrease the quality of and ability to prolong physical activity (Ravussin et al. [47]).

The views expressed by Mark Twain, that the only way to keep your health is to eat what you don't want, drink what you don't like, and do what you'd rather not, have no scientific foundation except that they point to an important principle that, taking into account the foregoing cautions, is still the leading nutritional doctrine to be advocated: Indulge moderately in what you like, partake of a great variety of foods, and keep your energy expenditure high.

# References

1. Wretlind, A. 1967. Nutrition problems in healthy adults with low activity and low caloric consumption. In: Blix, G., (ed): Nutrition and Physical Activity. Almquist and Wiksell, Uppsala.

2. Åstrand, P.O. 1979. Diet and exercise—How to secure an adequate intake of essential nutrients. Intern Med 1:23–26.

3. Brozek, J., Grande, F., Taylor, H.L. et al. 1957. Changes in body weight and body dimensions in men performing work on a low calorie carbohydrate diet. J Appl Physiol 10:412–420.

4. Yang, M.-U., Van Itallie, T.B. 1976. Composition of weight lost during short term weight reduction: Metabolic responses of obese subjects to starvation and low-calorie ketogenic and nonketogenic diets. J Clin Invest 58:722–730.

5. Van Itallie, T.B., Yang, M.-U. 1977. Diet and weight loss. N Engl J Med 297:1158–1161.

6. Benedict, F.G. 1915. A study of prolonged fasting, Pub. 203. Carnegie Institute, Washington, D.C.

7. Owen, O.E., Felig, P., Morgan, A.P. et al. 1969. Liver and kidney metabolism during prolonged starvation. J Clin Invest 48:574–576.

8. Garber, A.J., Menzel, P.H. et al. 1974. Hepatic ketogenesis and gluconeogenesis in humans. J Clin Invest 54:981–984.

9. Saudek, C.D., Felig, P. 1976. The metabolic events of starvation. Am J Med 60:117–126.

10. Stock, M.J., Morgan, N.G. et al. 1978. Effect of high altitude on dietary-induced thermogenesis at rest and during light exercise in man. J Appl Physiol 45:345–349.

11. Stock, M.J. 1980. Effects of fasting and refeeding on the metabolic response to a standard meal in man. Eur J Appl Physiol 43:35–40.

12. McLaren, D.S. 1974. Dietary protein in medical practice. Practitioner 212:441–447.

13. Felig, P. 1975. Amino acid metabolism in man. Ann Rev Biochem 44:933–956.

14. Lemon, P.W.R., Mullin, F.P. 1980. Effect of initial muscle glycogen levels on protein catabolism during exercise. J Appl Physiol 48:624–629.

15. Refsum, H.E., Gjessing, L.R., Strømme, S.B. 1979. Changes in plasma amino acid distribution and urine amino acids excretion during prolonged heavy exercise. Scand J Clin Lab Invest 39:407–413.

16. Consolazio, C.F., Johnson, H.L. 1972. Dietary carbohydrate and work capacity. Am J Clin Nutr 25:85–87.

17. Marable, N.L., Hickson, J.F. Jr. 1979. Urinary nitrogen excretion as influenced by a muscle-building exercise program and protein intake variation. Nutr Rep Int 19:795–805.

18. Linn, R., Stuart, S.L. 1976. The Last Chance Diet. Lyle Stuart Inc, Secaucus, N.J.

19. Isner, J.J., Sours, H.E., et al. 1979. Sudden, unexpected death in avid dieters using the liquid-protein-modified-fast diet. Observations in 17 patients and the role of the prolonged QT interval. Circulation 60:1401–1412.

20. Mayer, J.R. 1968. Overweight: Causes, Cost and Control. Prentice-Hall Inc, Englewood Cliffs, N.J.

21. Maiman, L.A., Wang, V.L. 1979. Attitudes toward obesity and the obese among professionals. J Am Diet Assoc 47:331–335.

22. Gollnick, P.D. 1977. Free fatty acid turnover and the availability of substrates as a limiting factor in prolonged exercise. In: The Marathon, Physiological, Medical, Epidemiological and Psychological Studies. Ann NY Acad Sci 301:64–71.

23. Costill, D.L., Coyle, E. 1977. Effects of elevated plasma FFA and insulin on muscle glycogen usage during exercise. J Appl Physiol 43:695–699.

24. Appenzeller, O., Schade, D.S. 1979. Neurology of endurance training. III. Sympathetic activity during a marathon race. Neurology 29:540.

25. Robison, G.A., Butcher, R.W., Sutherland, E.W. 1967. Adenyl cyclase as an adrenergic receptor. Ann NY Acad Sci 139:703–707.

26. Burns, T.W., Boyer, P.A., Terry, B.E. et al. 1979. The effect of fasting on the adrenergic receptor activity of human adipocytes. J Lab Clin Med 94:387–394.

27. Lithell, H., Orlander, J. et al. 1979. Changes in lipoprotein-lipase activity and lipid stores in human skeletal muscle with prolonged heavy exercise. Acta Physiol Scand 107:257–261.

28. Calkins, A. 1979. Observations on vegetarian dietary practice and social factors: The need for further research. J Am Diet Assoc 74:353–355.

29. Levin, B., Horwitz, D. 1979. Dietary fiber. Med Clin North Am 63:1043–1055.

30. How to evaluate medical information. 1978. Harvard Medical School Health Letters 3:6.

31. Herbert, V. 1979. Facts and fictions about megavitamin therapy. J Fla Med Assoc 66:475–481.

32. Anderson, R., Oosthuizen, R. et al. 1980. The effects of increasing weekly doses of ascorbate on certain cellular and humoral immune functions in normal volunteers. Am J Clin Nutr 33:71–76.

33. Visagie, M.E., DuPlessis, J.P., Laubscher, N.F. 1975. Effect of vitamin C supplementation on black mineworkers. S Afr Med J 49:889–892.

34. Horrobin, D.F., Oka, M., Manku, M.S. 1979. The regulation of prostaglandin $E_1$ formation: A candidate for one of the fundamental mechanisms involved in the actions of vitamin C. Med Hypoth 5:849–858.

35. Solomons, N.W., Jacob, R.A. et al. 1979. Studies on the bioavailability of zinc in man. III. Effects of ascorbic acid on zinc absorption. Am J Clin Nutr 32:2495–2499.

36. Treuherz, J. 1980. Zinc and dietary fibre: Observations on a group of vegetarian adolescents. J Hum Nutr 29:10A.

37. Wurtman, R.J., Cohen, E.L., Fernstrom, J.O. 1977. Control of brain neurotransmitter synthesis by precursor availability and food consumption. In: Usdin E., Hambur, D.A., Barchas J.D., (eds): Neuroregulators and Psychiatric Disorders. Oxford University Press, New York, pp. 103–121.

38. Anderson, G.H. 1979. Control of protein and energy intake. Role of plasma amino acids and brain neurotransmitters. Can J Physiol Pharmacol 57:1043–1057.

39. Morley, J. E. 1982. Food peptides. JAMA 247:2379-2380.

40. Sainani, G.S., Desai, D.B. 1979. Effect of dietary garlic and onion on serum lipid profile in Jain community. Indian J Med Res 69:776–780.

41. Masironi, R. 1979. Geochemistry and cardiovascular diseases. Philos Trans R Soc Lond [Biol] 288:193–203.

42. Bharadwaj, H. 1972. Effect of prolonged stay at high altitude on body fat content— an anthropometric evaluation. Human Biol 44:303–316.

43. Johnson, H.L., Consolazio, C.F. et al. 1971. Increased energy requirements of man after abrupt altitude exposure. Nutr Rep Int 4:77–82.

44. Jones, N.L., Robertson, D.G. 1971. Effects of hypoxia on fat metabolism in exercising humans. J Physiol [Lond] 222:30.

45. O'Hara, W.J., Allen, C., Shephard, R.J., Allen, G. 1979. Fat loss in the cold—a controlled study. J Appl Physiol 46:872–877.

46. Nestel, P.J., Podkolinski, M., Fidge, N.H. 1979. Marked increase in high density lipoproteins in mountaineers. Atherosclerosis 34:193–196.

47. Ravussin, E., Pahud, P. et al. 1979. Substrate utilization during prolonged exercise preceded by ingestion of $^{13}$C-glucose in glycogen depleted and control subjects. Pflügers Arch 382:197–202.

Chapter 6

# Effect of Sports on the Gastrointestinal Tract and Liver

by Nicholas A. Volpicelli

## Introduction

The emphasis of this chapter is on disorders of gastrointestinal and hepatic function, which may either adversely affect athletic performance or be precipitated by athletic activity and associated factors, such as diet and nutritional supplements. Moderate physical activity probably aids digestive function and prevents or treats certain digestive disturbances such as peptic ulcer and constipation. On the other hand, excessive training and effort or attempts to increase strength and endurance with "fad" diets, supplemental foodstuffs, and hormones may lead to serious and life-threatening medical illnesses.

## Abdominal Pain

Abdominal pain that occurs during strenuous physical activity, especially running, is referred to as a "stitch." This pain is transient and probably results from muscular spasm or trapped intestinal gas. Abdominal pain that persists after rest or that is chronic warrants medical investigation. It is particularly important to keep this in mind when evaluating athletes who participate in contact sports, since these individuals may have a ruptured spleen, liver, or pancreas that should be diagnosed and treated immediately. Chronic abdominal pain unrelated to trauma usually indicates an underlying disorder such as peptic ulcer and should be diagnosed and treated as in the nonathlete.

# Nausea and Vomiting

Nausea and vomiting in athletes may result from nervous tension. Strenuous exercise inhibits gastric emptying (Ramsbottom and Hunt [1]; Fordtran and Saltin [2]; Costill and Saltin [3]); food and liquids ingested shortly before and during an athletic event may therefore remain in the stomach and lead to nausea and vomiting. Nevertheless, it is often necessary to replace some fluid, electrolyte, and energy losses during long events. Dilute solutions of glucose or sodium chloride may be used for this, since these are emptied and absorbed during submaximal exercise (Fordtran and Saltin [2]; Costill and Saltin [3]). Glucose concentrations above 139 mM retard gastric emptying (Costill and Saltin [3]), as do amino acids or fats (Cooke [4]), and should therefore be avoided. Changes in intestinal blood supply and the effect of toxic metabolites on the vomiting center may also contribute to nausea and vomiting. Finally, head trauma is a cause of nausea and vomiting and can be an indication of increased intracranial pressure, a potential medical and surgical emergency. The occurrence of effect migraine (headache, nausea, and vomiting) in relation to competition is unusual. Forceful vomiting and retching can lacerate the mucosa at the esophagogastric junction (Mallory-Weiss syndrome) and produce hematemesis and shock.

# Diarrhea

Acute or chronic diarrhea is not uncommon in athletes. Acute diarrhea is usually of bacterial or viral origin. In most instances, the illness is self-limited and therapy is not indicated except to replace fluid and electrolytes. Nevertheless, acute diarrheal illness should be guarded against if possible since it decreases or prevents maximal physical performance. Special advice should be given to athletes traveling to countries where risk of exposure to diarrheal illness is high. The most common cause of acute infectious diarrhea contracted in foreign countries is enterotoxigenic *E. coli* (Gorbach et al. [5]), though shigella, salmonella, amebiasis, and giardiasis are still prevalent. Hygiene is the mainstay of prevention; athletes traveling to underdeveloped countries should avoid ingesting local water in any form, including ice cubes, uncooked vegetables, and fruits. Daily doxycycline prevents most toxigenic *E. coli* diarrheas and should be considered for use in those athletes at risk (Sack et al. [6]). This drug does not prevent diarrhea in all travelers and, if overused, may cause emergence of resistant organisms or untoward drug reactions (Merson [7]). Acute diarrhea in the "traveler" athlete may be relieved with bismuthsubsalicylate (Pepto-Bismol ®), 30-60 ml every 30 min for eight doses (total 240-480 ml) (Du Pont et al. [8]). If this brings no relief, fluids and electrolytes should be replaced. If gastrointestinal bleeding occurs or symptoms do not subside within a few days, the stool should be cultured and examined for parasites for appropriate treatment. Diarrhea frequently occurs in long-distance runners (Fogoros [9]; Volpicelli et al. [10]), especially during increased or more severe training and strenuous races. This usually subsides as training levels off or decreases. The cause of diarrhea in long-distance runners is unknown, but contributing factors may include 1) relative intestinal ischemia from shunting of blood away from the intestine to the heart and skeletal muscle; 2) changes in gut motility; 3) changes in intestinal secretion and absorption. Modifications in gut motility, secretion, and absorption are probably, at least in part, hormonally mediated. Endorphins are elevated in long-distance runners (Appenzeller et al. [11]), and increasing evidence indicates that these and related opioid compounds affect gastrointestinal motility, absorption, and secretion (Ambinder and Schuster [12]; McKay et al. [13]). Most long-distance runners with loose bowel movements take vitamin and iron supplements, which may contribute to changes in bowel habits (Volpicelli et al. [10]). Though most diarrheas in athletes are acute and self-limited, chronic diarrhea may also occur. When this is the case one should search for an underlying disorder such as ulcerative colitis, Crohn's disease, sprue, giardiasis, etc. A common but frequently unrecognized cause of bloating, chronic diarrhea and abdominal pain is lactase deficiency. This hereditary abnormality is especially common in Blacks, Orientals, Jews, Hispanics, and those of Southern Mediterranean origin. Avoidance of milk and milk products leads to cessation of symptoms. Recently, caffeine intake was touted as a possible aid to athletic endurance and performance (Ivy et al. [14]). Should this become accepted as a means of increasing endurance, it should be noted that caffeine produces diarrhea in some persons (Wald et al. [15]).

# Gastrointestinal Bleeding

Gastrointestinal bleeding in the athlete is probably from hemorrhoids, peptic ulcer, inflammatory bowel disease, polyps, cancer, etc., and the diagnosis and management of this is the same as in the nonathlete. Gastrointestinal bleeding in long-distance runners occurs during strenuous training or maximal effort and disappears when training declines or reaches a plateau (Fogoros [9]; Volpicelli et al. [10]). We have seen two long-distance runners with recurrent gastrointestinal bleeding presenting with melena. Neither was taking aspirin or other medications. In both instances, blood clotting radiologic and endoscopic studies of the upper and lower gastrointestinal tracts were normal. Bleeding ceased in each when training was reduced, but recurred when effort was increased to maximal levels. In one patient, bleeding did not recur when the total distance run was increased more gradually. In addition to these two cases, of 20 long-distance runners (15 men, 5 women) participating in races of marathon or greater distances, who were instructed to avoid all medications at least a week prior to the race, four (3 women and 1 man) had gastrointestinal blood loss (guaiac-positive stools) prior to and/or immediately after the race. Two of these (1 man, 1 woman) had a history of recurrent gastrointestinal hemorrhage that had been investigated medically and for which no source was found.

The cause of gastrointestinal bleeding in long-distance runners is unknown. It may be related to intestinal ischemia or possibly to jarring of the bowels during long runs. Whether or not this occurs in other athletes is not known. Gastrointestinal blood loss should not be attributed to strenuous activity in any athlete until appropriate studies are done to exclude the usual medical causes. Hemoglobin concentration declines after strenuous conditioning, such as in long-distance running (Bunch [16]). This is due to disproportionately increased plasma volume compared to red cell volume and should not be interpreted as evidence of gastrointestinal blood loss, unless there is blood in the stools or a low serum iron.

# Hepatitis

Both hepatitis A (infectious, short incubation) and hepatitis B (serum, Australian antigen-positive) may occur as a result of close association with a "community" of athletes.

## Hepatitis A

Hepatitis A is transmitted primarily by the fecal-oral route. Therefore, close personal contact with infected individuals or ingestion of contaminated water and/or food can lead to illness. (A devastating outbreak occurred in 1969 among members of the Holy Cross football team when they drank contaminated water (Morse et al. [17]; Chang and O'Brien [18]). Of 97 players, coaches, and trainers, 90 had evidence of acute hepatitis. A more usual circumstance confronting atheletes, trainers, and doctors is when one or more members of a team develop acute hepatitis A. In this instance, one must care for the affected individual(s), and for the potentially exposed team members. Medical management of the athlete with acute hepatitis A is no different than that of other individuals. Since specific treatment does not exist, care is supportive and should include a balanced diet and observation for increasing jaundice, encephalopathy, prolongation of the prothrombin time, and hypoglycemia, signs of hepatic failure. If the patient cannot eat, or if hepatic failure develops, hospitalization is necessary. There is no evidence that bed rest enhances healing, and, if the patient is able, "moderate" exercise may be allowed (Chalmers [19]; Repsher and Freehern [20]), though this recommendation is still controversial (Krikler and Zilberg [21]; Krikler [22]). Strenuous activity should be avoided during the acute stages. Certainly, when liver function studies are normal, the patient may gradually return to full activity. Hepatitis A does not lead to chronic hepatitis, and infection appears to confer life-long immunity. Individuals in close personal contact (roommates, household contacts, etc.) with hepatitis A patients should be passively immunized with immune globulin to prevent or decrease the severity of the acute illness. Passive immunization is not necessary unless all team members are in close personal contact. Furthermore, if a team was exposed to a common source of infection, such as contaminated water, attempts to immunize after an index case was recognized would probably be too late. Stool viral concentrations in affected individuals are highest during the incubation period and begin to fall with the onset of clinical hepatitis (Rakela and Mosly [23]). Therefore, the risk of transmitting infection is less if close personal contact occurs after the onset of jaundice, and is negligible once the patient recovers. Since most hepatitis A infections are subclinical (Azmuness [24]), it is necessary to measure liver function in each member of a team to determine who is already afflicted. In those with abnormal liver function, the presence of IgM antibody to hepatitis A confirms acute infection (Decker et al. [25]). The presence of IgG antibody without IgM antibody indicates remote infection and immunity.

# Hepatitis B

Hepatitis B is primarily transmitted by direct inoculation of infected blood or blood products into a susceptible host. In athletes, this is most likely to occur in contact sports in which open wounds are common. However, one of the largest reported outbreaks of hepatitis B occurred in Sweden among cross-country track-finders (Ringertz and Zetterberg [26]). In this noncontact sport, runners traverse a course along check points, in the shortest possible time. Frequently, they sustain open leg wounds from contact with surrounding obstacles and plants. After much investigation, it was concluded that hepatitis B was probably transmitted after the race by runners using common bathing sites where infected blood from one individual came in contact with open wounds of others who were susceptible. Runners were subsequently required to wear protective clothing, including leg shields, and arrangements were made for more sanitary conditions. Following these measures, the outbreak, which lasted from 1958 to 1962, disappeared. Although similar outbreaks of hepatitis B associated with athletics have not been reported, it should be kept in mind that transmission of blood from an open sore of one athlete to another should be avoided. Documentation of serum hepatitis has now been simplified by serologic tests sensitive and specific for hepatitis B surface antigen (HbsAg, HAA, Australian antigen). Transmission of blood positive for hepatitis B surface antigen into the blood stream of a previously uninfected individual, by whatever means including cuts and abrasions, can lead to infection. In these instances, the recipient of infected blood should be passively immunized with hepatitis B specific immune globulin, since ordinary immune globulin may not contain enough hepatitis B antibodies to be protective. The treatment of acute hepatitis B is the same as hepatitis A. However, unlike hepatitis A, hepatitis B infection may occasionally become chronic and lead to cirrhosis, for which there is no effective treatment. In addition, a small proportion of infected individuals may become chronic carriers of the hepatitis B virus, without evidence of ongoing disease. Therefore, those with acute hepatitis B should be followed medically until liver function is normal and hepatitis B surface antigen disappears from the serum in order to document complete recovery. Further evidence for complete recovery is the demonstration of antibody to hepatitis B surface antigen (HbsAb) in the serum of those previously infected. Whether to allow chronic carriers of hepatitis B to participate in sports in which they might transmit infection to others remains a major ethical problem. With the exception of the Swedish track-finders, major outbreaks of hepatitis B traced to sports have not been reported. Moreover, athletes might be infected with hepatitits B by close personal contact with non-athletes, sexual contacts, dental procedures, etc. It might be difficult to trace isolated cases to another "carrier" athlete. Until specific guidelines are established, the decision regarding athlete participation by a chronic carrier of hepatitis B virus must be individualized.

# Non-A, Non-B Hepatitis

Non-A, non-B hepatitis, presumably due to another virus or viruses, is now well-described (Feinstone et al. [27]) and accounts for most cases of post-transfusion hepatitis. The clinical illness and potential for chronic hepatitis (Knodell et al. [28]) is similar to hepatitis B, though the incubation period is shorter. There are no reports, as yet, to link this infection to athletes, but obviously the potential exists.

## Liver Function Tests

Occasionally, the physician is confronted with a well-trained, otherwise healthy athlete, who has "abnormal liver functions" including elevations in the bilirubin, serum glutamic-oxaloacetic transaminase (SGOT) and alkaline phosphatase. These abnormalities are particularly common in long-distance runners (Bunch [16]), but can occur in other athletes. Liver disease can be excluded if creatine phosphokinase (CPK) is also elevated and the serum gammaglutamyl transpeptidase (GGPT), glutamic-pyruvate transaminase (SGPT) albumin, and total protein are normal (Bunch [16]). If doubt still exists the athlete should stop strenuous exercise for a week, and serum enzymes will return to normal if underlying liver disease is not present (Bunch [16]). The use of androgenic-anabolic steroids to increase strength and endurance is another potentially serious cause of abnormal liver function in athletes and has been associated with peliosis hepatitis (dilated, blood-filled cystic spaces within the liver), and hepatocellular carcinoma (Johnson [29]). The use of these steroids is, therefore, undesirable. For the hundreds of other causes of abnormal liver function, the athlete should be evaluated and treated as the nonathlete.

## Chronic Hepatitis and Cirrhosis

There is no evidence that strenuous exercise aggravates chronic liver disease or cirrhosis. Patients usually avoid physical exertion, depending upon the severity and activity of the liver disease. Cirrhosis may be associated with pulmonary arteriovenous shunts (Bashour and Cochran [30]), leading to decreased arterial oxygen saturation; a decrease in available oxygen not only adversely affects athletic performance, but may also result in anoxia to vital organs during strenuous exercise.

# Exercise and Gastrointestinal Health

It has been shown epidemiologically that physical exercise reduces the chance of subsequent peptic ulcer (Paffenbarger et al. [31]). Though this might be explained by decreased alcohol and nicotine consumption by athletes, it is noteworthy that submaximal exercise reduces gastric acid secretion in normals (Ramsbottom and Hunt [1]) but not in those with established duodenal ulcers (Markiewiczk et al. [32]). This effect of exercise on peptic ulcer may be mediated humorally, since experimental ulcers in rats are inhibited by administration of sera from well-trained athletes (Frankl et al. [33]; Frankl [34]). Gastric carcinoma, on the other hand, may be increased in those with greater amount of physical activity, because they eat more and are consequently exposed to more potential gastric carcinogens (Stukonis and Doll [35]). Constipation is common in bedridden and hospitalized patients and disappears when they resume normal activity. As noted previously, many long-distance runners have loose and more frequent bowel movements during strenuous training. Therefore, chronic constipation in otherwise healthy individuals might respond to treatment with exercise such as jogging, and eliminate the need for cathartics. There is experimental evidence that regular exercise decreases the lithogenicity of bile in man and experimental animals (Simko [36]) and thus possibly decreases the incidence of cholesterol gallstones.

# Conclusion

Much needs to be learned regarding the effects of exercise and physical conditioning on gastrointestinal and hepatic function. Although gastrointestinal illness adversely affects athletic performance, it is unknown if certain inborn or acquired characteristics of gastrointestinal and hepatic function actually enhance athletic performance. Finally, it is commonly assumed that regular exercise improves gastrointestinal and hepatic function and eventually will be utilized to prevent and treat some functional disorders of these organs.

# References

1. Ramsbottom, N., Hunt, J.N. 1974. Effect of exercise on gastric emptying. Digestion 10:1-8.
2. Fordtran, J.S., Saltin, B. 1967. Gastric emptying and intestinal absorption during prolonged severe exercise. J Appl Physiol 23:331-335.
3. Costill, D.L., Saltin, B. 1974. Factors limiting gastric emptying during rest and exercise. J Appl Physiol 37:679-683.
4. Cooke, A.R. 1975. Control of gastric emptying and motility. Gastroenterology 68:804-816.
5. Gorbach, S.K., Kean, B.H., Evans, D.G., Evans, D.J., Bessudo D. 1975. Travelers' diarrhea and toxigenic Escherichia coli. N Engl J Med 292:933-936.
6. Sack, R.B., Froehlich, J.L., Zulich, A.W., Hidi, D.S., Kapikian, A.Z., Orskov, F., Orskov, I., Greenberg, H.B. 1979. Prophylactic doxycycline for travelers' diarrhea. Gastroenterology 76:1368-1373.
7. Merson, M.H. 1979. Doxycycline and the traveler. Gastroenterology 76:1485-1488.
8. Du Pont, H.L., Sullivan, P., Pichering, L.K., Haynes, G., Ackerman, P.B. 1977. Symptomatic treatment of diarrhea with bismuth subsalicylate among students attending a Mexican university. Gastroenterology 73:715-718.
9. Fogoros, R.N. 1980. "Runner's trots." Gastrointestinal disturbances in runners. JAMA 243:1743-1744.
10. Volpicelli, N.A., Levin, A., Appenzeller, O. Gastrointestinal bleeding in long distance runners. In preparation.
11. Appenzeller, O., Standefer, J., Appenzeller, J., Atkinson, R. 1980. Neurology of endurance training. V. Endorphins. Neurology 30:418-419.
12. Ambinder, R.F., Schuster, M.M. 1979. Endorphins: New gut peptides with a familiar face. Gastroenterology 77:1132-1140.

13. McKay, J.A., Linaker, B.D., Turnberg, L.A. 1981. Influence of opiates on ion transport across rabbit ileal mucosa. Gastroenterology 80:279-284.

14. Ivy, J.L., Costil, D.L., Fink, W.J., Lorver, R.W. 1979. Influence of caffeine and carbohydrate feedings on endurance performance. Med Sci Sports 11:6-11.

15. Wald, A., Back, C., Bayless, T.M. 1976. Effect of caffeine on the human small intestine. Gastroenterology 71:738-742.

16. Bunch, T.W. 1980. Blood test abnormalities in runners. Mayo Clin Proc 55:113-117.

17. Morse, L.J., Bryan, J.A., Chang, L.W., Hurley, J.P., Murphy, J.F., O'Brien, T.F. 1970. Holy Cross football team hepatitis outbreak. Antimicrob Agents Chemother 10:30-32.

18. Chang, L.W., O'Brien, T.F. 1970. Australian antigen serology in the Holy Cross football team hepatitis outbreak. Lancet 2:59-61.

19. Chalmers, T.C., Eckardt, R.K., Reynolds, W.E., Cigarroa, J.G., Neane, N., Reifenstein, R.W., Smith, C.W., Davidson, C.S. 1955. The treatment of acute infectious hepatitis. Controlled studies of the effects of diet, rest and physical reconditioning of the acute course of the disease and on the incidence of relapses and residual abnormalities. J Clin Inves 34:1163-1235.

20. Repsher, L.H., Freehern, R.K. 1969. Effects of early and vigorous exercise on recovery from infectious hepatitis. N Engl J Med 281:1393-1396.

21. Krikler, D.M., Zilberg, B. 1966. Activity and hepatitis. Lancet 2:1046-1047.

22. Krikler, D.M. 1971. Hepatitis and activity. Postgrad Med J 47:490-492.

23. Rakela, J., Mosly, W.J. 1977. Fecal excretion of hepatitis A virus in humans. J Infect Dis 135:933-938.

24. Azmuness, W., Dienstag, J.L., Purcell, R.H., Harley, E.J., Stevens, C.E., Wong, D.C. 1976. Distribution of antibody to hepatitis A in urban adults. N Engl J Med 295:755-759.

25. Decker, R.H., Overby, L.R., Ling, C.J., Frasner, G., Deinhardt, F., Boggs, J. 1969. Serologic studies of transmission of hepatitis A in humans. J Infect Dis 139:74-82.

26. Ringertz, O., Zetterberg, B. 1967. Serum hepatitis among Swedish track finders. N Engl J Med 276:540-546.

27. Feinstone, S.M., Kapikian, A.Z., Purcell, R.H., Alter, H.J., Holland, P.V. 1975. Transfusion associated hepatitis not due to viral hepatitis type A or B. N Engl J Med 292:767-770.

28. Knodell, R.G., Conrad, M.E., Ishak K.G. 1977. Development of chronic liver disease after acute non-A, non-B post-transfusion hepatitis: Role of gamma globulin prophylaxis in its prevention. Gastroenterology 72:902-909.

29. Johnson, F.L. 1975. The association of oral androgenic-anabolic steroids and life-threatening disease. Med Sci Sports 7:284-286.

30. Bashour, F.A., Cochran, P. 1966. Alveolar-arterial oxygen tension gradients in cirrhosis of the liver. Am Heart J 71(6):734-740.

31. Paffenbarger, R.S., Wing, A.L., Hyde, R.T. 1974. Chronic disease in former college students. XIII. Early precursors of peptic ulcer. Am J Epidemiol 100:307-315.

32. Markiewiczk, M., Cholwea, M., Lukin, M. 1975. Gastric basal secretion during exercise and restitution in patients with chronic duodenal ulcer. Acta Hepato-Gastroenterol 26:160-165.

33. Frankl, R., Csalay, L., Csakvary, G., Jako, P., Juhasz, J., Richter, A. 1969. Antiulcerogenic effect of blood sera from human subjects and from albino rats adapted to physical exercise and from inactive controls. Acta Med Acad Sci Hung 26(1):41-46.

34. Frankl, R. 1971. Humoral mechanism of ulcer-resistance of the organism adapted to physical exercise. Acta Med Acad Sci Hung 28(1):69-73.

35. Stukonis, M., Doll, R. 1969. Gastric cancer in man and physical activity at work. Int J Cancer 4:248-254.

36. Simko, V. 1978. Physical exercise and the prevention of artherosclerosis and cholesterol gall stones. Postgrad Med J 54:270-277.

# Chapter 7

# Fuel Metabolism
# in the Long Distance Runner

by Neil Kaminsky

The principles of fuel metabolism in the marathoner are poorly understood by the public and blatantly oversimplified by self-styled "experts" who lack knowledge of intermediary metabolism. Such "experts" have substituted hearsay and anecdotal information for reason and the scientific method in approaching the subject, thus promulgating absurd nutritional recommendations. Unfortunately, many of today's runners are unquestioningly following such recommendations without first investigating their validity.

There has been a great deal of investigation into fuel metabolism, primarily comparing normal human beings to the diabetic. A number of reliable laboratories have conducted solid scientific studies on energy utilization in the long-distance runner. Many of these studies are assembled in a "marathon issue" published by the New York Academy of Science (Milvy [1]). Other comprehensive summaries include Newsholme [2], Essen [3], Ahlborg et al. [4], Scheele et al. [5], and Locksley [6].

This chapter conveys information on substrate metabolism in the long distance runner and provides a basis for individuals to assess their nutritional needs. Nutritional recommendations, based on what is known, are also included.

## Fuel Utilization and Storage

To begin, one must compare substrate utilization and hormone fluxes in the fasting versus the fed states. (Cahill [7]; Randel et al. [8]). It soon becomes clear that running a marathon is a telescopic representation of a prolonged fast.

# Fed and Fasted States

Fig. 7–1 depicts processes at work in the fed and fasted states. As a meal is ingested, gut hormones are liberated that, in effect, tell the pancreas a meal is coming. As glucose begins to rise in the blood, the storage hormone, insulin, is released from the pancreatic beta cell. Glucose is absorbed by the liver, muscle, brain, etc., and any excess glucose not needed for (immediate) energy is stored in the liver and muscle as glucogen. Once glycogen stores in the muscle and liver have been saturated, further excess glucose is converted to fat in the liver. This fat is transported through the blood to fat depots, where it is stored as triglycerides. Fats that are ingested are likewise deposited in fat storage depots under the influence of insulin. Amino acids—breakdown products of protein formed in the gastrointestinal tract—are stored in muscle as protein, an action also enhanced by insulin. As with glycogen, muscle stores of protein also become saturated, and any protein taken in above the amount that muscle can accommodate loses "amino groups" and is stored as fat. (So much, then, for the "training table" and the high protein diet to put on more muscle mass.)

Insulin, therefore, is the storage hormone that in response to an ingested meal facilitates the storage of 1) carbohydrates as glycogen and fat, 2) fat in fatty depots, and 3) amino acids as proteins in muscle and other tissue. Some of the ingested glucose, also affected by the action of insulin, is used for immediate energy needs. On the other hand, the counter-regulatory hormones—glucagon from the pancreas, epinephrine, growth hormone, and corticotrophin-cortisol—are suppressed with the balanced meal or high carbohydrate meal.

## Fuel Mobilization

After fasting, the reversal of the "fed state" occurs as the body demands to be supplied with energy sources for metabolism (Fig. 7–1). Since fuel stores must be broken down, the storage hormone, insulin, falls to low levels; the counter-regulatory hormones rise and (with the decrease in insulin) the following sequence occurs: 1) glycogenolysis (breakdown of stored glycogen) initially, 2) gluconeogenesis (the making of new glucose), and 3) lipolysis (breakdown of stored fat). Fat, stored as triglycerides, yields fatty acids and glycerol. Thus, basic fuels for metabolism are provided in the fasted state. Specifically, glycogen breaks down in muscle and the liver to form glucose. Glucose from the liver is liberated into the blood stream, where it is taken up by other tissues and oxidized to $CO_2$ and water. During oxidation, high-energy phosphate bonds (e.g., ATP) for metabolism are formed (e.g., brain function, muscle contraction, etc.) (Fig. 7–2). The glucose derived from muscle glycogen acts locally in the muscle and does not enter the blood stream because of the absence of a certain enzyme (glucose-6-phosphatase) in muscle. However, lactate derived from muscle and other tissues, together with special amino acids from muscle stores, enter the liver and are transformed into new glucose.

Fat is the largest potential source of energy. It breaks down into glycerol and free fatty acids; the glycerol is then converted to glucose. Fatty acids have several possible metabolic pathways: for example, they can be taken up and directly metabolized by

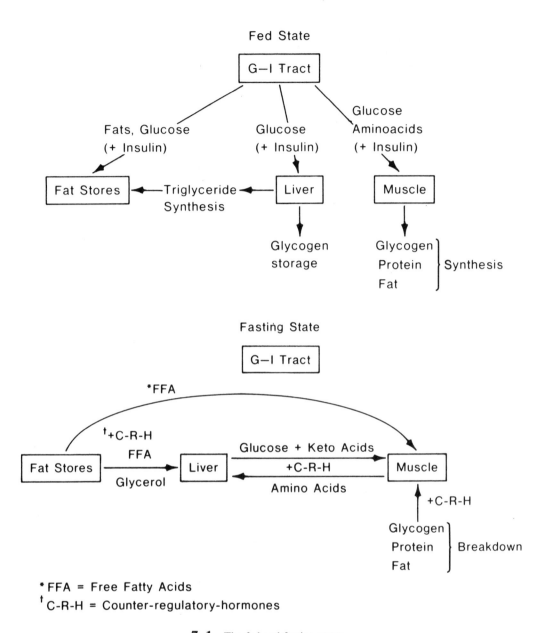

**7-1**   The fed and fasting states.

muscle, or they can travel to the liver where they are broken down and excreted back into the blood as ketoacids. These ketoacids can be directly used by muscle and brain as energy sources.

Therefore, going from the fed to the fasted state is a hormonal shift that allows for fuel storage in times of plenty and fuel mobilization in times of fasting. This metabolic shift is a finely tuned automatic continuum.

The hormonal profile and the metabolic events that occur in fasting are generally the same as those in a marathon run. However, in a marathon, the events in fasting are

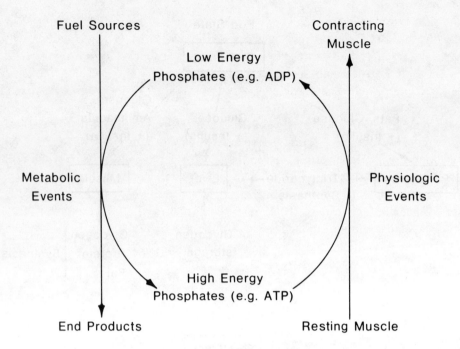

**7–2**  Coupling of energy production with utilization. High energy phosphates are produced from fuel sources. Physiologic events, such as muscle contraction, use high energy phosphates.

"telescoped" into 2 to 4 hours of maximum effort. There is no mystery to the fuel shifts, but considerable mystique surrounds attempts to improve the stores and the efficiency of their utilization.

# Fuel Metabolism in Exercise

## Use of Glycogen and Fat

In aerobic exercise, the production of high-energy phosphate bonds is able to keep pace with their utilization by exercising muscle (Fig. 7-2). Anaerobic metabolism occurs at the point where high energy phosphates are used in excess of those produced (this is in excess of 100% $\dot{V}o_{2max}$). (Newsholme [2]).

Carbohydrate is the preferred fuel source (Essen [3]). The simple explanation is that carbohydrate is totally combustible—there is an oxygen atom for every carbon atom. Regrettably, total body carbohydrate store is only about 200 g, two-thirds of which is in muscle. Muscle glucogen depletion occurs at about 20 to 25 miles and has been proposed as one of the causes of what is euphemistically called "hitting the wall" (Locksley [6]).

Why doesn't the body just switch to fat metabolism? Part (or maybe all) of the answer is that carbohydrate is a more combustible fuel, even though fat gives more energy per unit weight than carbohydrate. It is known that resting muscle in the fasting state uses principally fat. But, let that muscle work at 70% to 80% $\dot{V}O_2$ $_{max}$ and carbohydrate becomes the obligate fuel source until it runs out. Presumably, when the carbohydrate stores are depleted, fat cannot maintain the previous fast pace (Fig. 7–3).

Some excellent studies have been done by Newsholme [2], Essen [3], and Essen et al. [9] mapping fuel utilization at different levels of effort. Returning to the starvation analogy, nonexercising muscle uses principally fat (Randel et al. [8]). Even at levels of intensity up to 60% $\dot{V}O_2$ $_{max}$, lipids are the most important substrate for exercising muscle. The analogy breaks down at higher levels of effort as glycogen becomes the preferred substrate; the reason, in all likelihood, is the combustible nature of carbohydrate, but the mechanism for the shift to carbohydrate is unclear. Essen [3] and Randel et al. [8] have suggested that the fuel shift is tied in part to the accumulation of a product of glucose metabolism called citrate. In any event, it is clear that with more vigorous effort, relatively more carbohydrate is used than fat, and glycogen is depleted from muscle at a greater rate.

## Carbohydrate Loading

A great deal of effort has been expended to try to increase carbohydrate stores in muscle. J. Bergstrom and E. Hultman devised experiments correlating increased muscle glucogen stores and improved performance, thus providing the rationale for carbohydrate loading (Bergstrom et al. [10]; Karlsson and Saltin [11]; Bergstrom and Hultman [12]). Using a bicycle ergometer on one leg and the other nonexercising leg as the control, subjects rode the bicycle until the glycogen was depleted in the experimental leg muscle. After the subjects were refed carbohydrate-rich, carbohydrate-poor, or mixed diets, both muscles were-re-biopsied and the experimental leg was re-exercised. The experimenters were able to show that the carbohydrate-rich diet both increased the muscle glycogen stores and improved physical performance (Fig. 7–4). In applying the carbohydrate loading concept to distance running, Karlsson and Saltin [11] studied 10 athletes who ran two 30-km races separated by 3 weeks. Before each race they ate a mixed diet or followed a carbohydrate loading protocol consisting of a glycogen-depleting run, then 2 days of carbohydrate-poor feeding followed by a high carbohydrate diet for 3 days. The runners' leg muscles were biopsied before and after each run. The runners were found to have a higher muscle glycogen content and a better performance on the carbohydrate loading protocol than on a simple mixed diet without carbohydrate loading. Thus, there is experimental evidence suggesting that carbohydrate loading improves performance, that is, the *duration* of high performance, but not the speed.

## The "Glycogen Burst"

The biggest drain on glycogen stores occurs at the beginning of a marathon run (Essen et al. [9]), when approximately 20% of the available glycogen is used ("burst") in the first 5 minutes. Energy requirements are, obviously, instantaneous. Since glucose uptake early

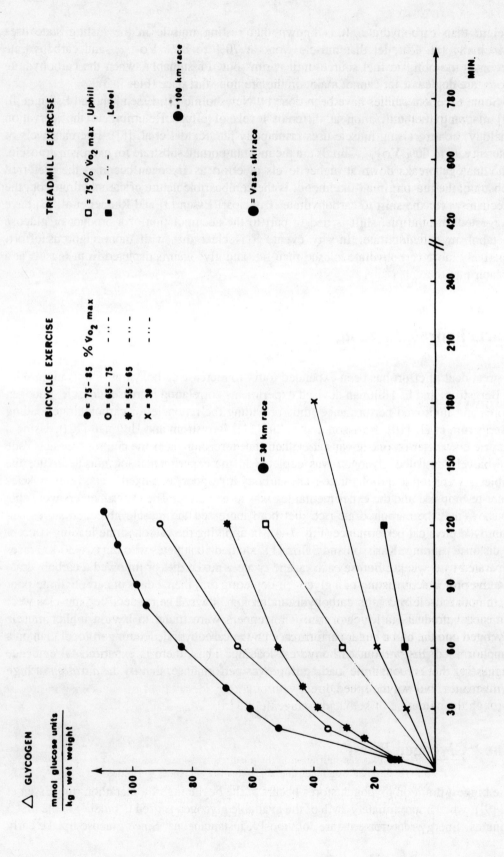

on is limited, the energy needs are supplied by glycogen breakdown. To utilize fat early and preserve glycogen, some investigators have recommended increasing triglycerides and fatty acids before a marathon. It has been shown that blocking fatty acid mobilization with nicotinic acid accelerates glycogen utilization, so it is assumed that the converse may be true, i.e., increasing fatty acid availability will spare glycogen. In fact, Newsholme [2] has shown that fatty acids slow glycolysis at several points in the breakdown of glycogen. Further, Costill et al. [13] have demonstrated a significant decrease in glycogen utilization during a 70% $\dot{V}_{O_2\ max}$ 30-min. treadmill run when subjects were given heparin immediately after a fatty meal. The heparin activates lipoprotein lipase and thereby increases fatty acids. Elevating free fatty acids may well be a reasonable suggestion for runners who begin their race relatively slowly with a $\dot{V}_{O_2\ max}$ below 70% to 80%, but is questionable at higher levels of effort.

The body's requirement for high energy phosphates is the final determinant of the fuel source, which is a function of the race's pace. The contractile process using ATP is coupled to the generation of ATP (Fig. 7-2). Given a continuum of preferred substrates (fatty acids to glycogen), if fatty acids are elevated at the beginning of effort, more fat will be utilized at the lower level of effort (where less ATP is needed), and perhaps less glycogen will be used at a higher level of effort. The elite marathoner would be using glycogen early since he or she has a greater demand for high energy phosphates.

## Lipolysis

In any event, fats break down either from fat depots or from fat stores in muscle itself (visually, "marbled" beef). Jones et al. [14] investigated fat utilization in light (36% $\dot{V}_{O_2\ max}$) versus heavy (70% $\dot{V}_{O_2\ max}$) exercise by having subjects pedal for 40 min. on a bicycle ergometer. Using plasma turnover rates of several fatty acids, it was found that light exercise was accompanied by mobilization of fat from peripheral adipose tissue stores. In heavy work, triglycerides within muscle broke down and the fatty acids were used directly by muscle. Glycerol, the other component of stored fat, was not used directly by muscle during heavy work and escaped into the blood stream to be taken up by the liver for gluconeogenesis.

In both muscle and liver, fatty acids are broken down to acetate, which is used directly for energy production. Much of the liver acetate is converted to ketoacids, which are then liberated into the blood stream and taken up by muscle, brain, and other tissues. Ketoacids function as a substrate for ATP synthesis. Fatty acids, therefore, whether liberated from peripheral stores, from muscle itself, or a combination of both, contribute to ATP synthesis in two ways: either directly through the metabolism of acetate or indirectly through the oxidation of ketoacids (Hagenfeldt [15]).

←——— **7–3**  Glycogen utilization in the quadriceps femoris (vastus lateralis) at different work intensities and with different modes and duration of exercises. Values taken from References 3, 4, 5, 6, 8, 9, 11, 18, and 26. (From Essen, B. 1977. Intramuscular substrate utilization during prolonged exercise. Ann N Y Acad Sci 301:30–44. Reprinted with permission.)

## Gluconeogenesis

So far, the discussion of metabolism has centered on fuel stored as glycogen and fat. The third major fuel source comes through the provision of new glucose from protein and from breakdown products of glycogen and glucose metabolism itself. The reader is referred to a recent outstanding review of amino acid metabolism in exercise by Lemon and Nagle [16].

With the onset of effort, glucose uptake by exercising muscle begins along with the other hormonally-induced metabolic events mentioned previously. Maximum gluconeogenesis rises many times above basal levels and provides roughly one-third of the fuel for ATP synthesis in Wahren's experimental model (Wahren [17]). More reliance is placed upon improved fat metabolism in conditioned runners, so glucose use is less (Fig. 7–5). The beginning substances for new glucose formation are lactate and pyruvate from muscle glycogen breakdown, the amino acid alanine from muscle, and glycerol from fat breakdown. It has also been suggested that ketoacids from fat can be converted to propanediol and then to glucose (Owen [18]). By a reversal of the anaerobic glycolytic pathway, lactate and pyruvate are converted to glucose through an energy-using process.

The glucose alanine cycle is represented in Fig. 7–6. Certain amino acids, perhaps coming from muscle, provide an amino group that combines with pyruvate in muscle to form alanine. Alanine travels through the blood to the liver where the amino group is shaved off, forming pyruvate again. Pyruvate is then converted to glucose, which enters the circulation for muscle, brain, and other tissue uptake.

Gluconeogenesis, therefore, provides a significant amount of carbohydrate as fuel for exercising muscle. Since training increases fat usage, less reliance is placed on gluconeogenesis.

# Effects of Training

The preceding section outlined the fuel sources that allow the marathoner to couple high-energy phosphate production to the ultimate goal of muscular contraction. Stored glycogen, lipids, and protein are converted to fuel substrates under hormonal influence. The following brief discussion, on the effects of training on substrate metabolism, is designed to show that training works—but anyone who has put on running shoes and kept them on, knows this.

Holloxyz et al. [19] and Costill et al. [20] have investigated training effects in detail. In addition to the salutory changes in heart function and the efficiency of skeletal muscular cellular respiration, training improves glycogen utilization and efficiency of fat use, thereby, in turn, sparing glycogen. Exactly which enzymes are involved in this adaptive and presumably inductive process are largely unknown, but there has been progress in their identification. For example, lipoprotein lipase activity has been known to be significantly higher in both male and female runners than in controls (Nikkila et al. [21]). Furthermore, insulin secretion is less in conditioned athletes than in age- and weight-matched controls (Lohman et al. [22]), presumably because of enhanced insulin binding

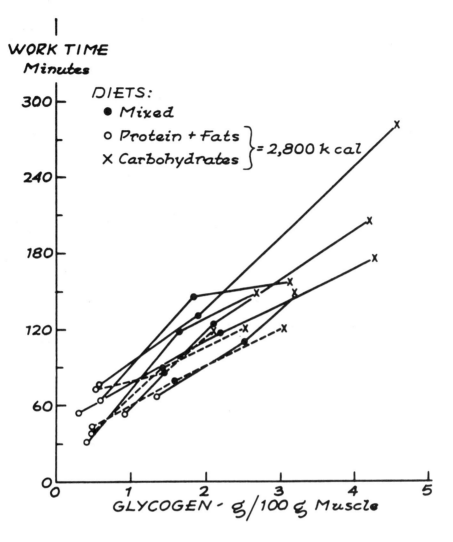

**7–4**  Effect of carbohydrate meals and duration of exercise—the carbohydrate loading effect. (From Bergstrom, J., Hermansen, et al. 1967. Diet, muscle glycogen and physical performance. Acta Physiol Scand 71:140–150. Reprinted with permission.)

to receptors (Pederson et al. [23]). Rahkila et al. [24] studied carbohydrate utilization in well-trained versus moderately trained subjects at the same level of effort. The well-trained group used approximately 11% less carbohydrate over the study period (Fig. 7–5).

The inference is that this efficiency is due to improved metabolism of fats, and is in accord with previous suggestions that training induces certain lipid-related enzymes to higher efficiency. Training is carbohydrate-sparing. Thus, because of these, as well as other metabolic alterations, training does improve performance. Hagan et al. [25] have found that marathon performance improves with low body mass, daily workouts, and training runs of long duration and distance.

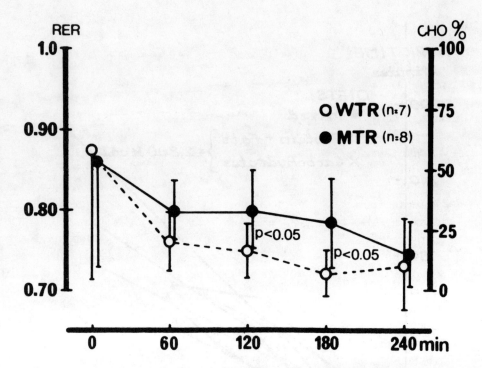

**7-5**  Respiratory exchange ratio (RER) and relative contribution of carbohydrates (CHO %) to the total energy production in well-trained (WTR) and moderately trained (MTR) groups of healthy men during a 4 h bicycle ergometry exercise. (From Rahkila, P., Soimajarvia, J. et al. 1980. Lipid metabolism during exercise II—respiratory exchange ratio and muscle glycogen content during four hour bicycle ergometry in two groups of healthy men. Eur J Appl Physiol 44:245–254. Reprinted with permission.)

# Nutritional Recommendations

There is no substitute for training in regard to ultimate performance. All the vitamins, carbohydrates, minerals, lack of red meat, etc., will not matter if the mileage has not been logged. The question therefore, is: If the training has been optimal, can nutrition influence performance?

## Ideal Body Weight

The first objective of the athlete-in-training is to project and strive for an ideal body weight. Determining ideal body weight cannot be done by "weight-height" charts, since they are approximations. The individual runner can look in a mirror and decide if he or she needs to lose weight and generally how much. If one wishes to be more scientific, body fat measurements can be obtained through a physiology laboratory. Generally, female runners should have a body fat composition of 15% or slightly lower, while males should

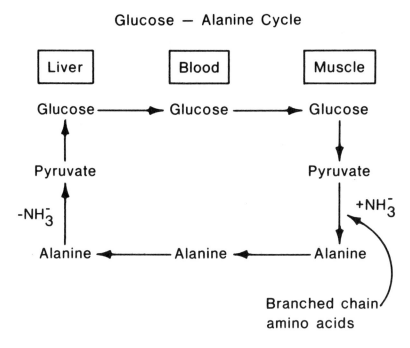

**7–6**  Glucose-alanine cycle.

have no more than 10% fat, perhaps ideally 5% to 8%. If a woman loses fat below a critical amount, she will become amenorrheic and have difficulty, furthermore, with thermoregulation.

Another caution: A balanced diet is important. As an example, after giving a lecture on fuel metabolism some time ago, I was approached by a fine runner who had just completed the Western States 100-Mile Endurance Run. During his training, he had serial body fat measurements performed and found that his percentage of body fat was rising while his weight remained stable. There is only one possible answer: He was in negative nitrogen balance and losing protein mass while replacing it with fat. On further questioning, he had a lactose intolerance and could not drink milk. He was simply not ingesting enough protein from other food sources to replace his muscle protein catabolism. Thus, if one keeps the body supplied with a balanced diet (roughly 55% carbohydrate, 25% protein, and 20% fat) and a liberal enough caloric intake, the body will deposit the fuel stores appropriately. The body is smarter than all of us who attempt to tamper with it. If one wishes to lose weight, then simply adjust the diet so that it is balanced and hypocaloric.

## To Carbohydrate-load or Not?

When the runner is at ideal body weight, what nutritional manipulations are reasonable prior to a marathon? With regard to carbohydrate loading, there is *some evidence* to *suggest* that one can supersaturate muscle with glycogen and, therefore, improve performance (Bergstrom et al. [10]); Karlsson and Saltin [11]; Bergstrom and Hultman [12]. Again, this author would emphasize the words "some evidence" and "suggest." On reviewing the evidence, one finds several problems: First, not one study has been performed over marathon distance; second, there are few appropriate statistical analyses in the studies done; and, third, the studies ignore the other beneficial effects of training, especially in the elite marathoner—that is, can adding more glycogen to an already fuel-efficient runner affect his or her performance positively? In addition, a ketogenic diet, which is identical to a carbohydrate-free diet, puts one in negative nitrogen balance, and muscle loss occurs. Given that the runner feels terrible due to electrolyte depletion, dehydration, and nausea, one wonders if carbohydrate loading prior to a marathon is worthwhile. A number of investigators are convinced absolutely of the value of carbohydrate loading. This author, however, would like to see more and better data before recommending it for every marathon competitor. One thing is certain: most people deplete and load incorrectly when eating excess carbohydrates for several days prior to a marathon. Granted, fluid balance is restored and carbohydrate reaccumulated, but excess carbohydrate is stored as unnecessary fat and, therefore, weight.

## Elevating Triglycerides

There may be some value in elevating triglycerides prior to a run in order to minimize glycogen loss during the "burst" at the beginning of a run. As discussed previously, fatty acids supply resting muscle and their level would fall abruptly with muscle uptake at the beginning of a run. Keeping the level of fatty acids high might force them to be used (Randel et al. [8]) early on in the race and thereby preserve muscle glucogen. Two cups of coffee will provide enough caffeine to raise fatty acids (Locksley [6]). Caffeine, a phosphodiesterase inhibitor, prevents the conversion of cyclic AMP to the inactive compound. Adrenalin (certainly circulating before a marathon) works through cyclic AMP to cause lipolysis, and thereby increases fatty acids. Caffeine keeps the fatty acids high.

## Running in the Post-absorptive State

One is often asked if a marathon should be run after ingesting carbohydrate or in the postprandial state. As noted in Fig. 7–1, insulin rises with a meal. The blood sugar rises initially, is usually back down within 2 hours, and then drops a little lower. In a marathon run, glucose will be taken up rapidly by muscle, and the normal tendency to hypoglycemia, which usually occurs at about 3 hours, will be exaggerated. The counter-regulatory hormones, suppressed by carbohydrate ingestion, will eventually be secreted but probably not before some unpleasant hypoglycemic symptoms have occurred. Insulin, of course, complicates the issue, since glycogenolysis, lipolysis, etc., do not occur until insulin has fallen to low levels despite the presence of counter-regulatory hormones. It is prudent, therefore, to run in the post-absorptive state, i.e., at least 4 hours after a meal.

Drinking carbohydrate-containing liquids toward the end of a marathon is of dubious value from a physiologic standpoint. Most of the liquids distributed during a race contain balanced or near-balanced solutions offering no more than 50 g glucose per liter. If a runner quickly drinks 4 oz, he or she is consuming about 25 cal, which is insignificant. Once one starts concentrating the carbohydrate into syrup consistency, however, nausea can result because of the osmotic load.

In summary, for the successful marathoner, achieving and maintaining ideal body weight is fundamental. There is no evidence to suggest that adding a battery of vitamins, minerals, or exotic concoctions, improves performance. The case for carbohydrate loading may be valid, but in the author's view, needs greater substantiation. Elevating fats prior to a run with black coffee is a reasonable, but unproven, physiologic suggestion and worth trying. The race should be run no sooner than 4 hours after ingesting a meal. Last, but more importantly, there is no substitute for training.

# The Diabetic Distance Runner

The diabetic distance runner is special, but there is no reason why diabetics cannot run a marathon. Their muscles adapt to training in the same way as nondiabetics (Costill et al. [26]). Almost all diabetic patients should exercise aerobically to lower their insulin requirements and perhaps to prevent cardiovascular complications (Richter et al. [27]). (Richter et al. [27], Vranic et al. [28], and Vranic and Berger [29] offer good reviews of diabetes and exercise.)

The problem with many exercise studies on diabetics is that they begin with the patient in the insulin-withdrawn state, that is, no insulin for 24 hours (Wahren [30]). No type I diabetic, however, should be treated with one insulin dose per day. The insulin withdrawal puts the diabetic metabolically at about 40 min into a run before he or she even takes a step. What happens is that with the low levels of insulin, the counter-regulatory hormones have caused glycogenolysis, gluconeogenesis, etc., to proceed to the point where a nondiabetic would be after some 40 min to exercise.

The ideal is to have diabetics begin a run with the same metabolic profile as their nondiabetic counterparts. The blood sugar should be between 80 and 120. The difference between the diabetic and the nondiabetic is that the diabetic will need a dose of insulin, albeit much smaller than usual and in the arm for slower absorption, and he or she will need to supply much of his or her fuel needs with ingested glucose. There are no formulas for doing this without knowing the blood sugar level, and the latter should be part of the diabetic's training process, requiring an occasional fingerstick blood sugar test. Appropriate "paraphernalia" and fluids can be carried during training and competition in a LiquiPac® or the like. Diabetics can balance fuel utilization with endogenous stores and exogenous sources, and thus run marathons successfully.

# References

1. Milvy, P. (ed). 1977. The Marathon: Physiological, Medical, Epidemiological and Psychological Studies. Ann N Y Acad Sci 301.
2. Newsholme, E.A. 1977. The regulation of intracellular and extracellular fuel supplied during sustained exercise. Ann N Y Acad Sci 301:81–91.
3. Essen, B. 1977. Intramuscular substrate utilization during prolonged exercise. Ann N Y Acad Sci 301:30–44.
4. Ahlborg, G., Felig, P. et al. 1974. Substrate turnover during prolonged exercise in man. J Clin Invest 53:1090–1090.
5. Scheele, K., Herzog, G. et al. 1979. Metabolic adaptation to prolonged exercise. Eur J Appl Physiol 41:101–108.
6. Locksley, R. 1980. Fuel utilization in marathons: Implications for performance. (Medical Staff Conference, University of California, San Francisco.) West J Med 133:493–502.
7. Cahill, G. 1981. Metabolism VI-1 to VI-14. In: Rubenstein, E., Federman, D., (eds): Medicine.
8. Randel, P.J., Garland, T.B. et al. 1966. Interaction of metabolism and the physiological role of insulin. Recent Prog Horm Res 22:1–48.
9. Essen, B., Hagenfeldt, L., Kaijser, L. 1977. Utilization of blood born and intramuscular substrates during continuous and intermittent exercise in man. J Physiol 265:489–506.
10. Bergstrom, J., Hermansen, L. et al. 1967. Diet, muscle glycogen and physical performance. Acta Physiol Scand 71:140–150.
11. Karlsson, J., Saltin, B. 1971. Diet, muscle glycogen and endurance performance. J Appl Physiol 31:203–206.
12. Bergstrom, J., Hultman, E. 1972. Nutrition for maximal sports performance. JAMA 22:999–1006.
13. Costill, D.L., Coyle, E. et al. 1977. Effects of elevated plasma FSA and insulin on muscle glycogen usage during exercise. J Appl Physiol 43:695–699.
14. Jones, N.L., Heigenhauser, C.J.F. et al. 1980. Fat metabolism in heavy exercise. Clin Sci 59:469–478.
15. Hagenfeldt, L. 1979. Metabolism of free fatty acids and ketone bodies during exercise in normal and diabetic man. Diabetes 28 (Suppl. I):66–70.
16. Lemon, P.W.R., Nagle, F.J. 1981. Effects of exercise on protein and amino acid metabolism. Med Sci Sports Exerc 13:141–149.
17. Wahren, J. 1977. Glucose turnover during exercise in man. Ann N Y Acad Sci 301:45–55.
18. Owen, O.E. 1982. Personal communication.
19. Holloxzy, J.O., Tennie, M.J. et al. 1977. Physiological consequences of the biochemical adaptations to endurance exercise. Ann N Y Acad Sci 301:440–454.
20. Costill, D.L., Fink, W.J. et al. 1979. Lipid metabolism in skeletal muscle of endurance trained males and females. J Appl Physiol 47:787–791.
21. Nikkila, E.A., Taskinen, M.R. et al. 1978. Lipoprotein lipase activity in adipose tissue and skeletal muscle of runners relation to serum lipoproteins. Metabolism 27:1661–1671.
22. Lohman, D., Liebold, F. et al. 1978. Diminished insulin response in highly trained athletes. Metabolism 27:521–524.
23. Pederson, O., Beck-Nielsen, H., Heding, L. 1980. Increased insulin receptors after exercise in patients with insulin dependent diabetes mellitus. N Engl J Med 302:886–892.
24. Rahkila, P., Soimajarvia, J. et al. 1980. Lipid metabolism during exercise II—respiratory exchange ratio and muscle glycogen content during four hour bicycle ergometry in two groups of healthy men. Eur J Appl Physiol 44:245–254.
25. Hagan, R.D., Smith, M.G., Gettman, L.R. 1981. Marathon performance in relation to maximal aerobic power and training indices. Med Sci Sports Exerc 13:185–189.

26. Costill, D.L., Cleary, T. et al. 1979. Training adaptations in skeletal muscle of juvenile diabetics. Diabetes 28:818–822.

27. Richter, E.A., Ruderman, M.B., Schneider, S.H. 1981. Diabetes and exercise. Am J Med 70:201–209.

28. Vranic, M., Horvath, S., Wahren, J. 1979. Proceedings of a Conference on Diabetes and Exercise 28 (Suppl I):1–113.

29. Vranic, M., Berger, M. 1979. Exercise and diabetes mellitus. Diabetes 28:147–163.

30. Wahren, J. 1979. Glucose turnover during exercise in healthy man in patients with diabetes mellitus. Diabetes 28 (Suppl I):1–113.

# Section 3
# Sports and Hormones, Fluids, and Electrolytes

Chapter 8

# Hormonal Regulation
# of Fluid and Electrolytes
# During Exercise[1]

by Maire T. Buckman and Glenn T. Peake

## Introduction

There are numerous studies on the effects of exercise on fluid and electrolyte balance in humans and substantial new information exists regarding the role of various hormones in these processes. This chapter reviews fluid compartment shifts and electrolyte changes, alterations in blood hormone levels, and associated effects during exercise. Clearly, results of a single study have limited generalized application since each exercise protocol is unique. Exercise has different effects, depending upon circumstances. For example, exercise acclimation at 39.8°C is associated with an increase in sweat rate, whereas acclimation at 23.8°C is associated with a decrease in sweat rate (Shvartz and Bhattacharya [1]). Thus, sweating and the associated water and electrolyte losses depend on environmental conditions and acclimation of the individual. Because variable exercise conditions have different effects on salt and water balance and potentially also on hormone secretion, the exercise milieu is precisely defined for each study discussed here.

The variables that characterize each exercise protocol can be divided into 1) environmental conditions, 2) exercise conditions, and 3) individual conditioning. Environmental conditions include temperature, humidity, wind factors, and altitude. Exercise conditions include position (supine, sitting, standing upright), type of exercise (weight lifting, running, climbing, cycling, swimming, etc.), and duration (5 min vs 8 h, for example). Individual conditioning is the level of exercise training of the participants. Thus, a person

[1]Supported by the Veterans Administration (Award to Dr. Maire T. Buckman) and NIH Grants 5-M01-RR 00997-07 and 5-R01-HD 05794-08.

who lives a semisedentary life without regular exercise beyond light walking may have a very different response to a given exercise protocol under defined environmental conditions from that of a highly trained person who, for example, jogs 10 miles each day. Likewise, sex and age may influence physiologic processes associated with exercise (Plowman, Drinkwater et al. [2]). Unfortunately, many exercise studies only partially define these variables, making integration of data difficult.

Serum or plasma hormone concentrations are frequently measured to determine hormonal secretory responses. However, other factors influence hormone concentrations independent of stimulus responsiveness. These include the size of the stored hormonal pool available for secretion, the volume for distribution of a hormone that may change under various conditions, and the clearance of the hormone. Since exercise in the heat, for example, is associated with a profound decrease in effective arterial blood volume, resulting in diminished renal blood flow, glomerular filtration rate, and splanchic blood flow, the effects on serum hormones may be anticipated to be independent of hormone secretion. These effects may result from hemoconcentration, altered hormone distribution, decreased renal excretion, or altered metabolism (Knochel [3]). Thus, an increase in hormone concentration after exercise may not result simply from enhanced release from its production or storage site. Furthermore, serum hormone concentration may not reflect biologic activity. Tissue or end-organ responsiveness also determines hormonal effects. For example, an increase in the number of aldosterone receptors at the distal renal tubule may enhance aldosterone activity without increased hormone concentrations. Conversely, decreased receptor numbers may diminish the activity at the same hormone concentration. Little is known about the effect of exercise on target-tissue responsiveness or receptor activity.

Two hormonal systems have a major impact on body fluid and electrolyte homeostasis: the renin-angiotensin-aldosterone system and the neurohypophyseal hormone, vasopressin. The anterior pituitary hormones, ACTH, growth hormone (GH), and prolactin may also affect water and electrolyte balance, but this is poorly defined.

# Renin-Angiotensin-Aldosterone System

The renin-angiotensin-aldosterone system is primarily regulated by the renal juxtaglomerular apparatus, which includes the renin-producing segment of the afferent arteriole and the proximal segment of the distal convoluted tubule, the macula densa. Renin secretion is inhibited by increased pressure on stretch receptors within the afferent arteriole and it is increased by decreased pressure or stretch (Tobian, Tomboulian et al. [4]). In addition, renin secretion is modulated by changes in tubular fluid composition at the macula densa (David and Freeman [5]). Volume expansion with sodium chloride has a profound inhibitory effect on renin secretion—more so than comparable expansion with dextran—presumably because of a specific effect of sodium chloride at the macula densa. In addition to these renal mechanisms, renin secretion is influenced by the sympathetic nervous system. This may occur directly via nerve terminals at the juxtaglomerular apparatus (Assaykeen and Ganong [6]) or by circulating catecholamines (Johnson et al. [7]). The neural component of renin secretion appears to be mediated by $\beta$-adrenergic

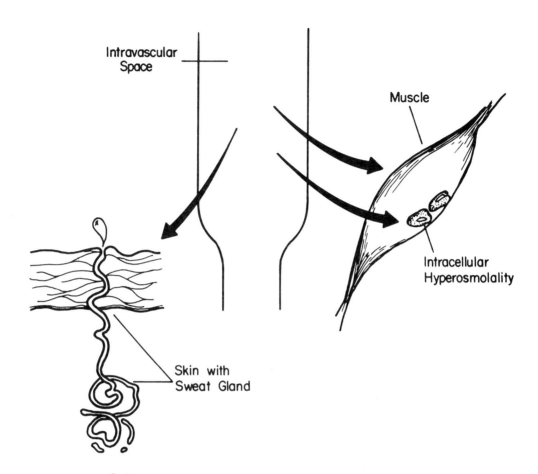

**8–1**   Mechanisms of fluid shifts during exercise. Blood is shunted to exercising muscle and skin. In muscle, intracellular hyperosmolality induces a shift of plasma water into the cells. Sweat production results in a hypotonic fluid loss. These fluid shifts result in contraction of plasma volume.

receptors (Reid and Morris [8]). Once renin is released from the juxtaglomerular cell into the systemic circulation, it cleaves an $\alpha2$-globulin substrate to form the decapeptide angiotensin I, which, in turn, is enzymatically converted to angiotensin II. Angiotensin II is a potent vasoconstrictor that stimulates aldosterone biosynthesis and secretion. Aldosterone stimulates sodium transport across a number of epithelial membranes, including kidney, sweat glands, salivary glands, and gastrointestinal tract (Knochel [9]; Sharp and Leaf [10]), and acts primarily in the kidney on the distal renal tubule, where it promotes resorption of sodium and secretion of potassium and hydrogen. Thus, the renin-angiotensin-aldosterone system is important in maintaining vascular tone and extracellular fluid volume by increasing sodium retention and plasma volume.

Strenuous exercise stimulates the renin-angiotensin-aldosterone cascade in humans. The initiating event in activating this cascade may be, in part, related to pronounced shifts in body fluids that occur with exercise (Fig. 8–1) (Costill [11]). These shifts are characterized by up to a 13% decrease in plasma and effective arterial blood volume occurring during the initial phase of strenuous exercise (Convertino et al. [12]; Geyssant et al. [13]; Melin et al. [14]). Activation of the renin-angiotensin-aldosterone system occurs after each acute bout of exercise, and heat acclimatization does not blunt this effect of exercise (Davies et al. [15]). Fluid replacement with physiologic saline blunted, but did not block renin release.

Several mechanisms account for the decreased blood volume. Muscular work, independent of environmental conditions, results in massive shunting of blood to skeletal muscle, so-called exercise hyperemia. Quantitatively, muscle blood flow varies almost directly with the degree of work and may increase 20–40 times above resting levels during intense exercise (Barcroft [16]). In addition to shunting of blood to skeletal muscle, a substantial shift of plasma water into muscle cells occurs during muscular contraction. This is due to increased osmolality within exercising muscle cells.

Glycogen, the major fuel for muscular contraction, is metabolized into smaller intermediary products; since the cell membrane is relatively less permeable to these substances than to water, water moves into the cells. During the early phases of exercise, 10% or more of the inflowing arterial blood may move from plasma into the cell (Schlein et al. [17]). Muscle water increases roughly 8% in active tissue during the early minutes of exercise, and this is associated with an equivalent decline in plasma water (Costill [11]). After the initial shifts, plasma and muscle water tend to be stable over 120 min of continued exertion. Thus, the major fluid shifts occur within the first 15 min of strenuous exercise and only minor changes are observed with continued exertion.

However, during the adaptation to continued bouts of exercise, plasma volume increases without a change in red blood cell mass (Convertino et al. [18]). Since plasma concentrations of $Na^+$, $K^+$, and albumin are maintained despite the increased plasma volume, the total blood content of these substances rises. With the increased plasma volume, an accompanying fall in hemoglobin concentration and hematocrit occurs.

Heat generated by muscle contraction and from the environment induces increased peripheral blood flow and sweating (Benzinger [19]), which are important in maintaining thermal equilibrium (Costill [11]). Sweating may further compromise effective arterial blood volume. Fluid and electrolyte losses in sweat depend on environmental conditions (temperature, humidity, wind speed) and on the degree and duration of physical exertion. Furthermore, acclimation modulates sweat losses (Shvartz et al. [1]). Maximum sweat rate in an untrained man may attain 1.5 L/h (Fasola et al. [20]), whereas, marathon runners may lose sweat in excess of 6 L (Costill [11]). Sweat is hypotonic to plasma. The principal ions in sweat are those from the extracellular compartment, i.e., sodium and chloride. Sodium in sweat ranges between 10 and 60 mEq/L (Shvartz et al. [1]). Sweat ion concentration is strongly influenced by sweat rate and the subject's state of heat acclimation. With increasing sweat, sodium and chloride concentrations increase (Shvartz et al. [1]). Thus, significant fluid and electrolytes can be lost by sweating and sweat-induced decrease in extracellular fluid volume may additionally stimulate renal renin secretion.

An exercise-associated decrease in blood volume, due to fluid shifts and sweat losses, results in reduced renal blood flow and glomerular filtration rate, thereby providing a potent stimulus for renin secretion. In addition, catecholamines increase with exercise (Fasola et al. [20]), and they, too, are potent stimulators for renin release. Catecholamine and renin responses during graded exercise suggest that renin secretion is related to enhanced sympathetic activity (Kotchen et al. [21]). Renin, in turn, activates the angiotensin system, which results in formation of active angiotensin II. Angiotensin II is a potent vasoconstrictor, but it has a minor role in blood pressure elevation with exercise (Fagard et al. [22]). More importantly, angiotensin II stimulates adrenal aldosterone secretion during exercise.

In addition to angiotensin II, ACTH and potassium also stimulate aldosterone secretion. Their role in exercise-induced increases in serum aldosterone has not been fully evaluated.

Aldosterone helps to maintain extracellular fluid volume by promoting sodium resorption in the kidney, the gastrointestinal tract, and sweat and salivary glands. The direct renal effect on distal tubular resorption of sodium and excretion of potassium begins 0.5–2 h after aldosterone administration and lasts 4–8 h (Barger et al. [23]; Ganong and Mulrow [24]; Ross et al. [25]; Sonnenblick et al. [26]). The delay in onset of aldosterone action on sweat, saliva, and gastrointestinal electrolytes is even longer (August et al. [27]), a fact implying that aldosterone secreted during short bouts of exercise may not become physiologically effective until after exercise is completed. Aldosterone seems to have a long-term homeostatic effect on the maintenance of plasma volume.

In one study, subjects were exposed to heat without exercise. This resulted in fluid shifts similar to those seen during exercise—shifts due to increased blood flow to the skin and to marked elevation in plasma aldosterone (Costill [11]). This study implied that during acute heat exposure, decreased plasma volume may stimulate aldosterone secretion. Studies of acute exercise and plasma aldosterone show that a single 60-min bout of exercise increased plasma renin and aldosterone nearly sevenfold above baseline (Follenius et al. [28]). Despite *ad libitum* water intake, aldosterone remained elevated for 11 h after exercise completion. The acute plasma aldosterone elevation, therefore, outlasts the exercise and may affect the long-term metabolic adaptation to exercise.

Aldosterone dynamics during graded exercise and plasma concentrations at sea level and high altitude were studied (Maher et al. [29]). Healthy males exercised rigorously for 6 wk on a mechanically braked bicycle ergometer for 20 min at 45% maximum oxygen consumption ($Vo_{2max}$), and after a 1-h rest again for 20 min at 75% $Vo_{2max}$. Plasma renin, angiotensin II, and aldosterone increased in a graded fashion at sea level, and after 11 days at 4300 M. In contrast, on the first day of altitude exposure, all three hormones were significantly lower, compared to those at sea level and after adaption to altitude. It was proposed that the acute hypoxemia of high altitude, known to increase renal blood flow, may signal a decrease in renin release and, secondarily, a decrease in aldosterone secretion (Hogan et al. [30]). This hypothesis is consistent with evidence suggesting that renal blood flow changes primarily activate the renin-angiotensin-aldosterone system during exercise (Fig. 8–2).

Prolonged exercise in heat results in large water and salt losses from sweating. This may further compromise intravascular volume and result in counter-regulatory sodium conservation by enhanced renal sodium resorption and by decreased sodium in sweat. Moderately conditioned normal men (average $Vo_{2max}$ 42 ml $O_2$/kg/min) exercised in a room maintained at 32°C and 45%–50% relative humidity to promote large salt and water losses from sweating. Activity consisted of cycling at 50% $Vo_{2max}$ for eight 15-min intervals spaced by 5-min rest periods. During rest periods, subjects ingested water equal to sweat losses. The change in plasma aldosterone paralleled that of plasma renin. Both hormones were significantly lower if water was replaced by an electrolyte solution containing 20 mEq/L sodium, 20 mEq/L potassium, and 23 g/L glucose. Ingestion of electrolytes offsets approximately 42% of the total body potassium (Francis and MacGregor [31]). This study suggests that sodium losses from sweating are a stimulus to aldosterone secretion, which can be partially reversed by sodium intake.

Under extreme conditions, during basic military training in hot climates, more than 12 L of fluid can be lost per day in sweat (Robinson and Robinson [32]). Sodium in sweat

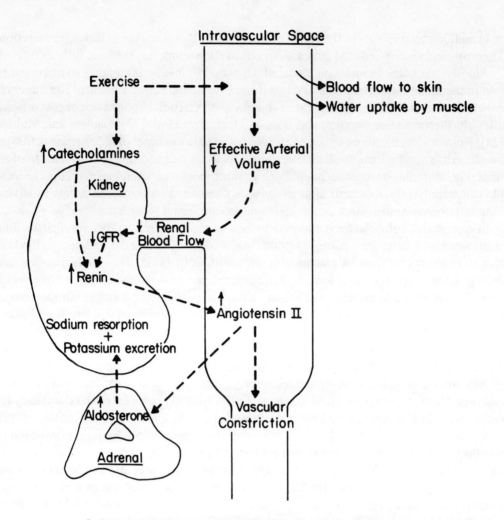

**8–2**   Proposed sequence of events leading to activation of the renin-angiotensin-aldosterone system during exercise. Significant sodium resorption and potassium excretion may occur at the sweat glands and in the kidney tubule.

averaged about 40–60 mEq/L, and potassium 4–9 mEq/L. Such training can, therefore, result in sodium losses in excess of 500 mEq and potassium losses of more than 100 mEq per day. These volume and electrolyte losses are potent stimuli for aldosterone secretion. Both aldosterone excretion and secretion are high compared to sodium intake in those engaging in intense physical conditioning in a hot climate (Knochel et al. [33]). Serial estimations of exchangeable $^{42}K$ showed a marked potassium deficit due to sweat and urinary losses. Inappropriately high urinary potassium losses for the potassium-depleted state occurred in those training in hot climates, an indication of an aldosterone effect on the kidney. Similar experiments in cooler climates did not show potassium depletion. Potassium deficits may be associated with rhabdomyolysis. Therefore, overproduction of aldosterone with exercise in the heat may be dangerous (Knochel et al. [33]).

# Vasopressin

Vasopressin is produced in the supraoptic and paraventricular nuclei of the anterior hypothalamus, and its granules are stored in the posterior pituitary gland (neurohypophysis). The primary function of vasopressin is to preserve tonicity of body fluids, and its secretion is regulated primarily by changes in plasma osmolality (Robertson et al. [34]). This is an exquisitely sensitive system; consequently, minute changes in plasma osmolality of 1%–2% result in significant changes in plasma vasopressin (Robertson et al. [34]). Increased plasma osmolality, with dehydration, results in increased vasopressin secretion and subsequent enhanced free-water resorption by the kidney. Decreased plasma osmolality after free-water intake, in contrast, causes suppression of vasopressin release and increased water excretion. Thus, small changes in extracellular fluid tonicity regulate vasopressin secretion, which, in turn, modulates renal handling of water in a way that restores extracellular fluid osmolality to normal.

The function of vasopressin to preserve body fluid tonicity is compromised only when hemodynamic factors reach threatening proportions. Blood volume must be decreased by 10%–15% before vasopressin release is significantly stimulated (Robertson and Athar [35]). At this level, tonicity may be increasingly compromised to conserve blood volume. When a normal adult was depleted of sodium by sweating in a heat chamber, body water tonicity did not decline until extracellular fluid volume was reduced by approximately 12% (McCance [36]). Major shifts in extracellular fluids may also be associated with alterations in vasopressin secretion. Increased ambient temperature from 25°C to 50°C was associated with increased plasma antidiuretic hormone; the hot environment dilates peripheral vascular beds and may decrease central blood volume (Moore [37]). Volume receptors regulate hypovolemic vasopressin secretion. Conversely, decreased ambient temperature from 26°C to 13°C was associated with decreased plasma vasopressin. Cooling caused peripheral vasoconstriction and increased central blood volume, which, in turn, decreased vasopressin secretion (Moore [37]). Thus, major changes in central blood volume, whether secondary to extracellular fluid loss or to redistribution, regulate vasopressin secretion.

Prolonged heavy exercise is associated with decreased urine formation (Castenfors [38]; Refsum and Stromme [39]). Increased shunting of blood to exercising muscle results in decreased splanchnic and renal circulation (Castenfors [38]). Decreased renal blood flow is proportional to the severity of exercise (Castenfors [38]). This causes decreased creatinine clearance ($C_{cr}$), which is quantitatively similar to decreased urine formation (Castenfors [38]). The significant correlation between decreased $C_{cr}$ and urine flow suggests that the diminished urine flow occurs, at least in part, secondary to decreased glomerular filtration. Maximum concentrating ability is decreased during exercise because of presumed reduction of interstitial sodium and urea secondary to decreased glomerular filtration. Nevertheless, the antidiuretic action of vasopressin may also be operative, and this possibility has recently been examined by several groups of investigators.

The effects of 7 days of hill-walking on fluid homeostasis and vasopressin concentration were examined (Williams et al. [40]). Serum electrolytes were stable, and plasma volume increased. Plasma vasopressin was also unchanged. In view of stable serum electrolytes and increased plasma volume during this type of exercise, one would not expect an increase in vasopressin secretion.

# Vasopressin Secretion

Plasma vasopressin increases in men 19–43 years of age with vigorous exercise. Vasopressin studies in women have not been published (Convertino et al. [12]). Plasma vasopressin in untrained men working on a cycle ergometer for 6 min at a time at work loads ranging from 100 W ($Vo_{2max}$ 40%) to 225 W ($Vo_{2max}$ 90%) did not increase at a work load performed at 40% $Vo_{2max}$; however, at higher work loads, vasopressin increased in a curvilinear fashion. Plasma volume decreased at each exercise level, with the maximum change of $-12.4\%$ occurring at the highest work load. Plasma osmolality increased in a curvilinear fashion from a mean resting level of 287 mOsm/kg to a mean maximum level of 302 mOsm/kg at the maximum work load. The change in osmolality correlated highly with the change in plasma sodium concentration. In order to examine the possible mechanisms of exercise-induced vasopressin release, correlation coefficients were examined. Vasopressin correlated best with changes in plasma osmolality and plasma sodium concentration and less well with changes in percent plasma volume. Thus, the investigators concluded that hyperosmolality is important in the regulation of vasopressin released during acute bouts of exercise (Convertino et al. [12]).

Effects of repeated exercise bouts on vasopressin secretion have also been studied in men working on a bicycle ergometer at approximately 160 W ($Vo_{2max}$ 65%) for 2 h/day for 8 days (Convertino et al. [18]). Increase in plasma volume to 112% above baseline occurred during the 8-day study period associated with maintenance of the resting plasma osmolality; this observation suggests that the exercise-associated volume expansion consisted of a corresponding isotonic increase in total solutes. Mean vasopressin increased eight-to ninefold over resting levels at completion of each exercise period, and the magnitude of the increase was similar on the first and last days of the exercise program, indicating that the increased plasma volume failed to exert an inhibitory influence on vasopressin secretion. As in the previous study, the increase in vasopressin correlated significantly with the acute increase in plasma osmolality and plasma sodium during exercise. Plasma volume decreased with each exercise bout to a similar degree at the beginning and end of the training program. Thus, the vasopressin response to acute exercise correlated with hyperosmolality and was unaffected by the 8-day training in this study.

Two groups of investigators studied the effect of chronic training on vasopressin. Geyssant et al. [13] examined the effect on plasma vasopressin concentrations in four untrained men who participated in a 5-month endurance program on a bicycle ergometer at 87% $Vo_{2max}$ four times per week to exhaustion. As in the previously mentioned study, baseline vasopressin values were similar throughout the training period, and a significant increase in vasopressin was observed before and after each training session. The magnitude of the increase was similar at the beginning and end of the 5-month program, but due to the small number of subjects, no statistical inference can be drawn.

The effect of training on vasopressin secretion was also studied by Melin et al. [14]. Subjects were divided into well-trained, trained, and untrained on the basis of $Vo_{2max}$ duration of exercise to exhaustion. The three groups then exercised on a bicycle ergometer at 80% $Vo_{2max}$ to exhaustion. Plasma vasopressin measured by bioassay increased significantly after exercise in all three groups to a comparable level. Thus, both of these studies showed that vasopressin responses to exercise did not depend on the level of physical training.

Wade and Claybaugh [41] studied the effect of hydration on vasopressin response in young men after 1 h of treadmill running at a heart rate approximately 35%, 70%, and 100% of predicted maximum rate. Subjects exercised following 10 h of water deprivation and after ingesting 300 ml of water. As in the previous studies, vasopressin changes correlated significantly with the work intensity. In addition, the increase in vasopressin after maximum exercise was greater following 10 h of water deprivation than after water supplementation. Plasma vasopressin returned to resting values 1 h after completion of exercise. Resting vasopressin levels, however, were similar in the two groups. In contrast to the previous studies, plasma vasopressin concentration did not correlate with plasma osmolality changes or plasma volume changes when correlations were examined during exercise. However, a positive correlation was observed between PRA and vasopressin, suggesting that angiotensin II influenced vasopressin secretion. Other investigators have reported conflicting results on the role of angiotensin II on vasopressin release (Schrier et al. [42]).

Several studies show that plasma vasopressin increases acutely with exercise and that the increase depends on work intensity and hydration status. Repetitive exercise does not alter the vasopressin response to acute exercise, and long-term training has no modulatory effect on this response. The mechanism of vasopressin increase with exercise may be related to the hyperosmolality that accompanies vigorous physical work and to a lesser extent on the hypovolemia associated with exercise. It has also been suggested that angiotensin II plays a role in exercise-associated vasopressin release. In addition, since vasopressin is primarily metabolized by the liver and the kidneys, decreased blood flow to these organs during exercise theoretically contributes to increased plasma levels of the hormone (Wade and Claybaugh [41]).

Physiologic consequences of increased plasma vasopressin have not been studied. Exercise has been associated with an increase in free-water clearance during exercise (Wade and Claybaugh [41]) and immediately after exercise (Melin et al. [14]). The decreased urine volume associated with exercise appears to be primarily due to a decrease in osmolar clearance associated with a decrease in negative free-water clearance. Since vasopressin decreases free-water clearance, the observed relative increase in free-water clearance with exercise suggests absence of a substantial role for vasopressin in the exercise-associated antidiuresis. However, since pre-exercise free-water clearance was already negative in these studies, ADH biologic effect could have already been maximal at the onset of exercise, and the decreased negative free-water clearance could represent exercise-associated changes in renal solute handling.

Other factors may modulate vasopressin activity at the renal tubule. Exercise increases renal prostaglandins, which may interfere with vasopressin action at the kidney (Oliw [43]; Share and Claybaugh [44]; Zambraski and Dunn [45]). Furthermore, norepinephrine released during exercise may play a role in the antidiuresis observed with exercise (Schrier et al. [42]). Norepinephrine administered by intravenous infusion increases renal water excretion in humans. This diuretic effect appears to be associated with alpha-adrenergic stimulating properties of norepinephrine. *In vitro* studies show that norepinephrine interferes with the cellular action of vasopressin. Serum cortisol increases with vigorous exercise and enhances free-water excretion. Although the precise respective roles of renal prostaglandins, norepinephrine, and cortisol in modulating the vasopressin effect on the renal tubule during exercise have not been studied, experimental data suggest that such interactions may be important in explaining the apparent contradictory findings of increased plasma vasopressin and enhanced free-water clearance with exercise.

# Anterior Pituitary Hormones

Corticotropin (ACTH) is the major determinant of adrenal cortisol secretion. Since exercise is associated with increased cortisol secretion, ACTH presumably rises during exercise (Few [46]). The function of the elevated cortisol is not clear, but it may help maintain or reestablish normal glomerular filtration and enhance water diuresis.

Growth hormone rises during exercise, but the effect is markedly blunted when exercise is performed in a cold environment (Frewin et al. [47]) and is potentiated in persons adapted to high altitude (Raynaud et al. [48]). In diabetic subjects, when blood glucose is increased, the growth hormone response to exercise is more marked, and this effect is no longer evident when blood glucose is chronically normal (Tamborlane et al. [49]). Since atropine will block the exercise-induced rise in plasma growth hormone, a cholinergic mechanism may mediate growth hormone release during exercise (Few and Davies [50]).

A potential role for opioid peptide neuroregulation of growth hormone secretion has been sought. In one study, administration of the opioid receptor blocker, naloxone, failed to alter the exercise-induced rise in growth hormone (Mayer et al. [51]), while Spiler and Molitch [52] found that naloxone blunted the rise in growth hormone induced by a similar bicycle ergometer work load. Further investigations are warranted to delineate a role for the opioids in the exercise-induced secretion of growth hormone.

Growth hormone has a variety of metabolic effects that might be involved in adaptation to exercise. It increases glomerular filtration, enhances renal resorption of sodium chloride, magnesium, and potassium, increases plasma volume, erythrocyte mass, and interstitial fluid volume, increases free fatty acid release from fat cells, and increases blood glucose and muscle glycogen stores (Daughaday [53]). Whether growth hormone is primarily responsible for these effects is not clear, since it may also modulate potent metabolic actions of other hormones.

Prolactin rises during exercise, but decreased ambient temperature blocks this effect of exertion (Frewin et al. [47]). Since pyridoxine is a coenzyme for dopa decarboxylase and has been shown to enhance exercise-induced growth hormone and decrease prolactin release, a role for dopaminergic neuroregulation in exercise-related release of these hormones has been suggested (Moretti et al. [54]). Metabolic actions of prolactin in the human subject, other than on breast milk production, are controversial. A role in renal salt and water retention has been proposed (Buckman et al. [55]), but prolactin may modulate the direct actions of other hormones on the kidney.

# Summary

Major secretory changes of anterior and posterior pituitary and adrenal hormones occur during exercise. These result from alterations in fluid distribution, catecholamine secretion, and other poorly understood mechanisms. The altered plasma hormones tend to restore effective intravascular volume by preventing salt and water loss through the kidneys and sweat glands. The renin-angiotensin-aldosterone system, according to extensive studies, has a primary influence on fluid and salt balance during exercise. Other hormones have been investigated, but their roles are not clearly defined. Growth hormone and possibly corticotropin, through regulation of cortisol secretion, may influence metabolic changes that occur during exercise, other than those associated with salt and water balance.

# References

1. Shvartz, R., Bhattacharya, A. et al. 1979. Deconditioning-induced exercise responses as influenced by heat acclimation. Aviat Space Environ Med 50:893–897.
2. Plowman, S.A., Drinkwater, B.L. et al. 1979. Age and aerobic power in women: A longitudinal study. J Gerontol 34:512–520.
3. Knochel, J.P. 1974. Environmental heat illness. Arch Intern Med 133:841–864.
4. Tobian, L., Tomboulian, A. et al. 1959. The effect of high perfusion pressures on the granulation of juxtaglomerular cells in an isolated kidney. J Clin Invest 38:605–610.
5. David, J.O., Freeman, R.H. 1976. Mechanisms regulating renin release. Physiol Rev 56:2–56.
6. Assaykeen, T.A., Ganong, W.F. 1971. The sympathetic nervous system and renin secretion. In: Martini, L., Ganong, W.F., (eds): Frontiers in Neuroendocrinology. Oxford University Press, London, pp 67–102.
7. Johnson, M.D., Fahri, E.R. et al. 1979. Plasma epinephrine and control of plasma renin activity: Possible extrarenal mechanisms. Am J Physiol 236:854–859.
8. Reid, I.A., Morris, B.J. 1978. The renin-angiotensin system. Ann Rev Physiol 40:377–410.
9. Knochel, J.P. 1977. Aldosterone. In: Kurtzman, N.A., Martinez-Maldonado, M., (eds): Pathophysiology of the Kidney. Charles C. Thomas, Springfield, pp 446–472.
10. Sharp, G.W.G., Leaf, A. 1973. Effects of aldosterone and its mechanism of action on sodium transport. In: Orloff, J., Berliner, R.W., (eds): Handbook of Physiology—Renal Physiology. American Physiological Society, Washington, D.C, pp 815–830.
11. Costill, D.L. 1977. Sweating: Its composition and effects on body fluid. Ann NY Acad Sci 301:160–170.
12. Convertino, V.A., Keil, L.C., Bernauer, E.M., Greenleaf, J.E. 1981. Plasma volume, osmolality, vasopressin, and renin activity during graded exercise in man. J Appl Physiol: 50(1):123–128.
13. Geyssant, A., Geelen, G., Denis, C., Allevard, A.M., Vincent, M., Jarsaillon, E., Bizollon, C.A., Lacour, J.R., Charib, C.I. 1981. Plasma Vasopressin, renin activity, and aldosterone: Effect of exercise and training. Eur J Appl Physiol 46:21–30.
14. Melin, B., Eclache, J.P., Geelen, G., Annat, G., Allevard, A.M. Jarsaillon, E., Zebidi, A., Legros, Charib, C.I. 1980. Plasma AVP, neurophysin, renin activity, and aldosterone during submaximal exercise performed until exhaustion in trained and untrained men. Eur J Appl Physiol 44:141–151.
15. Davies, J.A., Harrison, M.H., Cochrane, L.A., Edwards, R.J., Gibson, T.M. 1981. Effect of saline loading during heat acclimatization on adrenocortical hormone levels. J Appl Physiol 50(3):605–612.
16. Barcroft, H. 1963. Circulation in skeletal muscle. In: Hamilton, W.F. (section ed., Section 2): Circulation. In: Handbook of Physiology. A Critical Comprehensive Presentation of Physiologic Knowledge and Concepts, Vol. 3. Williams & Wilkins Co, Baltimore, pp 1353–1386.

17. Schlein, E.M., Jensen, D. et al. 1973. The effect of plasma water loss on assessment of muscle metabolism during exercise. J Appl Physiol 34:568–572.

18. Convertino, V.A., Brock, P.J., Keil, L.C., Bernauer, E.M. Greenleaf, J.E. 1980. Exercise training-induced hypervolemia: role of plasma albumin, renin, and vasopressin. J Appl Physiol: 48(4):665–669.

19. Benzinger, T.H. 1959. On physical heat regulation and the sense of temperature in man. Proc Natl Acad Sci USA 45:645–659.

20. Fasola, A.F., Martz, B.K. et al. 1966. Renin activity during supine exercise in normotensives and hypertensives. J Appl Physiol 21:1709–1712.

21. Kotchen, T.A., Hartley, L.H. et al. 1971. Renin, norepinephrine and epinephrine responses to graded exercise. J Appl Physiol 31:178–184.

22. Fagard, R.A., Reybrock, T. et al. 1978. Effect of angiotensin antagonism at rest and during exercise in sodium-depleted man. J Appl Physiol 45:403–407.

23. Barger, A.C., Berlin, R.D. et al. 1958. Infusion of aldosterone, 9-alpha-fluorohydrocortisone and antidiuretic hormone into the renal artery of normal and adrenalectomized, unanesthetized dogs: Effect on electrolyte and water excretion. Endocrinology 62:804–815.

24. Ganong, W.F., Mulrow, P.J. 1958. Rate of change in sodium and potassium excretion after injection of aldosterone into the aorta and renal artery of the dog. Am J Physiol 195:337–342.

25. Ross, E.J., Reddy, W.J. et al. 1959. Effects of intravenous infusions of dl-aldosterone acetate on sodium and potassium excretion in man. J Clin Endocrinol Metab 19:289–296.

26. Sonnenblick, E.H., Cannon, P.J. et al. 1961. The nature of the action of intravenous aldosterone: Evidence for a role of the hormone in urinary dilution. J Clin Invest 40:903–913.

27. August, J.T., Nelson, D.H. et al. 1958. Response of normal subjects to large amounts of aldosterone. J Clin Invest 37:1549–1555.

28. Follenius, M., Brandburger, G. et al. 1979. Plasma aldosterone, prolactin and ACTH: Relationships in man during heat exposure. Horm Metab Res 11:180–181.

29. Maher, J.T., Jones, L.G. et al. 1975. Aldosterone dynamics during graded exercise at sea level and high altitude. J Appl Physiol 39:18–22.

30. Hogan, R.P., Kotchen, T.A. et al. 1973. Effect of altitude on renin-aldosterone system and metabolism of water and electrolytes. J Appl Physiol 35:385–390.

31. Francis, K.T., MacGregor, R., III. 1978. Effect of exercise in the heat on plasma renin and aldosterone with either water or a potassium-rich electrolyte solution. Aviat Space Environ Med 49:461–465.

32. Robinson, S., Robinson, A.H. 1954. Chemical composition of sweat. Physiol Rev 34:202–220.

33. Knochel, J.P., Dotin, L.N. et al. 1972. Pathophysiology of intense physical conditioning in a hot climate. J Clin Invest 51:242–255.

34. Robertson, G.L., Athar S. et al. 1977. Osmotic control of vasopressin function. In: Andreoli, T.E., Grantham, J.J., Rector, F.C. (eds): Disturbances in Body Fluid Osmolality. American Physiological Society, Bethesda, pp 125–148.

35. Robertson, G.L., Athar, S. 1971. The interaction of blood osmolality and blood volume in regulating plasma vasopressin in man. J Clin Endocrinol Metab 42:613–620.

36. McCance, R.A. 1936. Experimental sodium chloride deficiency in man. Proc R Soc Lond [Biol] 119:245–268.

37. Moore, W.W. 1971. Antidiuretic hormone levels in normal subjects. Fed Proc 30:1387–1394.

38. Castenfors, J. 1977. Renal function during prolonged exercise. Ann NY Acad Sci 301:151–159.

39. Refsum, H.E., Stromme, S.B. 1978. Renal osmol clearance during prolonged heavy exercise. Scand J Clin Lab Invest 38:19–22.

40. Williams, E.S., Ward, M.P. et al. 1979. Effect of the exercise of seven consecutive days hill-walking on fluid homeostasis. Clin Sci Mol Med 56:305–316.

41. Wade, C.E., Claybaugh, J.R. 1980. Plasma renin activity, vasopressin concentration, and urinary excretory responses to exercise in men. J Appl Physiol 49(6):930–936.

42. Schrier, R.W., Berl, T., Anderson, R.J., McDonald, K.M. 1977. Nonosmolar control of renal water excretion. In: Andreoli, T.E., Grantham, J.J., Rector, F.C., Jr., (eds): Disturbances in Body Fluid Osmolality. pp 149–178, Williams and Wilkins, Baltimore.

43. Oliw, E. 1979. Prostaglandins and kidney function. Acta Physiol Scand [Suppl] 461:1–55.

44. Share, L., Claybaugh, R.J. 1972. Regulation of body fluids. Ann Rev Physiol 34:235–260.

45. Zambraski, E., Dunn, M. 1979. Renal prostaglandin (PG) secretion and excretion in exercising dogs. Fed Proc 38:893.

46. Few, J.D. 1974. Effect of exercise on the secretion and metabolism of cortisol in man. J Endocrinol 62:341–353.

47. Frewin, D.B., Frantz, A.G. et al. 1976. The effect of ambient temperature on the growth hormone and prolactin response to exercise. Aust J Exp Biol Med Sci 54:97–101.

48. Raynaud, J., Drouet, L., Martineaud, J.P., Bordachar, J., Coudert, J., Durand, J. 1981. Time course of plasma growth hormone during exercise in humans at altitude. J Appl Physiol: 50(2):229–233.

49. Tamborlane, W.V., Sherwin, R.S. et al. 1979. Normalization of the growth hormone and catecholamine response to exercise in juvenile-onset diabetic subjects treated with a portable insulin infusion pump. Diabetes 28:785–788.

50. Few, J.D., Davies, C.T.M. 1980. The inhibiting effect of atropine on growth hormone release during exercise. Eur J Appl Physiol 43:221–228.

51. Mayer, G., Wessel, J., Kobberling, J. 1980. Failure of naloxone to alter exercise-induced growth hormone and prolactin release in normal men. Clin Endocrinol 13:413–416.

52. Spiler, I.J., Molitch, M.E. 1980. Lack of modulation of pituitary hormones stress response by neural pathways involving opiate receptors. J Clin Endocrinol Metab 50:516–520.

53. Daughaday, W.H. 1981. The adenohypophysis. In: Williams R., (ed): Textbook of Endocrinology. W.B. Saunders Co, Philadelphia, pp 87–92.

54. Moretti, C., Fabbri, A., Gnessi, L., Bonifacio, V., Fraioli, F. 1982. Pyridoxine (B6) suppresses the rise in prolactin and increases the rise in growth hormone induced by exercise. N Engl J Med 8:444.

55. Buckman, M.T., Peake, G.T. et al. 1976. Hyperprolactinemia influences renal function in man. Metabolism 25:509–516.

Chapter 9

# Exercise
# and the Menstrual Cycle[1]

## by Karen A. Carlberg, Maire T. Buckman, and Glenn T. Peake

The recent increased popularity and quality of competition of women's athletics have drawn attention to the physiologic responses to exercise in women. Of special interest is the relationship between athletic training and female reproductive function. This chapter summarizes current knowledge about the effects of the menstrual cycle on athletic performance, and the effects of athletic training on the menstrual cycle. The first section describes physiologic responses to exercise throughout the normal menstrual cycle. The second section discusses the effects of regular strenuous exercise on premenstrual and menstrual symptoms. The third section deals with a topic that has attracted considerable research interest in the last few years: the disruption or cessation of the menstrual cycle that sometimes accompanies athletic training.

# Effects of the Menstrual Cycle
# on Exercise Performance

Whether or not the cyclic hormonal changes associated with the menstrual cycle, or menstruation itself, influence exercise performance depends on the individual woman and on the particular variables measured. Many investigators have asked athletes to subjectively evaluate their performance during different phases of the menstrual cycle. Erdelyi [1] reviewed several such studies, which revealed that during the menstrual flow, 42% to 48% of the athletes believed that their performance was worse, and 13% to 15% claimed to have a better performance. Erdelyi concluded that in most women, performance is best in the "postmenstrual" phase and poorest during the "premenstrual" phase and first 2

[1]Supported by the Veterans Administration and NIH Grants 5-M01-RR00997-07 and 5-R01-HD05794-08.

days of the menstrual period. Athletes competing in sports requiring a longer duration of effort were more affected by menstruation. Erdelyi attributed the variability in performance to both hormonal and psychologic factors.

Zaharieva [2] questioned 66 participants in the Tokyo Olympic Games about the effects of menstruation on their competitive performance. Thirty-seven percent of the women believed that there was no difference, 32% felt that their performance was worse during or prior to menses, 3% thought performance was better during menses, and 28% reported variable effects of menstruation on performance.

More recent studies have measured specific variables affecting exercise performance at different phases of the menstrual cycle. Jurkowski et al. [3] tested 9 nonathletic women during the mid-follicular and mid-luteal phases on a bicycle ergometer with light, heavy, and exhaustive work loads. There were no differences between the two phases in any variables reflecting oxygen delivery during the exercise, including exercise heart rate, stroke volume, ventilation, oxygen uptake, and carbon dioxide output. However, time to exhaustion at the highest work load was significantly longer during the luteal phase, and blood lactate was significantly lower during the luteal phase. A further study of disappearance rate for infused lactate revealed no differences between the follicular and luteal phases. The authors concluded that aerobic capacity and cardio-respiratory responses to exercise were not influenced by the phase of the menstrual cycle. But the length of time that exhaustive exercise could be maintained was increased during the lacteal phase, probably as a consequence of reduced lactate production that might result from the effects of estrogen and progesterone on carbohydrate metabolism.

Exercise performance and ventilatory drives during the mid-follicular and mid-luteal phases of the menstrual cycle were studied by Schoene et al. [4] in 6 highly trained athletes with normal menstrual cycles, 6 nonathletes with normal menstrual cycles, and 6 highly trained athletes with amenorrhea. During the luteal phase in the menstruating women, ventilatory drive increased, as shown by an increased resting minute ventilation, increased ventilatory equivalent ($V_E/\dot{V}_{O_2}$) during exercise, and increased ventilatory responses to hypoxia and hypercapnia. The increased ventilatory drive during the luteal phase was accompanied by a reduced maximal exercise response (total exercise time, maximum oxygen consumption, and maximum carbon dioxide production) in the nonathletes, but in the athletes, exercise performance did not decrease during the luteal phase. Responses of the amenorrheic athletes did not differ between the two testing periods.

Temperature regulation during exercise apparently is not affected by hormonal changes during the menstrual cycle. Wells and Horvath [5] studied thermoregulatory responses of 7 nonathletic women during treadmill walking in a hot environment in the early follicular, periovulatory, and mid-luteal phases of the menstrual cycle. There were no differences attributable to menstrual phase in rectal temperature, skin temperature, body heat content, sweat rate, weight loss, heart rate, oxygen uptake, oxygen pulse, expiratory volume, serum electrolytes, or electrolyte loss. Post-exercise lactate values were highest in the periovulatory phase and lowest during the early follicular phase. Frye et al. [6] conducted a similar study in a hot dry environment with 4 amenorrheic and 4 menstruating nonathletic women during the mid-follicular and mid-luteal phases of the menstrual cycle. In response to treadmill walking, both before and after heat acclimation, there were no differences between the mid-follicular, mid-luteal, and amenorrheic conditions in rectal temperature, skin temperature and tympanic temperature at onset of sweating, sweat rate, rate of heat storage, or heart rate.

In summary, most of the exercise responses for which there are objective measurements have not been influenced by the phase of the menstrual cycle. Where differences were seen, such as in ventilatory responses or blood lactate, results were contradictory. This probably reflects a large variability among individuals and the small magnitude of changes attributable to cyclic fluctuations in hormone levels.

# Effects of Exercise Training on Premenstrual and Menstrual Symptoms

Effects of regular physical exercise on premenstrual and menstrual symptoms have been studied. Most often the menstrual discomfort is diminished or unchanged by athletic training, but sometimes it is worsened.

Ingman [7] studied 107 Finnish athletes participating in 8 different sports. Thirteen percent reported that pain associated with menstruation was reduced or eliminated during athletic training and occasionally reappeared during intervals of rest. Three percent reported that menstrual pain was increased during training.

In 729 Hungarian athletes "unfavorable changes" in the menstrual cycle were associated with exercise in 18% of athletes under 18 years of age and in 7% of athletes 18 years and older. The most frequent complaint was dysmenorrhea (Erdelyi [1]).

Golub et al. [8] prescribed a program of calisthenic exercises for 302 junior high school students, and questioned them twice yearly for 3 years about premenstrual and menstrual symptoms and regularity in performing the exercises. By the end of the third year dysmenorrhea had developed in 61% of the girls who did not perform the exercises regularly and in 39% of the girls who continued to exercise.

Premenstrual and menstrual syndromes were compared in 136 physical education students and 612 university students by Timonen and Procope [9]. The athletic women reported less frequent: menstrual pelvic pain, low back pain, use of analgesics, premenstrual or menstrual headache, anxiety, depression, and fatigue. There were no differences between the groups in premenstrual dysmenorrhea or edema. The reduction in menstrual symptoms was attributed to an increased total capacity of the circulation.

Menstrual symptoms in 31 professional ballet dancers were similar to those in control subjects, except that intermenstrual bleeding was more common in the dancers. Twenty-seven percent of the dancers noted improvement of symptoms with increased dancing, 10% thought they were worse, and 63% noticed no change (Cohen et al. [10]).

Thus, the effects of regular strenuous exercise on premenstrual and menstrual symptoms vary among individuals, but the most common observations are improvement or no change. A mechanism for exercise-induced alterations in menstrual symptoms has not been investigated.

# Effects of Athletic Training on Menstrual Function

Recently the menstrual disturbances that accompany athletic training have attracted attention. This section discusses the types of dysfunction that occur and the associated factors. Endocrine studies in athletes and dancers with menstrual disturbances are described and tentative recommendations made for treatment of exercise-related menstrual dysfunction.

## Menstrual Disturbances Associated with Athletics and Dance

Prior to about 1970, the published reports on menstrual disturbances and athletic training concluded that menstruation was usually normal in athletes (Ingman [7]; Erdelyi [1]; Åstrand et al. [11]; Zaharieva [2]). In contrast, most studies published since 1970 indicate high incidence of amenorrhea, oligomenorrhea, and delayed menarche among athletic girls and women. This probably reflects increased strenuousness of women's training programs during the last decade.

**Amenorrhea and Oligomenorrhea**   A consensus exists that amenorrhea and oligomenorrhea are more common in athletes and dancers than in nonathletic women. Few investigators have actually compared large populations of athletic and nonathletic women, and definitions for the various menstrual disorders vary widely from one author to another. Nevertheless, the tendency toward a high incidence of menstrual irregularities among athletes and dancers is clear.

Among healthy, nonathletic women, 2% to 5% have secondary amenorrhea (Drew [12]; Pettersson et al. [13]; Singh [14]), and an additional 6% have oligomenorrhea (Singh [14]).

The incidence of secondary amenorrhea is consistently higher among athletes, although there is considerable variation in different populations of athletic women. Of 872 runners and joggers answering a newspaper questionnaire, 7% developed amenorrhea after they started running (Speroff and Redwine [15]). Of 83 runners, 15% had been amenorrheic for at least 4 months (Schwartz et al. [16]). Twenty-one percent of the 114 runners and joggers participating in another study reported 5 or fewer menstrual periods per year (Dale et al. [17]). Twenty-two percent of the 300 teenage athletes had secondary amenorrhea (Levenets [18]). In our own studies, 12% of 252 college varsity athletes had oligo/amenorrhea, defined as no menstrual periods in the previous 3 months or 4 or fewer periods in the previous year, compared to 2.6% of 426 nonathlete college students (Carlberg et al. [19]).

Dancers also experience amenorrhea frequently. Of 89 ballet students with a mean age of 16.8 years, 15% had secondary amenorrhea of at least 3 months' duration, and 22% had not yet begun to menstruate, including 9 girls who were at least 16 years of age

(Frisch et al. [20]). Among 30 professional ballet dancers with a mean age of 24.9 years, 37% had not menstruated in at least 3 months (Cohen et al. [10]).

**Luteal Phase Defects**   Regular strenuous exercise may alter the length of the luteal phase of the menstrual cycle. In an 18-month study of 1 ovulatory distance runner, a significant negative correlation between weekly mileage and luteal phase length was noted; as mileage increased from 0 to 53 mi/wk, luteal phase length declined from 14 to 4 days (Shangold et al. [21]). Four teenage swimmers had an average luteal phase length of 4.5 days, compared to an average of 7.8 days for 4 teenage control subjects (Bonen et al. [22]). Thus, athletes may be prone to shortened luteal phases, a condition sometimes associated with infertility (Strott et al. [23]).

**Delayed Menarche**   When athletic training begins before puberty, menarche may be delayed. Several investigators report significantly later menarche in athletes compared to age-matched controls: 13.6 yr ( $\pm 0.2$ SE) in 66 collegiate track and field athletes vs. 12.2 yr ( $\pm 0.3$) in 30 nonathletic college students (Malina et al. [24]); 14.2 yr ( $\pm 0.2$ SE) in 18 Olympic volleyball candidates and 13.1 yr ( $\pm 0.2$) in 53 college varsity athletes vs. 12.3 yr ( $\pm 0.1$) in 110 nonathletic college students (Malina et al. [25]); 15.1 yr ( $\pm 0.5$ SE) in 18 premenarcheal trained collegiate swimmers and runners vs. 12.7 yr ( $\pm 0.4$) in 10 nonathletic college students (Frische et al. [26]); and 15.2 yr ( $\pm 0.1$ SE) in 264 Indian sportswomen vs. 14.1 yr ( $\pm 0.1$) in 108 Indian college students (Sidhu and Grewal [27]). Frisch et al. [26] calculated that each year of training before menarche delayed menarche by 5 months. Menarche was later in 66 better swimmers (14.2 yr) than in 98 poorer swimmers (13.2 yr) (Stager et al. [28]).

   Dancers also reach menarche at a late age. Sixty-seven post-menarcheal ballet students began menstruating at an average of 13.7 yr (Frisch et al. [20]). A 4-year study of 15 ballet students showed a mean age of menarche of 15.4 yr, compared to 12.5 yr for 20 control subjects (Warren [29]). Two of these dancers had not yet begun to menstruate at age 18 yr. In 10 of the dancers the onset of menarche correlated with a decrease in exercise because of injury or other reasons.

   While it is likely that athletic training can delay pubertal development, girls who mature late may be more likely to excel in sports, both for physiologic and social reasons (Malina et al. [25]).

# Factors Associated with Exercise-Related Menstrual Disturbances

**Exercise Intensity and Duration**   The incidence of menstrual disturbances among athletes appears to be related to the type, intensity, and/or duration of the exercise performed. This probably accounts for much of the variability among athletic populations in the prevalence rate for amenorrhea. Several investigators note that menstrual disturbances are most common in athletes who are champions or who have the heaviest physical work loads (Erdelyi [30]; Chalupa [31]; Carlberg and Riedesel [32]). Distance runners appear to have more menstrual irregularities than women competing in other sports, although many sports have not been studied adequately. In our studies, oligo/amenorrheic distance runners ran significantly more miles per week than runners with regular menstruation or irregular menstruation (unpublished observations). Dale et al. [33] noted that runners with the most intensive training schedules and those who had been running for the longest time appeared to have the fewest menstrual periods. Feicht et al. [34] reported that the incidence of amenorrhea in runners ranged from 6% in those running the least to 43% in those running the most. However, in a subsequent study, the same investigators found that the incidence of amenorrhea was not related to weekly mileage among swimmers or bicycle racers (Feicht et al. [35]).

The importance of exercise intensity in the development of menstrual dysfunction is further emphasized by the appearance and disappearance of menstrual symptoms with increases and decreases in exercise. Many of the oligo/amenorrheic athletes in our studies reported changes in their menstruation that were associated with specific changes in their athletic training (unpublished observations). The changes included disruption of menstrual function associated with increased exercise, and normalization of menstrual function associated with reduced exercise. Some athletes were amenorrheic only during competitive seasons. Similarly, Cohen et al. [10] found that many ballet dancers had fewer menstrual periods during the ballet season and more periods during the off-season when training was reduced.

**Body Weight, Body Composition, and Weight Loss**    Extremely low body weight and weight loss are well-known causes of amenorrhea (Fries et al. [36]; Frisch and McArthur [37]; Knuth et al. [38]). A critical amount of stored fat is apparently necessary for the onset of menstruation and for maintenance of normal menstrual function (Frisch [39]). Female athletes often have between 5% and 20% body fat (Malina et al. [40]; Wilmore et al. [41]; Sinning [42], compared to an average of 20% to 29% body fat among nonathletic women (Young [43]; Sloan et al. [44]; Wilmore and Behnke [45]). Thus, one of the earliest hypotheses about exercise-related amenorrhea is that it might be attributed to the low percentage of body fat common among athletes (Wilmore et al. [41]).

The results of numerous published reports concerning body weight in amenorrheic athletes and dancers are contradictory. Several investigators measured significantly lower total body weight and percent ideal body weight in amenorrheic athletes and dancers compared to regularly menstruating athletes and dancers (Speroff and Redwine [15]; Schwartz et al. [16]; Cohen et al. [10]; Carlberg et al. [46]). We found that oligo/amenorrhea was much more common among underweight ahtletes than among athletes of normal weight, and that overweight athletes had menstrual patterns similar to those of nonathletic women (Carlberg et al. [47]). In addition, lower weight oligo/amenorrheic athletes participating in our studies tended to have more severe menstrual disturbances, i.e. amenorrhea, than heavier athletes, who tended to be oligomenorrheic rather than amenorrheic (Carlberg et al. [47]). On the other hand, some investigators report similar body weights in athletes with amenorrhea and normal menstruation (Feicht et al. [34]; Baker et al. [48]; Wakat et al. [49]).

Comparisons of body composition for athletes and dancers with amenorrhea and regular menstruation have also been contradictory. Some authors report that the percentage of body fat was similar in athletes and dancers with normal and abnormal menstruation (Baker et al. [48]; Hendrix and Lohman [50]; Calabrese et al. [51]; Reith et al. [52]; Wakat et al. [49]). Others have measured significantly lower values for percentages of body fat in amenorrheic athletes compared to menstruating athletes (Schwartz et al. [16];

Snyder et al. [53]). In our studies, oligo/amenorrheic athletes had slightly lower percentages of body fat than menstruating athletes, but the largest differences were in absolute fat weight and lean body weight, as well as in total body weight (Carlberg et al. [46]). Thus, the important variables may be the absolute amount of fat and the absolute amount of lean tissue, rather than the percentage of body fat.

Weight loss may also be an important factor in the etiology of menstrual disturbances in athletes. Many women become involved in sports, particularly running, for the purpose of losing weight. Amenorrheic runners reported significantly larger weight losses than runners who continued to menstruate normally (Schwartz et al. [16]). Many of the athletes we interviewed said that cessation or prolongation of their menstrual cycles accompanied weight losses ranging from 2 kg to 21 kg (unpublished observations).

Weight changes may influence menstrual function in athletes and dancers without changes in exercise regimen. Three amenorrheic professional ballet dancers regained normal menstrual cycles after intentionally gaining 4–7 kg (Cohen et al. [10]); 2 maintained a constant dancing work load and 1 increased her work load. Three oligo/amenorrheic distance runners identified a weight threshold for their menstruation that was around 90% ideal body weight in each case (unpublished observations). They menstruated sporadically when they weighed more than this threshold but not when they dropped below it, without changes in their weekly mileage.

On the other hand, changes in menstrual function can accompany changes in exercise regimen in the absence of weight or body composition change. Many of the ballet students first began menstruating during vacations or forced rest due to injury, and reverted to amenorrhea after resuming normal activity, all without significant changes in weight or body composition (Warren et al. [29]). Two amenorrheic infertile joggers did not ovulate in response to clomiphene citrate, but after discontinuing jogging both women conceived within two months, without a change in body weight (O'Herlihy [54]).

The mechanism of the interaction between low body weight and reproductive function is not clear. Nonathletic women suffering weight loss-related amenorrhea have numerous aberrations in hypothalamic function, including hypothalamic-pituitary regulatory mechanisms and thermoregulation (Vigersky et al. [55]). In addition, steroid hormones are metabolized to a considerable extent in adipose tissue, and, therefore, changes in body fat can alter endocrine function (Siiteri and MacDonald [56]; Fishman et al. [57]; Longcope et al. [58]; Longcope et al. [59]). Whether low body weight in oligo/amenorrheic athletes exerts its influence on the hypothalamus or on peripheral steroid metabolism, or both, has not been determined.

The role of low body weight, low body fat, and weight loss in production of exercise-related menstrual disturbances is still controversial. While body weight and body fat tend to be lower in oligo/amenorrheic athletes, some athletes continue to menstruate normally with very low levels of body fat. It is likely that factors related to body size contribute importantly to the menstrual dysfunction in some athletes, but are less important in others.

**Age, Menstrual Irregularity, and Other Factors**   Many other factors appear to be associated with exercise-related menstrual disturbances. One is age. Amenorrhea is more common in athletes who are under 30 years of age than in older women (Speroff and Redwine [15]; Baker et al. [48]). Other studies, however, indicate similar ages for athletes with amenorrhea and normal menstruation (Feicht et al. [34]; Wakat et al. [49]; Schwartz et al. [16]). Age appears to affect the incidence of secondary amenorrhea in nonathletic women as well (Pettersson et al. [13]).

A history of menstrual irregularity prior to initiation of athletic training may be present in many amenorrheic and oligomenorrheic athletes. Shangold [60] noted that most oligomenorrheic athletes had the same menstrual patterns before and after beginning intensive training. Schwartz et al. [16] reported that significantly more amenorrheic runners had a history of past irregularity than did normally menstruating runners. However, many of the amenorrheic athletes we interviewed had regular menstrual cycles before the initiation or intensification of training (unpublished observations). Baker et al. [48] noted that all the amenorrheic runners in their study had normal menstrual histories prior to regular running.

Prior pregnancy may protect a woman from exercise-related menstrual dysfunction. Several investigators found that amenorrhea is more common among nulliparous athletes than among parous athletes (Dale et al. [17]; Baker et al. [48]; Schwartz et al. [16]). This is also true for nonathletic women (Pettersson et al. [13]). Whether pregnancy somehow affects the hypothalamic-pituitary-ovarian axis to make menstrual disruption less likely, or whether women who are more susceptible to menstrual disturbances are less fertile and therefore less likely to become pregnant is not known.

Diet may influence the menstrual response to athletic training. A disproportionately large number of the oligo/amenorrheic athletes we interviewed were vegetarians (unpublished observations). A prospective 7-day dietary history administered by Schwartz et al. [16] showed that amenorrheic runners consumed a smaller percentage of their total intake as protein, although total protein intake was similar to that in menstruating runners because the amenorrheic women consumed more total calories. Frisch et al. [26] reported that premenarche-trained athletes, most of whom had irregular menstruation or amenorrhea, ate fewer total calories, less protein, less fat, and less calcium than postmenarche-trained athletes, who had a lower incidence of menstrual irregularities.

Serum chemical analyses showed no nutritional deficiencies in athletes with menstrual disturbances. Blood samples from 22 distance runners, many of whom had menstrual dysfunction, showed no abnormalities in protein, lipids, nitrogen, enzymes, or minerals (Dale et al. [17]). Similar analyses on blood samples from 5 underweight oligo/amenorrheic athletes (3 vegetarians) and 4 underweight regularly menstruating athletes by us were normal (unpublished observations).

Psychologic or emotional stress is a possible cause for exercise-related menstrual disturbances. Stress and amenorrhea or infertility are often associated in nonathletic women (Fava et al. [61]; Seibel and Taymor [62]). It might be that athletes, particularly college varsity athletes, are exposed to more stress than nonathletes from pressures associated with competition and time commitments. Runners rated the subjective stress associated with running, and the amenorrheic runners reported significantly more stress than the normally cycling runners (Schwartz et al. [16]). Depression, anxiety, obsessive/compulsive tendencies, hypochondriasis, and degrees of life stress assessed by four psychologic tests showed all runners were within the normal range, and revealed no difference between runners with amenorrhea and normal menstruation. Some of the athletes we interviewed said that psychologic stress contributed to their menstrual disturbances, but stress was cited less often than exercise as a cause for the menstrual changes (unpublished observations). Thus, psychologic stress may be important in production of menstrual disturbances in some athletes, but unimportant in others.

In summary, strenuous exercise can cause menstrual dysfunction, but many other factors may also be associated with athletic oligo/amenorrhea and thus increase a woman's susceptibility to this condition. Low body weight and low body fat are most commonly associated with exercise-related menstrual disturbances, but other factors, such as emotional stress and dietary changes, may also be important and deserve further study. In many women the combined effects of two or more stresses, as well as strenuous exercise, may disrupt cyclic menstrual activity.

# Endocrine Function in Athletes and Dancers with Menstrual Disturbances

Regardless of the importance of exercise quantity or the amount of body fat, menstrual dysfunction ultimately reflects a change in endocrine function. Changes might occur in hormone secretion, peripheral conversion of one hormone to another, hormone inactivation or catabolism, or target organ receptor function, and these alterations might occur in the hypothalamus, pituitary gland, ovary, uterus, or adipose tissue. This part of the chapter presents information available on endocrine function in athletes with menstrual disturbances.

**Hypothalamic-Pituitary Gonadotropin Function**   Amenorrhea with weight loss or emotional stress is associated with low to low-normal plasma concentrations or gonadotropins, reflecting diminished hypothalamic release of gonadotropin-releasing hormone (Frisch [39]; Lachelin and Yen [63]). Thus, women with exercise-related amenorrhea might have low levels of luteinizing hormone (LH) and follicle-stimulating hormone (FSH).

Basal plasma gonadotropins have been measured in amenorrheic athletes and dancers by a number of investigators, with contradictory results. Some reported gonadotropin levels below the normal range for the follicular phase of the menstrual cycle (McArthur et al. [64]; Warren [29]; Baker et al. [48]; Reith et al. [52]). LH was often more affected than FSH (McArthur et al. [64]; Reith et al. [52]). Others reported gonadotropins within the normal follicular range (Carlberg et al. [65]; Cohen et al. [10]; Fears et al. [66]), and some authors have measured basal LH levels that were higher than those in normal control subjects in the follicular phase (Bonen et al. [22]; Schwartz et al. [16]; Brisson et al. [67]). Weekly blood samples from anovulatory runners showed LH and FSH levels to be noncyclic (Dale et al. [17]). In teenage swimmers with short luteal phases, a normal mid-cycle LH surge occurred, but the FSH peak was absent (Bonen et al. [22]). Administration of gonadotropin-releasing hormone to amenorrheic athletes resulted in LH responses that ranged from low-normal to exceedingly high, and FSH responses that were higher than normal (McArthur et al. [64]; Fears et al. [66]).

In normal individuals, gonadotropin secretion occurs in pulses at approximately 1–4 hourly intervals (Yen et al. [68]). Pulsatile LH secretion is absent in women with some forms of secondary amenorrhea (Yen et al. [69]). In 3 amenorrheic athletes of normal body weight, pulsatile LH activity was normal (McArthur et al. [64]). However, in our studies, in 3 of 5 oligo/amenorrheic athletes tested, pulsatile LH secretion did not occur during a 5–6 h study period (Carlberg et al. [65]).

During acute bouts of exercise, plasma gonadotropins usually do not change in nonathletic women with normal menstrual cycles (Jurkowski et al. [70]; Bonen et al. [71]). Similar observations were made in athletes with primary (Brisson et al. [67]) and secondary amenorrhea (Carlberg et al. [65]; Fears et al. [66]). In contrast, (Cumming et al. [72]) reported increases in LH and FSH with exercise in both amenorrheic and normally cycling runners.

**Ovarian Hormones**   Plasma concentrations of estrogens and progesterone in women with amenorrhea due to weight loss or psychogenic disturbances may be below or within the normal range for the follicular phase of the menstrual cycle (Knuth et al. [38]; Lachelin and Yen [63]). In response to acute bouts of exercise in normally menstruating women, estrogen and progesterone levels often increase (Jurkowski et al. [70]; Bonen et al. [71]). These increases may result from reduced metabolic clearance of the hormones, due to diminished hepatic blood flow during exercise (Rowell [73]), rather than from increased hormone secretion.

In amenorrheic athletes, basal levels of 17-β-estradiol and estrone were either low (Baker et al. [48]; Reith et al. [52]) or within the normal range for the follicular phase of the menstrual cycle (Carlberg et al. [65]; Schwartz et al. [16]), and basal levels of progesterone and 17-α-hydroxyprogesterone were within the normal early follicular range in oligo/amenorrheic athletes (Carlberg et al. [65]).

In teenage swimmers with short luteal phases, estradiol was low throughout the menstrual cycle, particularly at mid-cycle and during the luteal phase (Bonen et al. [22]). Progesterone levels were slightly higher than controls during the follicular phase, but increased only minimally during the luteal phase. In one distance runner with luteal phase lengths inversely proportional to weekly mileage, luteal phase progesterone levels were lower during cycles when weekly mileage was high than when training was stopped (Shangold et al. [21]).

In response to acute bouts of exercise, concentrations of both estradiol and estrone increased in runners with amenorrhea and runners with normal menstrual cycles (Cumming et al. [72]). In our studies, significant increases during exercise in estradiol, estrone, progesterone, or 17-α-hydroxyprogesterone did not occur in athletes with oligo/amenorrhea or regular menstruation (unpublished observations).

The ratio of estrone to estradiol ($E_1/E_2$) reflects both ovarian function and peripheral steroid metabolism. While both hormones can arise from either source, estradiol is primarily of ovarian origin, whereas most estrone arises from peripheral conversion of androstenedione by adipose and possibly other tissues. In amenorrheic and menstruating runners, the $E_1/E_2$ ratio was significantly higher than in control subjects (Schwartz et al. [16]). We also observed an unusually high $E_1/E_2$ ratio due to high estrone levels in blood samples from resting athletes with oligo/amenorrhea and regular menstruation (unpublished observations). These findings suggest alteration in peripheral steroid metabolism in athletes that may contribute to menstrual disturbances in some women.

**Prolactin**   Hyperprolactinemia is a possible cause for exercise-related menstrual dysfunction. Plasma prolactin consistently rose during physical exercise, and during other stress in men and in women with normal or unspecified menstrual characteristics (Noel et al. [74]; Brisson et al. [75]; Shangold et al. [76]). Hyperprolactinemia is a well-known cause for amenorrhea and infertility in nonathletic women (Jacobs et al. [77]; Archer [78];

Bergh et al. [79]). Thus, it is reasonable to suggest an etiologic role for prolactin in athletic oligo/amenorrhea.

However, evidence from several studies fails to support this. Resting plasma prolactin is consistently within the normal range in athletes and dancers with menstrual dysfunction (Bonen et al. [22]; Schwartz et al. [16]; Cohen et al. [10]; Fears et al. [66]). Mean prolactin values may even be lower than those in control subjects, although differences were not always significant (Baker et al. [48]; Carlberg et al. [19]). During exercise, prolactin elevations have been the same or slightly lower in oligo/amenorrheic athletes compared to menstruating athletes (Carlberg et al. [19]; Fears et al. [66]; Wakat et al. [49]). Prolactin returned to near basal levels by 2 hours after exercise in athletes with oligo/amenorrhea and in regularly menstruating athletes (unpublished observations). Prolactin levels fell slightly during a dance workout in amenorrheic ballet dancers, but the work intensity was low (Cohen et al. [10]).

Thus, plasma prolactin is normal or below normal during rest and exercise in amenorrheic athletes, and during recovery from exercise high prolactin levels do not persist longer than in menstruating athletes. Therefore, it is not likely that hyperprolactinemia is responsible for athletic amenorrhea. This does not exclude the possibility of alteration in sensitivity of target organ receptors to the exercise-induced prolactin elevations.

**Androgens**   Experimental evidence suggests that one or more androgens contributes to exercise-related menstrual disturbances. Amenorrhea and infertility are associated with hyperandrogenism in nonathletic women (Ferriman and Purdie [80]; Rosenfield [81]; Smith et al. [82]). Physical exercise acutely increased plasma 17-ß-hydroxysteroids, testosterone, androstenedione, and dehydroepiandrosterone (DHEA) in women with normal (Cumming et al. [83]; Shangold et al. [76]) and unspecified (Sutton et al. [84]; Brisson et al. [85]) menstrual function. At this time, however, evidence is insufficient to support or dispute an association of moderate hyperandrogenism with athletic menstrual dysfunction.

Plasma androgens are normal or high-normal in resting amenorrheic athletes. Testosterone levels were significantly higher, although still within the normal range, in runners, many of whom were amenorrheic, compared to nonathletic controls (Dale et al. [33]). Testosterone and dehydroepiandrosterone-sulfate (DHEAS) were normal in amenorrheic runners, and androstendione and DHEA were slightly but not significantly elevated (Baker et al. [48]). Schwartz et al. [16] reported normal testosterone, androstenedione, and DHEAS in amenorrheic runners. In our studies, oligo/amenorrheic athletes had resting levels of testosterone and dihydrotestosterone (DHT) that were slightly but not significantly higher than those in regularly menstruating athletes (Carlberg et al. [86]). Testosterone and DHT responses to exercise were slightly but not significantly higher in the oligo/amenorrheic athletes. Cumming et al. [72] reported exercise-induced elevations in testosterone, androstenedione, and DHEA that did not differ between runners with amenorrhea and normal menstrual cycles.

Sex hormone-binding globulin (SHBG) is a plasma protein that binds much of the circulating androgens and estrogens. Only the free, unbound steroid hormones are biologically active, and thus SHBG levels determine the activity and balance between androgens and estrogens (Yen [87]). In amenorrheic runners SHBG levels were reduced compared to those in runners with regular menstrual cycles (Baker et al. [48]).

Thus, plasma concentrations of several androgens may be slightly elevated during rest and/or exercise in at least some athletes with menstrual disturbances. Subtle changes in androgen secretion, metabolism, or target organ sensitivity might contribute to exercise-related oligo/amenorrhea.

**Other Hormones**    Thyroid stimulating hormone (TSH), thyroxine ($T_4$), triiodothyronine ($T_3$), growth hormone, and cortisol have been measured in athletes and dancers with menstrual disturbances, but the available information is limited.

TSH was significantly reduced in amenorrheic runners compared to menstruating runners (Schwartz et al. [16]). $T_3$ levels were lower in very lean amenorrheic athletes than in lean menstruating athletes (Reith et al. [52]). In young ballet students with delayed menarche, TSH and $T_4$ levels were normal except for a low $T_4$ value in one girl (Warren [29]). Thus, thyroid function may be depressed in some athletes and dancers with menstrual abnormalities, but further studies are needed.

Growth hormone was within the normal range in resting amenorrheic professional ballet dancers, and during a dance practice it dropped slightly (Cohen et al. [10]). Cumming et al. [72] reported a rise in growth hormone during exercise in amenorrheic runners, but the values were not different from those in menstruating runners. Similar growth hormone levels were reported in oligo/amenorrheic and menstruating cross-country runners after a 5,000 m race (Wakat et al. [49]).

Cortisol may be normal or high-normal in amenorrheic athletes. Plasma cortisol concentrations were similar in resting amenorrheic and menstruating runners (Baker et al. [48]). In amenorrheic runners, cortisol levels were nearly the same as those in menstruating runners both at rest and post-exercise (Fears et al. [66]). Cumming et al. [72] reported that basal cortisol levels were significantly higher in runners than in nonrunners, but did not mention differences between runners with amenorrhea and normal menstrual cycles. In our studies, resting cortisol levels were significantly higher in oligo/amenorrheic athletes than in nonathletic women, while those in regularly menstruating athletes were intermediate (unpublished observations).

In summary, plasma gonadotropin, estrogen, and progesterone are apparently noncyclic in athletes with menstrual dysfunction, but are usually within or near normal follicular phase values and, therefore, are not as low as in other types of amenorrhea. Pulsatile gonadotropin activity apparently is absent in some, but not all, amenorrheic athletes. Prolactin physiology appears to be normal in athletes with menstrual disturbances, and, therefore, probably does not have an etiologic role in the dysfunction. Subtle changes in androgen secretion or metabolism in oligo/amenorrheic athletes may occur, but evidence for this is inadequate. Thyroid function may be depressed in some athletes with menstrual abnormalities. Thus far, most studies have merely measured the hormone in single basal blood samples. Circadian rhythms usually have not been considered. In order to understand more fully the endocrine correlate of exercise-related menstrual dysfunction, oligo/amenorrheic athletes should be studied for a longer time and should be subjected to more provocative testing that includes exercise testing and administration of drugs that will probe hypothalamic control of the pituitary-ovarian, -adrenal, and -thyroid axes.

## Clinical Management of Athletes and Dancers with Menstrual Disturbances

Recommendations for management of athletes and dancers with menstrual disturbances are difficult because the etiology of the dysfunction is not clear, and information is limited regarding the consequences of athletic amenorrhea for the future health of the individual. Menstrual function reverts to normal within 1 or 2 months in most women as a result of reduction in exercise, weight gain, or resolution of emotional stress.

Some sports medicine physicians advocate an aggressive approach to the treatment of amenorrheic athletes (Shangold [88]), while others believe that amenorrheic athletes usually require no treatment (Smith [89]). Most investigators would probably recommend a course of action between these two extremes. An athlete with menstrual irregularities should be evaluated to rule out other pathology. Most of these women seek medical attention, if only to be assured that significant physical problems do not exist. Hormonal treatment for athletic amenorrhea is, at this time, controversial.

The possibility of pregnancy in an amenorrheic athlete should not be discounted. Amenorrheic athletes have become pregnant without having menstruated in several months (unpublished observations).

# References

1. Erdelyi, G.J. 1962. Gynecological survey of female athletes. J Sports Med Phys Fitness 2:174–179.
2. Zaharieva, E. 1965. Survey of sportswomen at the Tokyo Olympics. J Sports Med Phys Fitness 5:215–219.
3. Jurkowski, J.E.H., Jones, N.L., Toews, C.J., Sutton, J.R. 1981. Effects of menstrual cycle on blood lactate, $O_2$ delivery, and performance during exercise. J Appl Physiol 51:1493–1499.
4. Schoene, R.B., Robertson, H.T., Pierson, D.J., Peterson, A.P. 1981. Respiratory drives and exercise in menstrual cycles of athletic and nonathletic women. J Appl Physiol 50:1300–1305.
5. Wells, C.L., Horvath, S.M. 1974. Responses to exercise in a hot environment as related to the menstrual cycle. J Appl Physiol 36:299–302.
6. Frye, A.J., Kamon E., Webb, M. 1982. Responses of menstrual women, amenorrheal women, and men to exercise in a hot, dry environment. Eur J Appl Physiol 48:279–288.
7. Ingman, O. 1952. Menstruation in Finnish top class sportswomen. In: Karvonen, M.J., (ed): Proceedings of the International Symposium of the Medicine and Physiology of Sports and Athletics at Helsinki. Finnish Association of Sports Medicine, pp 96–99.
8. Golub, L.J., Menduke, H., Lang, W.R. 1968. Exercise and dysmenorrhea in young teenagers: A 3-year study. Obstet Gynecol 32:508–511.
9. Timonen, S., Procope, B.J. 1971. Premenstrual syndrome and physical exercise. Acta Obstet Gynecol Scand 50:331–337.
10. Cohen, J.L., Kim, C.S., May, P.B., Ertel, N.H. 1982. Exercise, body weight, and amenorrhea in professional ballet dancers. Physician Sportsmed 19(4):92–101.
11. Åstrand, P.O., Eriksson, B.O., Nylander, I., Engstrom, L., Karlberg, P., Saltin, B., Thoren, C. 1963. Girl swimmers, with

special reference to respiratory and circulatory adaptation and gynaecological and psychiatric aspects. Acta Paediatr Scand [Suppl] 147:1–75.

12. Drew, F.L. 1961. The epidemiology of secondary amenorrhea. J Chronic Dis 14:396–407.

13. Pettersson, F., Hans, F., Nillius, S.J. 1973. Epidemiology of secondary amenorrhea. I. Incidence and prevalence rates. Am J Obstet Gynecol 117:80–86.

14. Singh, K.B. 1981. Menstrual disorders in college students. Am J Obstet Gynecol 140:299–302.

15. Speroff, L., Redwine, D.B. 1980. Exercise and menstrual function. Physician Sportsmed 8(5):41–52.

16. Schwartz, B., Cumming, D.C., Riordan, E., Selye, M., Yen, S.S.C., Rebar, R.W. 1981. Exercise-associated amenorrhea: A distinct entity? Am J Obstet Gynecol 141:662–670.

17. Dale, E., Gerlach, D.H., Martin, D.E., Alexander, C.R. 1979. Physical fitness profiles and reproductive physiology of the female distance runner. Physician Sportsmed 7(1):83–95.

18. Levenets, S.A. 1979. Peculiar features of physical and sexual development of girls regularly going in for sport. Gig Sanit (1):25–28.

19. Carlberg, K.A., Buckman, M.T., Peake, G.T. 1981. Prolactin responses to exercise in oligo/amenorrheic and menstruating athletes. Int J Sports Med 2:272 (abstract).

20. Frisch, R.E., Wyshak, G., Vincent, L. 1980. Delayed menarche and amenorrhea in ballet dancers. N Engl J Med 303:17–19.

21. Shangold, M., Freeman, R., Thysen, B., Gatz, M. 1979. The relationship between long distance running, plasma progesterone, and luteal phase length. Fertil Steril 31:130–133.

22. Bonen, A., Belcastro, A.N., Ling, W.Y., Simpson, A.A. 1981. Profiles of selected hormones during menstrual cycles of teenage athletes. J Appl Physiol 50:545–551.

23. Strott, C.A., Cargille, C.M., Ross, G.T., Lipsett, M.B. 1970. The short luteal phase. J Clin Endocrinol Metab 30:246–251.

24. Malina, R.M., Harper, A.B., Avent, H.H., Campbell, D.E. 1973. Age at menarche in athletes and non-athletes. Med Sci Sports 5:11–13.

25. Malina, R.M., Spirduso, W.W., Tate, C., Baylor, A.M. 1978. Age at menarche and selected menstrual characteristics in athletes at different competitive levels and in different sports. Med Sci Sports 10:218–222.

26. Frisch, R.E., Gotz-Welbergen, A.V., McArthur, J.W., Albright, T., Witschi, J., Bullen, B., Birnholz, J., Reed, R.B., Hermann, H. 1981. Delayed menarche and amenorrhea of college athletes in relation to age of onset of training. JAMA 246:1559–1563.

27. Sidhu, L.S., Grewal, R. 1980. Age of menarche in various categories of Indian sportswomen. Br J Sports Med 14:199–203.

28. Stager, J.M., Robertshaw, D., Miescher, E. 1982. Age of menarche, athletic performance, and age at the initiation of training in women swimmers. Fed Proc 41:1750.

29. Warren, M.P. 1980. The effects of exercise on pubertal progression and reproductive function in girls. J Clin Endocrinol Metab 51:1150–1157.

30. Erdelyi, G.J. 1976. Effects of exercise on the menstrual cycle. Physician Sportsmed 4(3):79–81.

31. Chalupa, M. 1978. Some results gained by a gynecologist during a follow-up of female top-sportswomen (champions). Cesk Gynekol 43:268–270.

32. Carlberg, K.A., Riedesel, M.L. 1979. Athletic training and body composition as factors in secondary amenorrhea. Physiologist 22:17 (abstract).

33. Dale, E., Gerlach, D.H., Wilhite, A.L. 1979. Menstrual dysfunction in distance runners. Obstet Gynecol 54:47–53.

34. Feicht, C.B., Johnson, T.S., Martin, B.J., Sparkes, K.E., Wagner, W.W., Jr. 1978. Secondary amenorrhea in athletes. Lancet 2:1145–1146 (letter).

35. Feicht, C.B., Martin, B.J., Wagner, W.W., Jr. 1980. Is athletic amenorrhea specific to runners? Fed Proc 39:371 (abstract).

36. Fries, H., Nillius, S.J., Pettersson, F. 1974. Epidemiology of secondary amenorrhea. II. A retrospective evaluation of etiology with special regard to psychogenic factors and weight loss. Am J Obstet Gynecol 118:473–479.

37. Frisch, R.E., McArthur, J.W. 1974. Menstrual cycles: Fatness as a determinant of minimum weight for height necessary for their maintenance or onset. Science 185:949–951.

38. Knuth, U.A., Hull, M.G.R., Jacobs, H.S. 1977. Amenorrhea and loss of weight. Br J Obstet Gynaecol 84:801–807.

39. Frisch, R.E. 1977. Food intake, fatness, and reproductive ability. In: Vigersky, R.A., (ed): Anorexia Nervosa. Raven Press, New York, pp 149–161.

40. Malina, R.M., Harper, A.B., Avent, H.H., Campbell, D.E. 1971. Physique of female track and field athletes. Med Sci Sports 3:32–28.

41. Wilmore, J.H., Brown, C.H., Davis, J.A. 1977. Body physique and composition of the female distance runner. Ann N Y Acad Sci 301:764–776.

42. Sinning, W.E. 1978. Anthropometric estimation of body density, fat, and lean body weight in women gymnasts. Med Sci Sports 10:243–249.

43. Young, C.M. 1961. Body fatness in normal young women. N Y State J Med 61:1928–1931.

44. Sloan, A.W., Burt, J.J., Blyth, C.S. 1962. Estimation of body fat in young women. J Appl Physiol 17:967–970.

45. Wilmore, J.H., Behnke, A.R. 1970. An anthropometric estimation of body density and lean body weight in young women. Am J Clin Nutr 23:267–274.

46. Carlberg, K.A., Buckman, M.T., Peake, G.T., Riedesel, M.L. Body composition of oligo-amenorrheic athletes. Med Sci Sports Exerc. In press.

47. Carlberg, K.A., Buckman, M.T., Peake, G.T., Ricdesel, M.L. 1981. Low body weight increases susceptibility to athletic oligo/amenorrhea. Med Sci Sports Exerc 13:105 (abstract).

48. Baker, E.R., Mathur, R.S., Kirk, R.F., Williamson, H.O. 1981. Female runners and secondary amenorrhea: Correlation with age, parity, mileage, and plasma hormonal and sex-hormone-binding globulin concentrations. Fertil Steril 36:183–187.

49. Wakat, D.K., Sweeney, K.A., Rogol, A.D. 1982. Reproductive system function in women cross-country runners. Med Sci Sports Exerc 14:263–269.

50. Hendrix, M.K., Lohman, T.G. 1981. Incidence of menstrual disorders in female collegiate athletes and its relation to body fat content. Med Sci Sports Exerc 13:104 (abstract).

51. Calabrese, L., Kirkendall, D., Floyd, M., Rapoport, S., Weiker, G., Bergfeld, J. 1982. Menstrual abnormalities and body composition in professional female ballet dancers. Med Sci Sports Exerc 14:145 (abstract).

52. Reith, P., Byrd, P., Silver, B., Kyner, J., Thomas, T.R. 1982. Premenarchial hormonal pattern in lean athletic women with secondary amenorrhea. Med Sci Sports Exerc 14:145.

53. Snyder, A.C., Froehlich, M.P., Lamb, D.R. 1981. Body fat and menstrual history of college athletes. Med Sci Sports Exerc 13:104–105 (abstract).

54. O'Herlihy, C. 1982. Jogging and suppression of ovulation. N Engl J Med 306:50–51 (letter).

55. Vigersky, R.A., Andersen, A.E., Thompson, R.H., Loriaux, D.L. 1977. Hypothalamic dysfunction in secondary amenorrhea associated with simple weight loss. N Engl J Med 297:1141–1145.

56. Siiteri, P.K., MacDonald, P.C. 1973. Role of extraglandular estrogen in human reproduction. In: Greep, R.O., (ed): Handbook of Physiology. American Physiological Society, Washington, D.C. pp 615–629.

57. Fishman, J., Boyar, R.M., Hellman, L. 1975. Influence of body weight on estradiol metabolism in young women. J Clin Endocrinol Metab 41:989–991.

58. Longcope, C., Pratt, J.H., Schneider, S.H., Fineberg, S.E. 1976. In vivo studies on the metabolism of estrogens by muscle and adipose tissue of normal males. J Clin Endocrinol Metab 43:1134–1145.

59. Longcope, C., Pratt, J.H., Schneider, S.H., Fineberg, S.E. 1976. The in vivo metabolism of androgens by muscle and adipose tissue of normal men. Steroids 28:521–533.

60. Shangold, M.M. 1980. Sports and menstrual function. Physician Sportsmed 8(8):66–70.

61. Fava, G.A., Fava, M., Kellner, R., Serafini, E., Mastrogiacomo, I. 1981. Depression, hostility and anxiety in hyperprolactinemic amenorrhea. Psychother Psychosom 36:122–128.

62. Seibel, M.M., Taymor, M.L. 1982. Emotional aspects of infertility. Fertil Steril 37:137–145.

63. Lachelin, G.C.L., Yen, S.S.C. 1978. Hypothalamic chronic anovulation. Am J Obstet Gynecol 130:825–831.

64. McArthur, J.W., Bullen, B.A., Beitins, I.Z., Pagano, M., Badger, T.M., Klibanski, A. 1980. Hypothalamic amenorrhea in runners of normal body composition. Endocr Res Commun 7:13–25.

65. Carlberg, K.A., Peake, G.T., Buckman, M.T., Srivastava, L.S. 1981. Pituitary-ovarian axis in oligo/amenorrheic athletes. Fed Proc 40:396 (abstract).

66. Fears, W.B., Yu, J., Ferguson, E., Glass, A.R., Vigersky, R.A. 1982. Mechanism of exercise-induced secondary amenorrhea. In: Program and Abstracts. (The Endocrine Society, 64th Annual Meeting, June 16–18, 1982). Williams & Wilkens, Baltimore, p 86 (abstract).

67. Brisson, G.R., Dulac, S., Ledoux, M., Peronnet, F., Decarufel, D., Proteau, L. 1982. Blood gonadotrophic hormone levels in ovarian dysfunction of athletes. Med Sci Sports Exerc 14:145 (abstract).

68. Yen, S.S.C., Tsai, C.C., Naftolin, F., Vandenberg, G. Ajabor, L. 1972. Pulsatile patterns of gonadotropin release in subjects with and without ovarian function. J Clin Endocrinol 34:671–675.

69. Yen, S.S.C., Rebar, R., Vandenberg, G., Judd, H. 1973. Hypothalamic amenorrhea and hypogonadotropinism: Responses to synthetic LRF. J Clin Endocrinol Metab 36:811–816.

70. Jurkowski, J.E., Jones, N.J., Walker, W.C., Younglai, E.V., Sutton, J.R. 1978. Ovarian hormonal responses to exercise. J Appl Physiol 44:109–114.

71. Bonen, A., Ling, W.Y., MacIntyre, K.P., Neil, R., McGrail, J.C., Belcastro, A.N. 1979. Effects of exercise on the serum concentrations of FSH, LH, progrestrone, and estradiol. Eur J Appl Physiol 42:15–23.

72. Cumming, D.C., Strich, G., Brunsting, L., Greenberg, L., Ries, A.L., Yen, S.S.C., Rebar, R.W. 1981. Acute exercise-related endocrine changes in women runners and nonrunners. Fertil Steril 36:421–422 (abstract).

73. Rowell, L.B. 1974. Human cardiovascular adjustments to exercise and thermal stress. Physiol Rev 54:75–159.

74. Noel, G.L., Suh, H.K., Stone, J.G., Frantz, A.G. 1972. Human prolactin and growth hormone release during surgery and other conditions of stress. J Clin Endocrinol Metab 35:840–851.

75. Brisson, G.R., Volle, M.A., DeCarufel, D., Desharnais, M., Tanaka, M. 1980. Exercise-induced dissociation of the blood prolactin response in young women according to their sports habits. Horm Metab Res 12:201–205.

76. Shangold, M.M., Gatz, M.L., Thysen, B. 1981. Acute effects of exercise on plasma concentrations of prolactin and testosterone in recreational women runners. Fertil Steril 35:699–702.

77. Jacobs, H.S., Franks, S., Murray, M.A.F., Hull, M.G.R., Steele, S.J., Nabarro, J.D.N. 1976. Clinical and endocrine features of hyperprolactinaemic amenorrhoea. Clin Endocrinol 5:439–454.

78. Archer, D.F. 1977. Current concepts of prolactin physiology in normal and abnormal conditions. Fertil Steril 28:125–134.

79. Bergh, T., Nillus, S.J., Wide, L. 1977. Hyperprolactinaemia in amenorrhoea—incidence and clinical significance. Acta Endocrinol 86:683–694.

80. Ferriman, D., Purdie, A.W. 1965. Association of oligomenorrhoea, hirsuties, and infertility. Br Med J 2:69–72.

81. Rosenfield, R.L. 1973. Relationship of androgens to female hirsutism and infertility. J Reprod Med 11:87–95.

82. Smith, K.D., Rodriguez-Rigau, L.J., Tcholakian, R.K., Steinberger, E. 1979. The relation between plasma testosterone levels and the lengths of phases of the menstrual cycle. Fertil Steril 32:403–407.

83. Cumming, D.C., Brunsting, L., Greenberg, L., Strich, B., Ries, A.L., Yen, S.S.C., Rebar, R.W. 1981. Patterns of endocrine response to exercise in normal women. In: Programs and Abstracts, The Endocrine Society, 63rd Annual Meeting, June 17–19, 1981. Williams and Wilkens, Baltimore, p 465 (abstract).

84. Sutton, J.R., Coleman, M.J., Casey, J., Lazarus, L. 1973. Androgen responses during physical exercise. Br Med J 1:520–522.

85. Brisson, G.R., Volle, M.A., Desharnais, M., Brault, J., Audet, A., DeCarufel, D. 1978. Δ⁴-androstenedionemie a l'effort chez la femme. Can J Appl Sport Sci 3:183 (abstract).

86. Carlberg, K.A., Peake, G.T., Buckman, M.T., Srivastava, L.S. 1981. Androgen response to exercise in oligo/amenorrheic and menstruating athletes. In: Program and Abstracts, The Endocrine Society, 63rd Annual Meeting, June 17–19, 1981. Williams and Wilkens, Baltimore, p 351 (abstract).

87. Yen, S.S.C. 1978. Chronic anovulation due to inappropriate feed-back system. In: Yen, S.S.C., Jaffe, R.B., (eds): Reproductive Endocrinology: Physiology, Pathophysiology and Clinical Management. W.B. Saunders Co., Philadelphia, pp 297–323.

88. Shangold, M.M. 1982. Evaluating menstrual irregularity in athletes. Physician Sportsmed 10(2):21–22 (editorial).

89. Smith, N.J. 1980. Excessive weight loss and food aversion in athletes simulating anorexia nervosa. Pediatrics 66:139–142.

# Chapter 10

# Stress Hormone Response to Exercise[1]

by David S. Schade

## Introduction

Exercise requires major changes in metabolic fuels to maintain increased muscle contraction and to supply adequate glucose for the central nervous system. In the basal state, muscle metabolizes lipid exclusively and the central nervous system uses glucose. During exercise, lipid metabolism by muscle increases, but after 90 min, glucose metabolism accounts for 41% of oxygen uptake by leg muscles (Ahlborg et al. [1]), potentially depriving the nervous system of its metabolic fuel (Felig and Wahren [2]). The physiological adaptation that ensures adequate fuel to muscles and the central nervous system is the subject of this chapter.

Energy expended by muscle during exercise is derived from ATP, generated from ADP and high-energy phosphate bonds from creatine phosphate. Sufficient supplies of ATP and creatine phosphate depend upon oxidative phosphorylation of two- and three-carbon molecules from lipid and carbohydrate precursors in muscle mitochondria. When these precursors are not available, ATP decreases and muscle contraction ultimately ceases. Substrates for muscle metabolism are derived from muscle and extramuscular sources, mainly fat and liver cells. The quantities of carbohydrate and lipid precursors in various tissues in man (Havel [3]) are presented in Table 10–1, which shows that most energy substrate is lipid, stored outside of muscle. Glycogen and triglycerides are the two major storage forms (Fig. 10–1). These are relatively stable and remain in storage sites unless stimulated for release by hormones secreted during exercise. Enzymes involved in making energy available differ and function in a number of reactions for both carbohydrate and

[1]Supported in part by a grant from The Sugar Association. The author is the recipient of NIH Research Career Development Award #1KZ4AM00260-03.

**Table 10–1**   Fuel Stores in a 70-kg Man in Kilocalories and Percent of Total Stored

| Site | Tissue | Glycogen Kcal | % | Triglyceride Kcal | % |
|------|--------|---------------|---|-------------------|---|
| Muscular | Muscle | 1600 | 1.4 | 2,300 | 2 |
| | Liver | 300 | 0.2 | 90 | 0.1 |
| Extramuscular | Fat | 100 | 0.1 | 108,000 | 96 |
| Total | | 2000 | 1.7 | 110,390 | 98.1 |

lipid precursors. The amount of energy released must meet, but not greatly exceed, the immediate needs of the organism.

Protein, mostly from muscle, can also be used as energy substrate. It is broken down to amino acids, which are converted to glucose in the liver. Alanine and glutamine from this source are the main amino acids used for gluconeogenesis, hence the designation, glucose-alanine cycle (Felig [4]). Although muscle is a potential substrate for glucose production, conservation of muscle protein during exercise is the rule. In spite of this, muscle breakdown during exercise occurs to some extent (Dill et al. [5]). During prolonged fasting, use of carbohydrate and lipid stores precedes muscle catabolism.

Muscle contains small amounts of carbohydrate and lipid, which provide fuel for rapid exercise of short duration (Table 10–1). Continuous exercise for longer periods requires extramuscular sources of energy. Inadequate energy substrate rarely limits muscle contraction in man.

The hormones that mobilize energy during exercise (Fig. 10–2) are called "stress" hormones and include catecholamines, glucagon, cortisol, and growth hormone. They are also called "counter-regulatory" hormones because their effects are opposite to the anabolic effects of insulin (Eaton and Schade [6]).

There are four "stress" hormones that elevate blood sugar, but only insulin reduces blood sugar. The reasons for four stress hormones are 1) a deficiency of any one may result in hypoglycemia; 2) each stress hormone has a characteristic onset and duration of action, and each affects different cells; 3) there is synergism between the stress hormones (Eigler et al. [7]). Thus, this system emphasizes the importance of maintaining adequate blood glucose at all times.

In a runner participating in the 1978 Albuquerque Marathon, all four stress hormones increased acutely (Fig. 10–3a). However, the largest rise in catecholamines occurred between 19 and 26 miles, which might relate to increased fatigue associated with the last 6 miles of the race, or to the excitement of approaching the finish line. In spite of increased uptake of glucose by muscle, plasma glucose rose (Fig. 10–3b) because of increased hepatic glucose production. Plasma nonesterified fatty acids also doubled, and ketone bodies (acetoacetate and 3-hydroxybutyrate) increased ninefold. Although blood flow to muscle may more than triple during strenuous exercise, the lack of energy substrates for muscle metabolism was not limiting this runner. Furthermore, plasma glucose was sufficient for optimal central nervous system function.

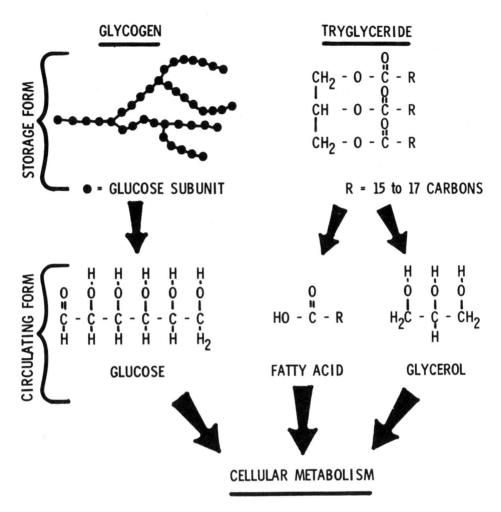

**10–1**    Storage and circulating forms of metabolic fuels. Carbohydrate is stored as glycogen. Glycogenolysis in liver results in release of glucose into the circulation. Lipid is stored as triglyceride, principally in adipose tissue. Triglyceride is catabolized by a hormone-sensitive lipase, resulting in release of fatty acids and glycerol into blood. Fatty acid is used directly for muscle metabolism, and glycerol is converted to glucose by liver.

# The Individual Stress Hormones

## Catecholamines

The catecholamines are structurally related and have potent effects during exercise. Epinephrine originates in the adrenal medulla, and norepinephrine is synthesized in postganglionic sympathetic nerve terminals. These two hormones have similar, but not identical, metabolic functions. They cause vasoconstriction and mobilization of lipids and

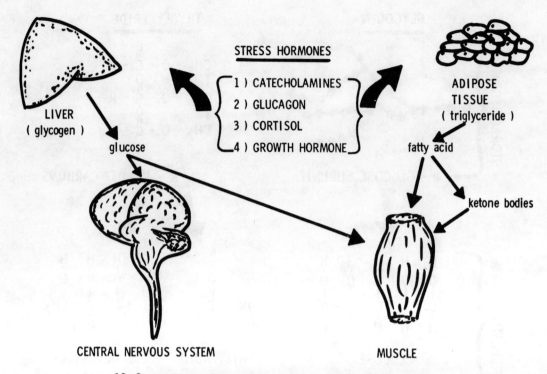

**10–2**   Metabolic activity of stress hormones. Each mobilizes glucose from liver and fatty acids from adipose tissue. Glucose is used by brain and muscle during exercise. Fatty acids are used by muscle directly or indirectly after their hepatic conversion to ketone bodies. In the absence of stress hormones, circulating energy substrates could not maintain muscle contraction and nervous system function.

carbohydrates during exercise. Catecholamines enhance phosphorylation of liver glycogen, which is subsequently hydrolyzed to glucose. Gluconeolysis is particularly important during exercise, when increased muscle use of glucose tends to cause hypoglycemia. Catecholamines may also stimulate gluconeogenesis.

Catecholamines are the most potent lipolytic hormone known. At concentrations of less than $10^{-6}$ M (one molecule of catecholamine per million molecules of water), these compounds stimulate conversion of fat to fatty acids (Schade and Eaton [8]), which are the main energy source for muscle. Among the other effects of catecholamines (Fig. 10–4) is the suppression of insulin, a potent inhibitor of both glycogenolysis and lipolysis. Suppression occurs during exercise by direct effect of catecholamine on the pancreas in spite of elevated plasma glucose (Iverson [9]). Catecholamines concurrently stimulate pancreatic glucagon, the most potent gluconeogenic hormone in man. Thus, these compounds are probably the most important of the stress hormones.

## Glucagon

Glucagon was discovered as a contaminant of insulin. When insulin was injected into an animal, elevation of plasma glucose occurred (glucagon effect) prior to its expected

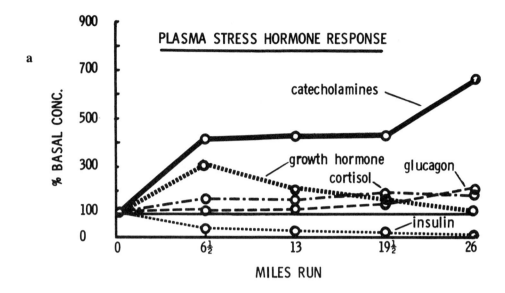

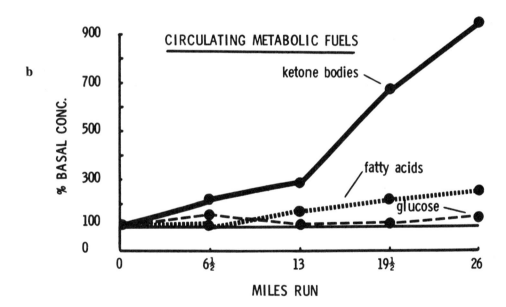

**10–3**  Elevated plasma stress hormones (a) and energy substrates (b) in a marathon runner. The greatest increase in stress hormones occurred in the catecholamines, which were responsible for the suppression of insulin throughout the 26-mile race. Coincident with the rise in stress hormones, plasma glucose, fatty acids, and ketone bodies also rose in spite of increased use during exercise (b). Plasma levels of these metabolic fuels were never less than basal, suggesting that their availability was not limiting exercise tolerance.

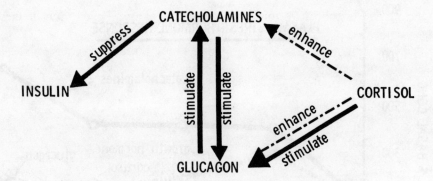

**10–4**   Hormonal-hormonal interactions during exercise. In addition to their effects on cellular metabolism, each hormone alters concentration or activity of the other stress hormones. Most important of these interactions is suppression of insulin by catecholamines, permitting catabolic activity of all four stress hormones.

decline (insulin effect). Glucagon is four times more potent in raising plasma glucose than insulin is in decreasing it. Glucagon produces changes in hepatic gluconeogenic hormones in man within minutes of administration (Greene et al. [10]). It is secreted by pancreatic alpha cells, which adjoin beta cells (insulin-secreting cells) in the islets of Langerhans.

Several studies show that strenuous exercise is a potent stimulus for glucagon secretion in man, and mild exercise may not induce its release. Glucagon acts mainly on the liver, but when insulin is sufficiently suppressed, it may stimulate lipolysis in adipose tissue. Glucagon enters the portal vein directly after secretion, exposing the liver to elevated plasma concentrations that stimulate gluconeogenesis and glycogenolysis, thus increasing hepatic glucose production. Glucagon stimulates cellular cyclic AMP, which increases hepatic enzyme activity, rather than promoting synthesis of new enzyme protein.

During the last decade, it was shown that glucagon promotes conversion of fatty acids to ketone bodies in the liver and suppresses their conversion to triglycerides (Schade et al. [11]). This is important during exercise, when fatty acids in plasma exceed the capacity of muscle to use them. Glucagon-mediated conversion of fatty acids to ketone bodies, readily oxidized by muscle cells, ensures additional fuel for muscle. In contrast, triglycerides require hydrolysis before becoming available for muscle oxidation.

Glucagon also exerts hormone-to-hormone interaction. Unlike catecholamines, glucagon stimulates insulin secretion during exercise. However, glucagon also stimulates catecholamine secretion from the adrenal, thereby enhancing glycogenolysis *in vivo* (Gerich et al. [12]). Thus, glucagon, both at hepatic and adrenal levels, helps prevent hypoglycemia during exercise.

## Cortisol

Exercise is a potent stimulus for corticotropin secretion which, in turn, stimulates adrenal production of cortisol. Plasma cortisol rises approximately 15 min after initiation of exercise. Increased plasma cortisol, unlike glucagon and the catecholamines, causes metabolic changes in about 90 min, and the effects are prolonged (Schade et al. [13]). This delay reflects the mechanism by which cortisol affects cellular events. Glucagon and catecholamines stimulate cyclic AMP in the cell membrane, and cortisol stimulates new nuclear RNA and protein synthesis. Specific proteins in the cytoplasm transport cortisol from the cell surface to the nucleus. The delay in its metabolic effects is due to the time necessary for cortisol transport to the nucleus.

Cortisol affects carbohydrate metabolism by promoting synthesis of hepatic enzymes involved in gluconeogenesis. Recent studies show that cortisol activity is synergistic with that of glucagon and catecholamines. During exercise, when all three hormones are elevated, hepatic glucose production is greatly increased. In addition, cortisol stimulates the release of alanine from muscle, an important gluconeogenic substrate, and inhibits glucose uptake by peripheral tissue, by blocking insulin-dependent and independent pathways.

Corticotropin and cortisol increase plasma nonesterified fatty acids by promoting lipolysis, thus providing additional energy for muscle. Cortisol may also alter hepatic lipid metabolism. Cortisol and other hormones are not known to have synergistic effects on lipid metabolism, but cortisol may affect lipid metabolism indirectly by stimulating glucagon secretion (Marco et al. [14]).

## Growth Hormone

Exercise is a major stimulus for growth hormone secretion, and this is used clinically for the hormone's evaluation. Of the four stress hormones, the metabolic activity of growth hormone is least understood. It is both glucogenic and lipolytic, thereby enhancing availability of metabolic fuels during exercise, and it is similar to cortisol in the delay that occurs between elevation in plasma and metabolic effects (Schade et al. [15]). Like cortisol, the delay is related to new protein synthesis.

The lipolytic effect of growth hormone occurs both *in vitro* and *in vivo* (Schade et al. [15]). Furthermore, growth hormone causes elevation of plasma ketone bodies and thus increases fuel for muscle during exercise (Schade et al. [15]). Growth hormone also induces hyperglycemia when insulin is suppressed during exercise by catecholamines.

# Summary

This chapter reviewed the hormones that provide adequate fuel for muscle and nervous system during exercise. The hormones responsible for raising plasma nonesterified fatty acids, ketone bodies, and glucose are: 1) catecholamines from the adrenal medulla and sympathetic nerve terminals, 2) glucagon from the pancreas, 3) cortisol from the adrenal cortex, and 4) growth hormone from the pituitary gland. These hormones have distinctive actions and temporal profiles of their metabolic effects.

Adequate fuel for muscle contraction is provided by four stress hormones that raise plasma nonesterified fatty acids, and ketone bodies, metabolic fuels that are rapidly used by muscle, sparing muscle glycogen and increasing exercise tolerance. These hormones also raise plasma glucose, which tends to decrease during exercise as muscle blood flow and glucose uptake increases. The avid use of glucose by muscle is partially counteracted by three of the four stress hormones (catecholamines, cortisol, and growth hormone), which inhibit the uptake of glucose by peripheral tissues, thus ensuring an adequate glucose for the central nervous system. This intricate hormonal system usually functions well, since exercise-induced hypoglycemia is rare, and limitation of exercise due to inadequate substrate is almost nonexistent.

# References

1. Ahlborg, G., Felig, P., Hagenfeldt, L. et al. 1974. Substrate turnover during prolonged exercise in man: Splanchnic and leg metabolism of glucose, free fatty acids, and amino acids. J Clin Invest 53:1080–1090.
2. Felig, P., Wahren, J. 1975. Fuel homeostasis in exercise. N Engl J Med 293:1078–1084.
3. Havel, R.J. 1972. Caloric homeostasis and disorders of fuel transport. N Engl J Med 287:1186–1192.
4. Felig, P. 1973. The glucose-alanine cycle. Metabolism 22:179–207.
5. Dill, D.B., Edwards, H.T., deMeio, R.H. 1935. Effects of adrenalin injection in moderate work. Am J Physiol 3:9–16.
6. Eaton, R.P., Schade, D.S. 1978. Modulation and implications of the counterregulatory hormones: Glucagon, catecholamines, cortisol, and growth hormone. In: Katzen, H.M., Mahler, R.J., (eds): Advances in Modern Nutrition. Diabetes, Obesity, and Vascular Disease, Vol 2. Hemisphere Publishing Corporation, Washington, D.C., pp 341–366.
7. Eigler, N., Sacca, L., Sherwin, R.S. 1979. Synergistic interactions of physiologic increments of glucagon, epinephrine, and cortisol in the dog. J Clin Invest 63:114–123.
8. Schade, D.S., Eaton, R.P. 1979. The regulation of plasma ketone body concentration by counter-regulatory hormones in man. III. Effects of norepinephrine in normal man. Diabetes 28:5–10.
9. Iverson, J. 1973. Adrenergic receptors and the secretion of glucagon and insulin from the isolated, perfused canine pancreas. J Clin Invest 52:2102–2116.
10. Greene, H.L., Taunton, O.D., Stifel, F.B., Herman, R.H. 1974. The rapid changes of hepatic glycolytic enzymes and fructose-1, 6-diphosphatase activities after intravenous glucagon in humans. J Clin Invest 53:44–51.
11. Schade, D.S., Woodside, W., Eaton, R.P. 1979. The role of glucagon in the regulation of plasma lipids. Metabolism 28:874–886.
12. Gerich, J.E., Karam, J.H., Forsham, P.H. 1973. Stimulation of glucagon secretion by epinephrine in man. J Clin Endocrinol Metab 37:479–481.
13. Schade, D.S., Eaton, R.P. Standefer, J. 1977. Glucocorticoid regulation of plasma ketone body concentration in insulin deficient man. J Clin Endocrinol Metab 44:1069–1079.
14. Marco, J., Calle, C., Roman, D., Diaz-Fierros, M., Villaneuva, M.L., Valverde, I. 1973. Hyperglucagonism induced by glucocorticoid treatment in man. N. Engl J Med 288:128–131.
15. Schade, D.S., Eaton, R.P., Peake, G.T. 1978. The regulation of plasma ketone body concentration by counter-regulatory hormones in man. II. Effects of growth hormone in diabetic man. Diabetes 27:916–924.

# Chapter 11

# Fluid and Electrolytes in Endurance Training

## by Dale G. Erickson

Why does the marathon runner often experience the sequence of events depicted in Figure 11–1?

"Hitting the wall," a poorly defined entity, may result from interrelated metabolic events that include electrolyte losses, volume depletion, exhaustion of glycogen stores, acidosis, and other phenomena. Much of the evidence that provides us some understanding of this occurrence comes from D. Costill and B. Saltin, several of whose reports are cited in this chapter.

Large sweat losses can impair performance of endurance athletes (Costill et al. [1]) by reducing plasma volume and work capacity. Dehydration influences performance by its effect on muscle water. In this chapter body water, sweat composition, fluid compartment shifts with dehydration, and hormonal and renal mechanisms that protect the circulation of the endurance athlete are reviewed, with guidelines for fluid and electrolyte replacement during endurance training.

# Water

The human body resides in a "sea of water." In a 70-kg person, two-thirds of body weight, or approximately 45 kg, is water. Body water exists in separate but continually interacting compartments. Two-thirds of total body water (about 30 kg) is intracellular. The remaining one-third is extracellular. The extracellular fluid (ECF) is divided into interstitial and plasma spaces that comprise three-fourths and one-fourth of the ECF, respectively. In a 70-kg person, interstitial volume is approximately 11 L, and the plasma volume, 4 L. The electrical charge of plasma proteins provides the attractive force or oncotic pressure for water, which maintains plasma volume. The leaner athlete has proportionally more total body water, perhaps 70% of body weight, and conversely, the more obese individual has less body water.

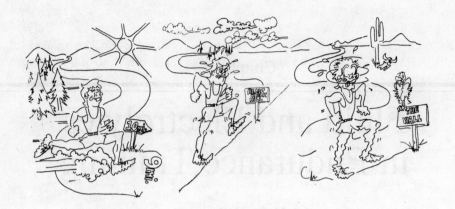

**11–1**  Hypothetical events related to fluid and electrolyte balance. (Reproduced with permission, Ken Wilson, artist.)

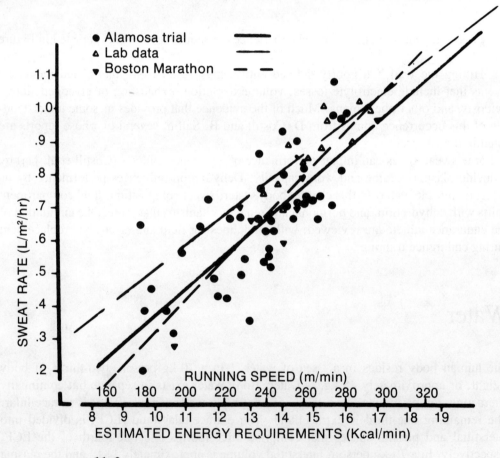

**11–2**  Relationship between running speed (energy expenditure) and sweat rate during treadmill (2 h) and marathon running. (From Costill, D.L. 1977. Sweating: Its composition and effects on body fluids. Ann NY Acad Sci 301:160–173. Reproduced with permission.)

Body water is, in a sense, the most critical "nutrient." Most essential nutrients may be absent from the diet for days or months without serious effects. Not so with water. Without it one cannot survive for more than a few days, and without adequate hydration, an athlete cannot compete an endurance event such as a marathon run. Most problems encountered by marathon runners are the result of inadequate water replacement. Hormones, nutrients (amino acids, glucose, free fatty acids), antibodies, and waste products (urea, creatinine, $CO_2$) are all transported in plasma to water that surrounds individual cells, and the body's more important chemical reactions are carried out in water and are less efficient when body water is depleted (Smith [2]).

Water is of critical importance in regulating body temperature. Excessive heat produced with exercise is dissipated by sweating, which can function only if ample water is supplied to sweat glands. If the body is completely covered or if environmental heat and humidity are high, body heat loss by sweat evaporation is decreased.

Nathan Smith points out that one of the earlier attempts to climb Mt. Everest failed because of inadequate water (Smith [2]). A Swiss climbing team carried only enough fuel to melt snow for a pint of water per day per climber during the last 3 days of the climb, and this was inadequate in the face of the enormous energy expended at high altitude. Sir Edmund Hillary later succeeded, in part, because each member of the team was given 7 pints of water per day.

Daily water losses are great with strenuous physical activity. Body water is entirely replaced every 11–13 days (Smith [2]). Most adults require 2.5 L of water per day, which is supplied in food and fluids. In addition, carbohydrates, protein, and fats are metabolized to $CO_2$ and water, contributing about one-fifth of the daily water requirement (Smith [2]).

The greatest water loss is in urine and sweating. Water lost from lungs in expired air and from the skin without obvious perspiration is called "insensible" water loss. The lower the humidity, the greater the insensible water loss.

Body water and plasma osmolality are regulated primarily by antidiuretic hormone (ADH), which effectively maintains extracellular fluid volume but is severely stressed during water deficits. Thirst cannot always be relied upon to stimulate adequate water replacement (Smith [2]; Saltin [3]). During strenuous physical activity, athletes should be encouraged to drink well beyond thirst satisfaction to insure adequate hydration.

# Sweating

Heat dissipation depends upon vaporization of sweat, and sweat production is proportional to the rate of energy expended (i.e., running speed) (Fig. 11–2). With high energy expenditures, sweating approaches 1 liter/$m^2$/h which may result in a 5-L sweat loss for an average-sized man during a 3-h marathon. A warm environment further increases sweat volume. Despite fluid intake during the race, sweat may produce a 12% reduction in body water and an 8% reduction in body weight (Costill [4]). Greater than 2% weight loss from exercise-induced sweating places severe demands on the thermoregulatory and cardiovascular systems (Saltin [5]).

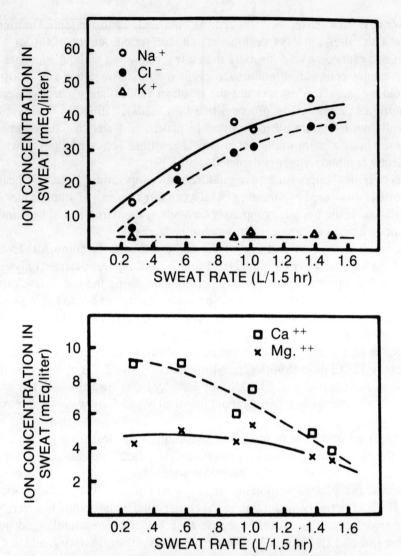

**11–3**   Relationship between sweat rate and concentration of Na⁺, Cl⁻, and K⁺ (top) and Ca⁺⁺ and Mg⁺⁺ (bottom). (From Costill, D.L. 1977. Ann NY Acad Sci 301:160–173. Reproduced with permission.)

Sodium ($Na^+$), potassium ($K^+$), chloride ($Cl^-$), and magnesium ($Mg^{++}$) concentrations in sweat vary considerably from person to person and are influenced by sweat rate and heat acclimatization. Sodium is generally 40–60 mEq/liter; $Cl^-$ 30 mEq/L; $K^+$ is 4–5 mEq/L; and $Mg^{++}$ is 1.5–5 mEq/L (Costill [4]). Sweat is hypotonic and the ions lost are principally sodium and chloride. As the sweat rate rises with increasing energy expenditure, the sodium and chloride in sweat increase; potassium and magnesium remain about the same, and calcium decreases (Fig. 11–3) (Costill [4]). A 4.1-liter sweat loss with a 5.8% reduction in body weight results in losses of 155 mEq/L $Na^+$, 16 mEq/L $K^+$, 137 mEq/L $Cl^-$, and 13 mEq/L $Mg^{++}$ (Costill et al. [6]). This approximates a 5%–7% total body deficit of sodium chloride. Potassium and magnesium losses are minimal, about 1.2%. The major ionic deficits are those of the extracellular fluid space, particularly sodium chloride.

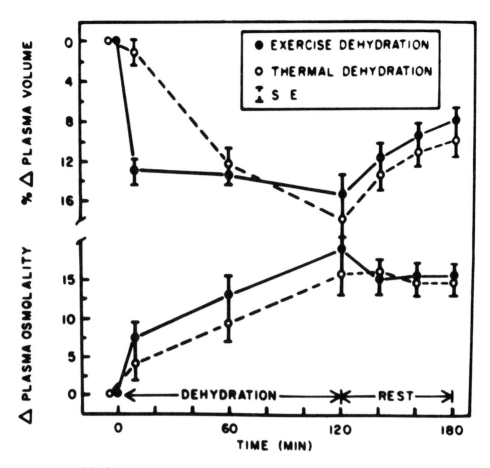

**11–4**  Changes in plasma volume and osmolality during exercise and thermal (sauna) dehydration. The subjects were dehydrated 4% at the end of both exercise and heat exposures. (From Costill, D.L. 1977. Sweating: Its composition and effects on body fluids. Ann NY Acad Sci 301:160–173. Reproduced with permission.)

# Fluid Compartment Shifts

The understanding of plasma and interstitial and intracellular fluid compartment changes during continuous exercise and progressive dehydration has been facilitated by studies (Saltin [5]; Costill [7]) in which water and electrolyte content of muscle cells was determined (Bergstrom [8]).

Costill [4] states: "If we assume that the changes in plasma water and electrolytes during exertion are representative of interstitial fluids, it is then possible to describe the influence of acute exercise and subsequent dehydration on various body fluid compartments". The changes induced by prolonged exercise on plasma volume and osmolality (Fig. 11–4) occur early in strenuous exercise. Muscle hyperosmolality accounts for the movement of water from plasma into muscle. Plasma volume then remains fairly constant after a 13% decrement for the remaining 2 h of exercise. Increased plasma osmolality is the protective mechanism that maintains plasma volume without a further drop, a fact

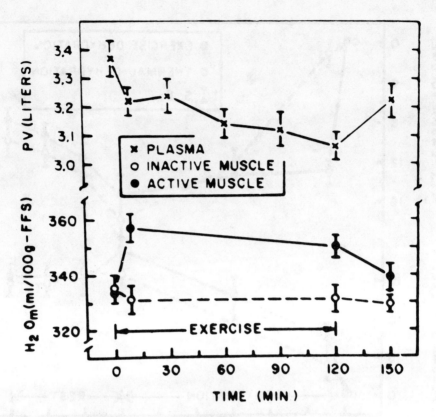

**11–5** Changes in plasma volume and water content of inactive (deltoid) and active (vastus lateralis) muscles during 2 h of exercise. (From Costill, D.L. 1977. Sweating: Its composition and effects on body fluids. Ann NY Acad Sci 301:160–173. Reproduced with permission.)

suggesting that body water lost during exercise comes from interstitial and/or the intracellular spaces. Water moves into active muscle but not into inactive muscle (Fig. 11-5) (Costill [4]). This may be due to hydrostatic pressure forcing water into exercising muscles, and also to increased muscle osmolality. Water in exercising muscle increased 8%, or about the amount that was lost from plasma.

What is the origin of water in sweat? In 2 h of exercise (Fig. 11–5), the subject lost 2.33 kg in body weight, and approximately 150 ml of that was from plasma. If the change in plasma volume is proportional to interstitial fluid loss, then another 580 ml, or 0.58 kg, of fluid is accounted for. Additional water came from glycogen breakdown (approximately 370 ml), oxidation (approximately 460 ml), metabolism (approximately 160 g), and 500 ml from muscle. This totals 2.22 kg and is close to the 2.33-kg actual weight loss.

With progressive exercise and dehydration, proportionally more fluid is lost from the extracellular space (Fig. 11–6) (Costill [7]). Fluid leaving the interstitial space is proportionally greater at 2.2% dehydration, but is less at 4.1% dehydration. Water derived from plasma is about the same at all levels of dehydration, approximately 10%. The absolute water loss in more profound dehydration is drawn equally from both the extra- and intracellular spaces, but it should be remembered that the intracellular compartment contains two-thirds of total body water.

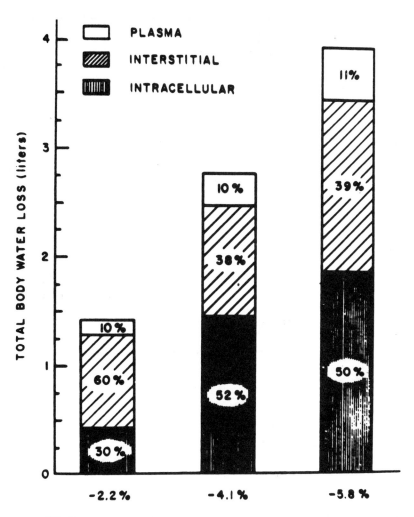

**11–6** Distribution of water loss from plasma, interstitial, and intracellular compartments during varying levels of dehydration. (From Costill, D.L. 1977. Sweating: Its composition and effects on body fluids. Ann NY Acad Sci 301:160–173. Reproduced with permission.)

# Ionic Losses with Dehydration

From seven men studied before, during, and after 2 h of continuous cycling at 60%–70% maximum oxygen uptake (Costill [7]), muscle biopsies were taken after 10 and 120 min exercise, and 30 min after exercise. Potassium, sodium, chloride, magnesium and osmolality were measured in venous blood at various time intervals and these values reflected plasma volume. Muscle glycogen decreased 64 $\mu$mol/kg during exercise, but remained the same during rest. The combined loss of body water via sweating, urination, and respiration was responsible for 3.2% reduction in body weight. Electrolyte losses (urine and sweat) averaged 96 mEq $Na^+$, 22 mEq $K^+$, 04 mEq $Cl^+$, and 4.6 mEq $Mg^{++}$.

The major ion loss was from the extracellular fluid compartment; therefore, it is not surprising that water came disproportionately from plasma and interstitial spaces. Early in

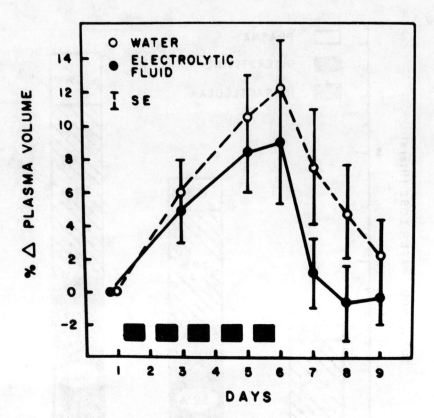

**11–7**    Percentage change in plasma volume during 5 days of repeated dehydration (3% per day). During one series the subjects were permitted to drink only water. In the second series thirst was satisfied by *ad libitum* ingestion of an electrolyte drink. (From Costill, D.L. 1977. Sweating: Its composition and effects on body fluids. Ann NY Acad Sci 301:160–173. Reproduced with permission.)

exercise, $K^+$ left muscle and later reentered active muscle. Magnesium moved into exercising muscle slowly and was associated with a gradual decline in plasma $Mg^{++}$. The $Mg^{++}$ transfer was likely due to metabolic need, but the mechanism for this is not known. This study confirmed only small losses of $K^+$ and $Mg^{++}$ with continuous exercise. The findings in this study are controversial; other investigators have reported extreme $K^+$ losses during exercise, particularly in hot climates (Knochel [9, 10]).

# Metabolic Effects of Repeated Exercises

The foregoing discussion concerned the acute effects of exercise. The metabolic effects of repeated exertion for 5 successive days, a situation which closely mimics endurance training, were studied in 12 subjects (Costill [7]). All ate and drank *ad libitum,* but water, $K^+$, $Na^+$, $Cl^-$, and calories were monitored. Sweat and urinary water and electrolytes were measured each 24 h (Fig. 11–7).

A net increase in plasma volume occurred, greater if water only were permitted and slightly less if an electrolyte-containing drink were allowed. Plasma renin and aldosterone

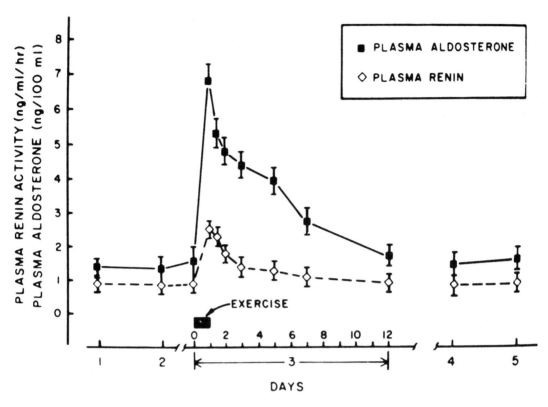

**11–8**  Alterations in plasma renin activity and aldosterone concentration as a result of one 60-min exercise bout. (From Castenfors, J. 1977. Renal function and prolonged exercise. Ann NY Acad Sci 301:151–159. Reproduced with permission.)

increased with exercise, sodium was resorbed, and plasma volume expanded (Fig. 11–8). The subjects stored an average of 392 mEq Na⁺ in 5 days, an amount accounting for the increased plasma volume. Thus, the regularly exercising athlete produces a protective "cushion" against extracellular fluid losses.

Why does the "electrolyte drink" not provide as great a cushion as plain water? The answer, presumably, is that sodium-containing solutions expand extracellular volume enough to blunt the stimulus for renin production, thus resulting in smaller amounts of aldosterone and decreased volume expansion.

# Renal Function During Prolonged Exercise

Prolonged exercise is associated with an increase in the renal filtration fraction, which results from a relatively smaller drop in glomeruli filtration than in renal blood flow (Castenfors [11]) (Fig. 11–9). Thus, more of the decreasing renal blood is filtered. Urinary output is decreased by about 30%, as a result of decreased glomerular filtration and of antidiuretic hormone effect (Fig. 11–10) (Castenfors [11]). Erythrocytes and protein may be found in the urine. The proteinuria suggests that glomerular capillary

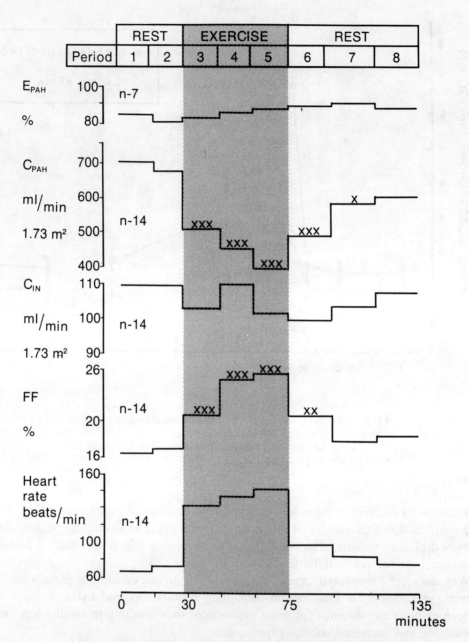

**11–9**   Effect of supine exercise on renal hemodynamics in normal subjects. Mean values of PAH extraction ($E_{PAH}$), $C_{PAH}$, C, FF, and heart rate are shown. X denotes a statistically significant difference compared with Period 2. (From Castendors, J. 1977. Renal function and prolonged exercise. Ann NY Acad Sci 301:151–159. Reproduced with permission.)

permeability is increased during exercise. A possible mechanism for this is hyperthermia, which is known to produce proteinuria, and core body temperature rises with exercise.

Hematuria with exercise was initially described as "exercise pseudonephritis" (Gardner [12]), but red cell casts are not usually found in the urine of athletes. Cystoscopic examinations in runners with hematuria frequently show a hemorrhagic posterior bladder wall, presumably from repeated bladder trauma (Glassock [13]). There is no evidence that

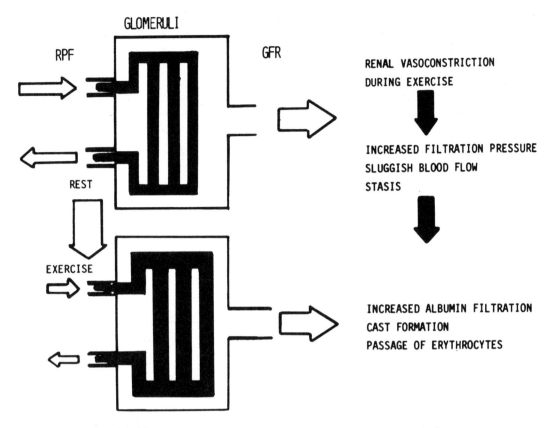

**11–10**   Effect of exercise on glomerular circulation-hypothetical scheme. (From Castenfors, J. 1977. Renal function and prolonged exercise. Ann NY Acad Sci 301:157. Reproduced with permission.)

exercise hematuria or proteinuria is associated with permanent damage to the kidneys or bladder. If gross hematuria with exercise continues when exercise is reduced, one should look for other causes.

# Restoration of Fluid Losses

Fluid replacement beyond the demands of thirst should be encouraged with prolonged exercise. Most studies indicate that the athlete who drinks just to satisfy thirst will not replenish fluid losses. Fluid replacement is important throughout the exercise period to correct losses from the plasma space and to provide the water necessary for evaporative cooling (sweating); but are the water, sugar, and electrolytes ingested during exercise absorbed? Gastric emptying of 14 mEq NaCl and 56 mol of glucose was decreased as maximum oxygen consumption ($\dot{V}O_{2max}$) increased with exercise. However, the decreased gastric emptying was inconsequential until $\dot{V}O_{2max}$ reached 75% (Fig. 11–11) (Costill and Saltin [14]). Therefore, with increasing intensity of exercise, gastric empty-

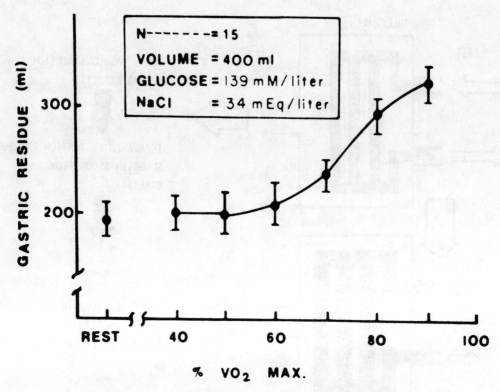

**11–11**   Effect of intensity of exercise on volume remaining in stomach 15 min after test meal of 400 ml. (From Costill, D.L., Saltin, B. 1974. Factors limiting gastric emptying during rest and exercise. J Appl Physiol 37:679–683. Reproduced with permission.)

ing is inhibited, but not completely. The fluid meal is delivered slowly to the intestine, and relatively high concentrations of glucose solution can be emptied from the stomach of an exercising athlete (Fig. 11–12) (Pederson [15]).

Once the meal is in the intestine, the absorption of water, sodium, potassium, chloride, and glucose is not impaired until exercise intensity reaches 70% of maximal oxygen uptake (Fordtran and Saltin [16]). Radioisotope studies above 70% $\dot{V}_{O2max}$ suggest that glucose continues to be absorbed (Costill et al., [17]), but definitive studies of this are not available (Saltin [3]).

Glucose ingested during exercise helps to preserve glycogen stores (Fig. 11–13) (Ahlborg and Felig [18]) and, irrespective of whether glucose is taken before or during exercise, it tends to decrease free fatty-acid release and glycerol production. Oral glucose taken during prolonged exercise, therefore, is utilized for energy (Saltin [3]). Further studies by Cade, et al. [19] demonstrated that glucose-electrolyte fluid ingestion had a positive benefit on endurance performance.

What is recommended for replenishment? 1) The athlete should be encouraged to drink water in excess of thirst. Water is the most important "nutrient" that needs replenishing. 2) Glucose-containing solutions are beneficial and are emptied from the stomach and absorbed during exercise, to some degree preserving glycogen stores for later use. 3) It is not necessary to replenish potassium during exercise since losses are minimal. Muscle

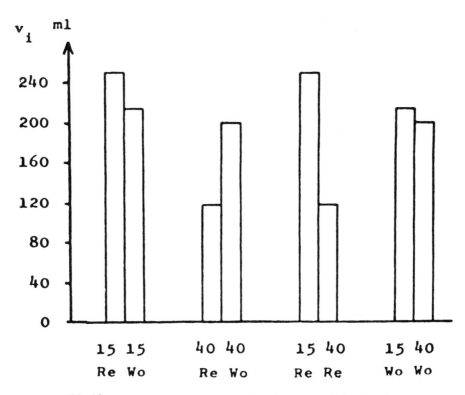

**11–12**   Volume emptied to the intestine ($V_1$) at rest (Re) and work at 60% of $\dot{V}_{O_{2max}}$ for 60 min (Wo) comparing a 15% and 40% glucose solution. The interesting finding is the bar to the right, indicating that a 40% glucose solution can be emptied as quickly as a 15% solution. (From Pederson, E.F. 1975. Glucose uptake in the stomach, Report No. 79. Krogh Institute, Copenhagen. Reproduced with permission.)

potassium is increased with exercise whether the athlete is on a low-or high $K^+$ diet (Costill [7]). Sodium chloride should be replaced but given only in hypotonic solutions. The ingestion of salt without water during exercise should never be practiced. Plasma is already relatively hypertonic because of water loss from it to exercising muscles. Magnesium replacement is possibly helpful because of the increasing metabolic need for magnesium in exercising muscle.

Electrolyte-sugar solution suitable for replenishment in endurance training should contain sugar, sodium chloride in hypotonic concentrations, and very little, if any, potassium. The available solutions are presented in Table 11–1. All of them have sugar. Only two have low concentrations of potassium (Gatorade and Body Punch). Gatorade

**Table 11–1**   Solutions Suitable for Replenishment in Endurance Training

| Product | Sodium (mg/100 ml) | Potassium (mg/100 ml) |
|---|---|---|
| ERG | 32 | 42 |
| Gatorade | 48 | 9 |
| Brake-time | 48 | 39 |
| Sportade | 62 | 56 |
| Body Punch | 11 | 9.1 |

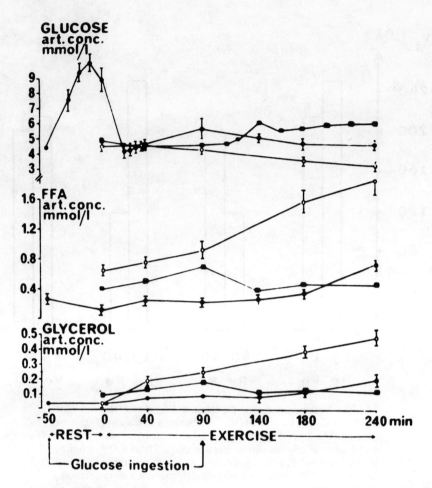

**11–13** Arterial concentration of glucose, free fatty acids, and glycerol in three different series of experiments. Each experiment consisted of a rest period (50 min) and exercise for 240 min at 30% $\dot{V}_{O_{2max}}$. In one series no glucose was given (0) and in the other 200 g glucose was administered either 50 min before exercise or after 90 min of exercise. (Adapted from Ahlborg, G., Felig, P. 1977. Substrate utilization during prolonged exercise preceded by ingestion of glucose. Am J Physiol 233:188. Reproduced with permission.)

has a higher concentration of sodium but is still hypotonic. The American College of Sports Medicine recommends that the most popular solutions, Gatorade and Gookinaid ERG, be diluted to less than 50% concentration when used for actual competition, to further decrease the sodium content [20]. The College further recommends a 0.5 L fluid ingestion per half-hour for the marathon runner [20].

Plain water should be heavily emphasized for replenishment. Far and away, this is the most critical issue. However, replenishment with glucose and *hypotonic* NaCl solutions during exercise may be of benefit.

Finally, the advice given to the depleted football player may be given with slight variation to all endurance athletes: "What you need is a lot of water and a little salt."

# References

1. Costill, D.L., Krammer, W.F., Fisher, A. 1970. Fluid ingestion during distance running. Arch Environ Health 21:520–525.
2. Smith, N.J. 1976. The athlete's need for water and salt. In: Food for Sport. Bull Publishing Company, Palo Alto, pp 91–103.
3. Saltin, B. 1978. Fluid, electrolyte, and energy losses and their replenishment in prolonged exercise. In: J. Parizkova, J., Rogozkin, V.A., (eds): Nutrition, Physical Fitness, and Health, Vol. 7. University Park Press, Baltimore, pp 77–97.
4. Costill, D.L. 1977. Sweating: Its composition and effects on body fluids. Ann NY Acad Sci 301:160–173.
5. Saltin, B. 1964. Circulatory responses to submaximal and maximal exercise after thermal dehydration. J Appl Physiol 19:1119–1124.
6. Costill, D.L., Cote, R., Fink, W. 1976. Muscle water and electrolytes following varying levels of dehydration in man. J Appl Physiol 40:6–11.
7. Costill, D.L. 1978. Muscle water and electrolytes during acute and repeated bouts of dehydration. In: Pariskova, J., Rogozkin V.A., (eds): Nutrition, Physical Fitness, and Health, Vol. 7. University Park Press, Baltimore, pp 98–115.
8. Bergstrom, J. 1962. Muscle electrolytes in man. Determination by neutron activation analysis on needle biopsy specimens. A study done on normal subjects, kidney patients, and patients with chronic diarrhea. Scand J Clin Lab Invest 18:16–20.
9. Knochel, J.P. 1975. Dog days and siriasis: How to kill a football player. JAMA 233:513–515.
10. Knochel, J.P. 1977. Potassium deficiency training in the heat. Ann NY Acad Sci 301:174–181.
11. Castenfors, J. 1977. Renal function and prolonged exercise. Ann NY Acad Sci 301:151–159.
12. Gardner, K.D. 1956. Athletic pseudonephritis-alteration of urinary sediment by athletic competition. JAMA 167:807–813.
13. Glassock, R. 1980. Personnal communication.
14. Costill, D.L., Saltin, B. 1974. Factors limiting gastric emptying during rest and exercise. J Appl Physiol 37:679–683.
15. Pederson, E.F. 1975. Staerke glucose-oplosnigers virkning PA mavesekken optagelse AF glucose, PA legemets vaeskevdbytte OG PA blod glucose koncentrationen, I hvile OG under arbejde. [Glucose uptake in the stomach], Report No. 79. Krogh Institute, Copenhagen.
16. Fordtran, J.S., Saltin, B. 1967. Gastric emptying and intestinal absorption during prolonged severe exercise. J Appl Physiol 23:331.
17. Costill, D.L., Bennett, A., Broman, G., Eddy, D. 1973. Glucose ingestion at rest and during prolonged exercise. J Appl Physiol 34:764.
18. Ahlborg, G., Felig, P. 1977. Substrate utilization during prolonged exercise preceded by ingestion of glucose. Am J Physiol 233:188.
19. Cade, R., Spooner, G., Schlein, E., Pickering, M., Dean, R. 1972. Effect of fluid, electrolyte, and glucose replacement during exercise on performance, body temperature, rate of sweat loss, and compositional changes of extracellular fluid. J Sports Med Phys Fitness 12:150–156.
20. Heat peril in distance runs spurs ACSM guideline alert. 1975. Phys Sportsmed 3(7):85–7.

# Section 4
# Heart, Blood Vessels, Pulmonary and Hematologic Adaptation to Exercise

# Chapter 12

# Cardiovascular Adaptations to Sustained Aerobic Exercise

by Jerry E. Goss

Sustained aerobic exercise requires increased oxygen delivery to muscle cells. Improved aerobic performance comes about mainly through changes in the cardiovascular system, which improves oxygen transport, and through adaptation in skeletal muscles. These changes are modified by coronary artery disease and aging.

This chapter reviews the cardiovascular adaptations that develop with aerobic training and explores the modifications produced by coronary artery disease and aging.

## Heart Rate and Stroke Volume

The easiest physiologic function to measure and compare longitudinally in individuals or between groups of subjects is heart rate. Whether a person is an elite marathoner or a quality middle-aged distance runner, his or her resting heart rate is 15–20 beats per minute slower than average heart rate (Kasch [1]; Paolone et al. [2]; Morganroth et al. [3]). This has been attributed to alterations in the autonomic nervous system (Lin and Horvath [4]; Scheuer and Tipton [5]). The sinoatrial node in the right atrium is influenced by the autonomic nervous system, which controls intrinsic heart rate. Controversy exists concerning relative changes in parasympathetic and sympathetic activity to the heart as a result of training, but in the resting state, increased parasympathetic activity and reduced sympathetic activity are most likely (Scheuer and Tipton [5]). Increased parasympathetic activity or increased vagal tone explain some of the atrioventricular conduction changes seen in the resting electrocardiogram of endurance athletes (Lichtman et al. [6]).

Reduction in maximal heart rate from endurance training (Scheuer and Tipton [5]; Rowell [7]; Ekblom [8]) has been attributed to: 1) changes in autonomic control; 2) increased stroke volume; and 3) reduction in circulating catecholamines (Scheuer and Tipton [5]; Hartley et al. [9]). Endurance training decreases heart rate for a submaximal work load and increases stroke volume (Scheuer and Tipton [5]; Froelicker [10]). Peripheral responses to training are also important in the exercise/heart-rate response. It has been shown in bicycle ergometer studies that the reduced heart-rate response to a work load occurs only when using trained muscles (Clausen et al. [11]). One group of subjects used arms and one group used legs. After training, the subjects were tested with alternate arm and leg exercises. The lower heart rate response to exercise load was seen only when the trained limb was used.

Stroke volume also increased with endurance training (Morganroth et al. [3]; Hanson et al. [12]; Rowell [7]; Ekblom [8]; Hartley et al. [13]). Echocardiographic techniques were used to compare 15 long-distance runners to a control group of noncompetitive students (Morganroth et al. [3]). A statistically significant increase in stroke volume ($p < 0.01$) in the endurance-trained athletes was found. Seven elite runners who had a mean stroke volume of 189 ml at maximal oxygen consumption ($\dot{V}O_{2max}$) were studied by dye dilution techniques (Ekblom [8]). Less well trained endurance runners at $\dot{V}O_{2max}$ had a stroke volume of 149 ml, and 8 untrained subjects at $\dot{V}O_2{}^{max}$ had a stroke volume of 122 ml. Endurance training, therefore, increased stroke volume by 55% in elite runners compared to untrained subjects.

# Maximal Oxygen Consumption

Endurance training significantly increased the maximal work capacity, commonly expressed as maximal $\dot{V}O_{2max}$ (Scheuer and Tipton [5]; Hanson et al. [12]). Sedentary middle-aged men had $\dot{V}O_{2max}$ of 30 ml/kg/min; football defensive linemen, trained in strength and not endurance, had an average $\dot{V}O_{2max}$ of 45 ml/kg/min (Wilmore [14]), soccer stars had $\dot{V}O_{2max}$ of 58 ml/kg/min; and elite distance runners had $\dot{V}O_{2max}$ of 79 ml/kg/min (Gettman and Pollock [15]). Values as high as 85 ml/kg/min were reported in endurance runners (Saltin and Astrand [16]).

Increased maximal oxygen consumption is a function of increased maximal cardiac output and increased arteriovenous difference in oxygen concentration (Ekblom [8]; Froelicker [10]). Stroke volume is greater in trained athletes both at rest and during exercise (Rowell [7]). Since the heart rate in trained athletes at $\dot{V}O_{2max}$ is not increased, the increased maximal cardiac output is due to increased stroke volume. In 7 well-trained distance runners, an average cardiac output of 36 L/min was recorded, the highest value being 42.3 L/min. Eight untrained males had maximum cardiac output of 23.9 L/min (Ekblom [8]), i.e., endurance-trained athletes had about 50% greater maximal cardiac output than did untrained controls. Enhanced oxygen extraction, i.e., widening arteriovenous oxygen difference, during maximum exercise accounts for the other 50% of increased oxygen supplied to cells of endurance-trained athletes (Rowell [7]). In those whose cardiac output can be only minimally increased with training, oxygen extraction by the tissues is the major factor in increasing oxygen supply and maximal work capacity. A patient with limited left ventricular function and an artificial pacemaker would be an example. The mechanism for increased extraction is primarily redistribution of blood flow from the areas of low extraction, such as the splanchnic bed, to areas of high extraction, i.e., skeletal muscles (Rowell [7]). Submaximal work loads require the same oxygen consumption after training so that total body efficiency is unchanged (Froelicker [10]). Therefore, cardiac output and arteriovenous oxygen differences are unchanged at submaximal work loads by aerobic training in normal subjects (Scheuer and Tipton [5]; Hartley et al. [9]; Froelicker [10]; Mitchell [17]).

# Blood Pressure

In studies of more than 3000 men, the resting systolic and diastolic blood pressures were significantly lower in physically fit persons than in those in poor physical condition (Cooper et al. [18]), and both resting systolic and diastolic blood pressures in 66 middle-aged men were significantly lower after 1 year of modest aerobic training (Paolone et al. [2]). Similar observations of less magnitude were made in untrained men, ages 52–88 years, after only 6 weeks of aerobic training (de Vries [19]). Others have noted no decrease in blood pressure with endurance training (Hanson et al. [12]; Ekblom et al. [20]; Frick et al. [21]), but significant reduction in blood pressure of hypertensive patients placed in exercise programs was found (Boyer and Kusch [22]; Choquette and Ferguson [23]). Personal observation supports the concept of variation in blood pressure response to endurance training. The importance of initial blood pressures was pointed out (Hellerstein et al. [24]). If a person had low blood pressure before training, the pressure did not change, but if initially elevated, both resting systolic and diastolic pressures decreased significantly after aerobic conditioning, perhaps explaining some contradictory observations.

The mean arterial pressure in trained athletes at $\dot{V}O_{2max}$ may be increased, unchanged, or slightly decreased (Scheuer and Tipton [5]). Reduction in systolic blood pressure at $\dot{V}O_{2max}$ with aerobic training occurred in middle-aged men (Paolone et al. [2]), and significant ($p < 0.01$) decrease in the diastolic pressure from 86 mm Hg to 76 mm Hg was noted after 1 year of training, with further decline to 66 mm Hg after 2 years of modest aerobic training. With exercise, systolic pressure increases in normal subjects, but usually not above 210 mm Hg, and the diastolic pressure remains the same or is decreased (Hellerstein et al. [24]). If systolic blood pressure exceeds 220 mm Hg and the diastolic is above 95, the response to exercise is considered to be abnormal and suggests underlying hypertension (Hellerstein et al. [24]).

The mechanism for blood pressure change with exercise is based on the relationship of arterial blood pressure (BPa) to cardiac output (CO) and peripheral resistance (PR) (BPa = CO × PR). When exercise commences, skeletal muscle activation increases venous return and cardiac output. At the same time, the arterioles supplying the exercising muscles dilate, and peripheral vascular resistance decreases. The net result of these initial changes is decreased blood pressure. Early activation of the sympathetic nervous system and withdrawal of parasympathetic tone increases heart rate, stimulates the myocardium, and constricts splanchnic and renal arterial and venous beds, which raise cardiac output and peripheral vascular resistance. The overall result is increased arterial pressure or no change (Hellerstein et al. [24]). During exercise, plasma norepinephrine increases with the intensity of work, but in well-trained athletes the sympathetic response is less than in untrained individuals for the same work load (Hellerstein et al. [24]).

# Myocardial Contractility and Perfusion

Endurance training improves myocardial contractility, shown by increased mean ventricular ejection rate and maximal first derivative of the pressure pulse by as much as 35% (Hanson et al. [12]). Several studies of aerobically untrained rats showed increased cardiac actomyosin ATPase activity, which provides metabolic support for hemodynamic alterations implying improved myocardial contractility (Penpargkul and Scheuer [25]; Scheuer and Stezoski [26]; Bhan and Scheuer [27]).

Aerobic training appears to improve myocardial perfusion. The diameters of main coronary artery lumens were up to three times their usual width in necropsy studies of great endurance athletes (Currens and White [28]). Coronary arterial beds, estimated by the weight of vinyl acetate corrosion casts, were increased in aerobically trained rats (Tepperman and Pearlman [29]), and the ratio of the cross-sectional area of the coronary artery capillary lumen to ventricular muscle fibers was also increased with exercise (Mitchell [17]). The capillary:ventricular fiber ratios in exercise-trained rats from youth to old age were significantly increased for trained animals in another study (Tomanek [30]). Hypoxia produced by restriction of coronary blood flow in dogs caused increased collateral flow (Eckstein [31]). Mild circumflex coronary artery narrowing produced increased collateral blood flow only in the aerobically trained animals. In those with moderate to severe narrowing, both the trained and untrained animals showed increased collateral flow, but the effect was enhanced by endurance training. These studies support the concept that aerobic training improves both macro- and micro-coronary blood flow.

# Cardiac Hypertrophy

In contrast to skeletal muscle, cardiac muscle does not increase its respiratory capacity, but does hypertrophy in response to endurance training; therefore, trained athletes have larger hearts than sedentary controls of similar body weight (Morganroth et al. [3]; Holloszy [32]; Blair et al. [33]). Echocardiograms on college swimmers, runners, wrestlers, and control subjects showed that swimmers and runners had significantly ($p < 0.001$) larger left ventricular volumes. The swimmers, runners, and wrestlers had significantly ($p < 0.001$) larger left ventricular size, but only wrestlers had a significantly ($p < 0.001$) thicker ventricular wall. This finding indicates that endurance-trained athletes develop increased cardiac volume in contrast to wrestlers, whose exercise is mainly isometric and consequently leads to mural cardiac hypertrophy (Morganroth et al. [3]). When male national and international standard aerobically trained athletes were compared to matched untrained controls, both ventricles were significantly larger in the trained athletes. Left ventricular volume was 43% larger ($p < 0.002$), and right ventricular volume was 24% larger ($p < 0.005$) (Blair et al. [33]). Increased left ventricular size increases work capacity since positive correlation exists between heart size and maximal cardiac output (Holloszy [32]; Blair et al. [33]).

# Myocardial Oxygen Consumption

Myocardial oxygen consumption is determined by 1) basal oxygen requirement, 2) electrical activity, 3) internal work (tension × heart rate), 4) external work (load × shortening), and 5) the contractile state (Mitchell [17]; Sonnenblick et al. [34]). The basal oxygen requirement (Mitchell [17]) and oxygen consumed by electrical activity are low (Klocke et al. [35]). Oxygen consumption induced by internal work is about twice that induced by external work (Coleman et al. [36]; Sonnenblick et al. [37]). Tension, heart rate, and contractile state are the principal determinants of myocardial oxygen consumption (Mitchell [17]; Sonnenblick et al. [34]). Measurement of myocardial oxygen consumption is difficult at rest and almost impossible during exercise. For that reason a number of calculations that approximate myocardial oxygen consumption are used (Froelicker [10]; Mitchell [17]). The double product (peak systolic blood pressure × heart rate), the triple product (peak systolic blood pressure × heart rate × ejection time), and the tension-time index (area under the left ventricular or aortic pressure curve during systole × heart rate) are all used as estimates of myocardial oxygen consumption (Froelicker [10]; Hanson et al. [12]; Mitchell [17]).

Hanson et al. [12] demonstrated a significant reduction in tension-time index (myocardial oxygen consumption) with aerobic training in a group of middle-aged men at rest and at all levels of exercise; the greatest decrease occurred in the mid-range of exercise intensity. After 1 year of modest aerobic training, 45 middle-aged men had an 18% reduction in double product (myocardial oxygen consumption) (Paolone et al. [2]), which is important when the modest intensity of the program is considered. Although myocardial oxygen consumption is difficult to measure, aerobic training in man appears to reduce myocardial oxygen consumption both at rest and during exercise.

# Adaptations in Coronary Artery Disease

In patients with coronary artery disease (CAD), aerobic training produces many of the same cardiovascular adaptations that occur in normal people (Mitchell [17]; Hartley et al. [38]; Frick and Katila [39]; Lueker and Atterbom [40]), but the severity of CAD and the amount of functional cardiac muscle that is present may limit adaptation. Viable cardiac muscle and, to some extent, ischemic cardiac muscle (Scheuer and Stezoski [26]) can adapt, but areas of dyskinetic scar cannot. Regeneration of myocardial cells does not occur. Heart rate, at rest and with submaximal work, is decreased in patients with CAD after aerobic training (Frick and Katila [39]; Lueker and Atterbom [40]; Varnauskas et al. [41]; Clausen and Trap-Jensen [42]; Redwood et al. [43]). Stroke volume has not been consistently improved by aerobic training, a finding that is probably related to the extent of left ventricular scarring (Hartley et al. [38]). Frick and Katila [39] showed significant (p < 0.05) increase in stroke volume at submaximal work loads in 7 patients who had undergone modest aerobic training after suffering myocardial infarction, but the findings of Detry et al. [44] did not support this. Mean systemic blood pressure reduction at submaximal work load in aerobically trained patients with CAD was noted in several studies summarized by Hartley et al. (38). A significant reduction ($p < 0.02$) in systolic blood pressure from 153 to 137 mm Hg with modest aerobic training using stationary bicycle ergometers has also been found (Redwood et al. [43]).

Aerobic training almost uniformly improved $\dot{V}_{O_{2max}}$ (aerobic power) in patients with CAD (Mitchell [17]; Lueker and Atterbom [40]; Redwood et al. [43]; Detry et al. [44]). In patients with CAD but without angina, $V_{O_{2max}}$ increased by 18%, and in those with angina $V_{O_{2max}}$ increased by 30% after aerobic training (Detry et al. [44]). Four middle-aged male patients with extensive myocardial infarction complicated by left ventricular dysfunction and two patients with cardiogenic shock, all with severe diffuse coronary atherosclerosis and moderate reduction in left ventricular function, increased average predicted $\dot{V}_{O_{2max}}$ from 16 to 32 ml/kg/min, or 100%, after 9 months of aerobic training (Leuker and Atterbom [40]). When patients with left ventricular dysfunction and ejection fractions of 30% or less (normal $> 50\%$) were exercised on a treadmill, 50% had normal exercise tolerance in spite of significant left ventricular dysfunction, and some had incredible exercise capacity considering their degree of dysfunction. One such patient had an ejection fraction of only 14%, but was able to exercise on graded treadmill for 15.5 min (Sheffield protocol; normal $> 11$ min) (Benge et al. [45]).

Certain patients with CAD can perform high levels of aerobic work. Seven patients with previous myocardial infarctions completed the Boston Marathon after training (Kavanagh et al [46]). Their average race speed was 5.4 mph, corresponding to 81% of their $\dot{V}_{O_{2max}}$. Since most patients with CAD do not perform at maximal work loads, an increased $\dot{V}_{O_{2max}}$ allows the aerobically trained patient to work at submaximal loads at a lower percentage of maximal work capacity. Aerobic training improves exercise capacity before appearance of angina pectoris. Seven patients with previous myocardial infarction and angina pectoris increased the average $\dot{V}_{O_{2max}}$ at the onset of anginal pain from 9.6 to 15 ml/kg/min ($p < 0.01$), allowing them to cycle 6.8 min longer with 6 weeks of training (Redwood et al. [43]).

The mechanism by which patients with CAD improve exercise performance with aerobic training is unclear (Froelicker [10]; Mitchell [17]; Frick and Katila [39]; Varnauska et al. [41]; Clausen and Trap-Jensen [42]; Detry et al. [44]). Patients with CAD showed increased arteriovenous oxygen difference after aerobic training in one study (Detry et al. [44]) and no change during submaximal exercise load in another study (Frick and Katila [39]). No significant change in cardiac output, but increased stroke volume, was reported by two groups of investigators (Frick and Katila [39]; Clausen and Trap-Jensen [42]) while others (Varnauskas et al. [41]; Detry et al. [44]) reported decreased cardiac output during submaximal exercise after training. Cardiac output and arteriovenous oxygen difference at submaximal work loads are usually unchanged by training in normals. The increased arteriovenous oxygen difference during submaximal work in patients with CAD after training, therefore, supports the concept that improved peripheral extraction is more important than cardiac function in increasing work capacity of the trained CAD patient (Froelicker [10]). The relative importance of cardiac function and peripheral circulatory changes in exercise capacity after aerobic training varies from patient to patient, depending upon the extent of left ventricular dysfunction.

Several studies of CAD patients after exercise training suggest that there is reduced myocardial oxygen consumption at submaximal work loads (Frick and Katila [39]; Redwood et al. [43]; Detry et al. [44]). One study used the tension-time index (TTI) to show this (Frick and Katila [39]). In another study the exercise load required to produce angina pectoris was defined in 7 patients with CAD, and the triple product at that load was calculated (Redwood et al. [43]). The subjects then trained for 6 weeks and were retested at the same work load that had previously produced angina. Only 1 of the 7 experienced angina, and the triple product decreased from 4300 to 3521 (p < 0.025). The same subjects continued training with progressively increasing work loads until angina pectoris reappeared. A significant increase in triple product occurred at the onset of angina (4885 vs 4300; p < 0.05). These findings suggest that training reduces myocardial oxygen requirement at a given exercise load and may enhance myocardial oxygen delivery in patients with coronary artery disease.

# Adaptations with Aging

Aging is a progressive process that results in decline in work capacity, loss of flexibility, poor balance, and delayed reaction time. Obesity is also an accepted part of aging in many parts of the world. Fig. 12–1, an adaptation from Cantwell [47], illustrates the progressive decline in $\dot{V}_{O_{2max}}$ that occurs at all levels of physical fitness with aging. Fifty percent decline in $\dot{V}_{O_{2max}}$ occurs from age 30 to 70 years for the average fit person. This decline may be greater if the person is well-trained as a youth but not fit when older. The loss of work capacity is primarily due to reduction in maximal heart rate (Kasch [1]; Gertenblith et al. [48]; Kavanagh and Shephard [49]; Pollock [50]; Granath et al. [51]), stroke volume (Granath et al. [51]), and cardiac output (Kasch [1]; Granath et al. [51]). Increased systemic blood pressure (Kavanagh and Shephard [49]; Pollock [50]; Granath et al. [51]) and peripheral resistance (Kasch [1]) also occur, and both require increased left ventricular work.

Right heart catheterizations during recumbent exercise showed $O_2$ consumption of 1.46 L/min in men 60–83 years of age, compared to 2.06 L/min in men, average age 23 years (Granath et al. [51]). Cardiac output was also lower (13.1 L/min) in the older group compared to 18.5 L/min in the younger group. Heart rate and stroke volume were reduced in the older group, compared to the younger group. Systolic blood pressure was 39 mm Hg higher in the older group at maximal work load. Average pulmonary artery wedge pressure was 7 mm Hg higher in the older group. Higher pulmonary artery wedge pressures and left ventricular end-diastolic pressures were found in another study of older subjects during exercise (Tartulier et al. [52]). This suggests that the ventricle in the older person is less compliant and has increased resistance to filling at heavy work loads.

Since reduction in physical work capacity ($\dot{V}_{O_{2max}}$) is a recognized indicator of physiologic aging, it can be used to assess the effect of aerobic training on the aging process. Sedentary males 40–50 years of age have $\dot{V}_{O_{2max}}$ of 29–35 ml/kg/min (Kasch [1]; Pollock [50]), which places them in the low- to average-fitness category (Fig. 12-1). Comparison with Table 12-1 indicates that the older endurance runners have a high maximal work capacity for age (Pollock [50]). Even runners over 70 years of age had a 14% higher maximal work capacity than the sedentary 40- to 50-year-old men. Reduction in maximal work capacity (aerobic power) occurs with age, even in endurance-trained athletes, with the largest decrease appearing after the age of 70 (Kavanagh and Shephard

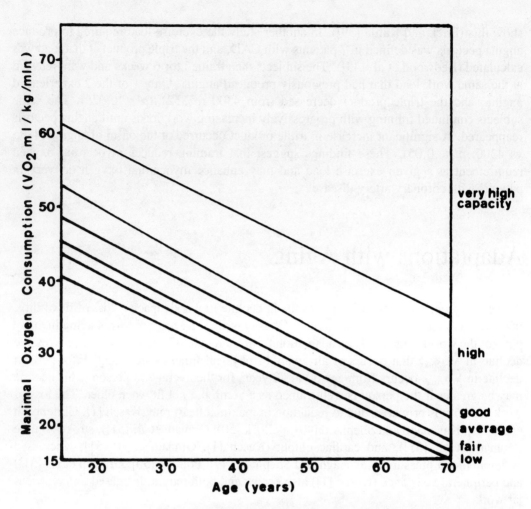

**12–1**   Decline in cardiopulmonary fitness with aging in untrained individuals. (Adapted from Cantwell, J.D. 1977. Stress testing indicated in a variety of complaints. Physician Sportsmed 5(2):70–74).

**Table 12-1**   Maximal $Vo_2$ (ml/kg/min) of Older Endurance Runners*

| Age (yr) | Kavanagh and Shephard (1977) | Pollock (1974) | Asano et al. (1976) | Grimby and Saltin (1966) |
|---|---|---|---|---|
| 40–50 | 49.9 | 57.5 | 49.7 | 57 |
| 50–60 | 46.0 | 54.4 | 45.1 | 53 |
| 60–70 | 41.6 | 51.4 | 42.2 | 43 |
| >70 | 29.0 | 40.0 | 38.9 | — |

*Adapted from Kavanagh, J., and Shephard, R.J. 1977. The effects of continued training on the aging process. Ann NY Acad Sci 301:656–670.

[49]; Pollock [50]). In older endurance competitors, a decrease of about 8 ml/kg/min of $\dot{V}O_{2max}$ (aerobic power) occurred from 35 to 65 years of age, compared to a steady decline in the average person of 4–5 ml/kg/min per decade from age 25 to 65 years (Kavanagh and Shephard [49]). The rate of decline of $\dot{V}O_{2max}$ is, therefore, 33%–45% slower in endurance-trained competitors compared to the average population. These studies were of competitive endurance athletes. What about the recreational aerobic runner? Sixteen active men, 45 years old, ran 24 km/wk for 10 years (Kasch [1]). At age 45 their average $\dot{V}O_{2max}$ was 43.1 ml/kg/min, placing them in the high maximal work capacity for age (Fig. 1). After 10 years of training, their average $\dot{V}O_{2max}$ was not significantly changed (44.4 ml/kg/min), but they were now in the very high work capacity range for age. Basically, these men kept their maximal work capacity stable over a 10-year period while maximal work capacity for the general population was declining.

Whether increased survival of older people or animals occurs as a result of exercise is not clear (Goodrick [54]). Mean longevity of 6-week-old male and female Wistar rats in either standard laboratory cages or in cages with activity wheels was 11.5% longer in female rats allowed voluntary exercise than in control female rats (p<0.01), and was 19.3% longer in male rats allowed voluntary exercise than the male controls (p<0.01) (Goodrick [54]). Although endurance training does not allow the immortality hoped for by some (Scaff [55]), it modifies many aspects of aging.

# References

1. Kasch, F.W. 1976. The effects of exercise on the aging process. Physician Sportsmed 4(6):64–69.

2. Paolone, A.M., Lewis, R.R., Lanigan, W.T., Goldstein, M.J. 1976. Results of two years of exercise training in middle-aged men. Physican Sportsmed 4(12):72–77.

3. Morganroth, J., Maron, B.J., Henry, H.L., Epstein, S.E. 1975. Comparative left ventricular dimensions. Ann Intern Med 82:521–524.

4. Lin, T., Horvath, S.M. 1972. Autonomic nervous control of cardiac frequency in the exercise-trained rat. J Appl Physiol 33:796–799.

5. Scheuer, J., Tipton, C.M. 1977. Cardiovascular adaptations to physical training. Ann Rev Physiol 39:221–251.

6. Lichtman, J., O'Rourke, R.A., Klein, A., Karliner, J.S. 1973. Electrocardiogram of the athlete. Arch Intern Med 132:763–770.

7. Rowell, L.B. 1974. Human cardiovascular adjustments to exercise and thermal stress. Physiol Rev 54:75–159.

8. Ekblom, B. 1969. Effect of physical training on oxygen transport system in man. Acta Physiol Scand [Suppl] 328:5–45.

9. Hartley, L.H., Mason, J.W., Hogan, R.P., Jones, L.G., Kotchen, T.A., Mougey, E.H., Wherry, F.E., Pennington, L.L., Ricketts, P.T. 1972. Multiple hormone responses to prolonged exercise in relation to physical training. J Appl Physiol 33:607–610.

10. Froelicker, V.F. 1976. The hemodynamic effects of physical conditioning in healthy young men and middle-aged individuals, and in coronary heart disease. In: Naughton J.P., Hellerstein H.K., (eds): Exercise Testing and Exercise Training in Coronary Heart Disease. Academic Press, New York, pp 63–77.

11. Clausen, J.P., Trap-Jensen, J., Lassen, N.A. 1971. Evidence that the relative exercise bradycardia induced by training can be caused by extra cardiac factors. In: Larsen O.A., Malmborg R.P., (eds): Coronary

Heart Disease and Physical Fitness. University Park Press, Baltimore, pp 27–28.

12. Hanson, J.S., Tabakin, B.S., Levy, A.M., Nedde, W. 1968. Long term physical training and cardiovascular dynamics in middle-aged men. Circulation 38:783–788.

13. Hartley, L.H., Grimby, G., Kilbom, A., Nilsson, N.J., Astrand, I., Bjure, J., Ekblom, B., Saltin, B. 1969. Physical training in sedentary middle-aged and older men. III. Cardiac output and gas exchange at submaximal and maximal exercise. Scand J Clin Lab Invest 24:335–344.

14. Wilmore, J.H. 1976. Football pros' strengths and CV weakness—charted. Physician Sportsmed 4(10):44–54.

15. Gettman, L.R., Pollock, M.L. 1977. What makes a superstar? A physiological profile. Physician Sportsmed 5(5):64–68.

16. Saltin, B., Astrand, P.O. 1967. Maximal oxygen uptake in athletes. J Appl Physiol 23:353–358.

17. Mitchell, J.H. 1975. Exercise training in the treatment of coronary heart disease. Adv Intern Med 20:249–272.

18. Cooper, K.H., Pollock, M.L., Martin, R.P., White, S.R., Linnerud, A.C., Jackson, A. 1976. Physical fitness levels vs. selected coronary risk factors. JAMA 236:166–169.

19. de Vries, H.A. 1970. Physiological effects of an exercise training regimen upon men aged 52 to 88. J Gerontol 25:325–336.

20. Ekblom, B., Astrand, P.O., Saltin, B., Steinberg, J., Wallstrom, B. 1968. Effect of training on circulatory responses to exercise. J Appl Physiol 24:518–528.

21. Frick, M.H., Konttinen, A., Sarajas, H.S.S. 1963. Effects of physical training on circulation at rest and during exercise. Am J Cardiol 12:142–147.

22. Boyer, J.L., Kasch, F.W. 1970. Exercise therapy in hypertensive men. JAMA 211:1668–1671.

23. Choquette, G., Ferguson, R.J. 1973. Blood pressure reduction in "borderline" hypertensives following physical training. Can Med Assoc J 108:699–703.

24. Hellerstein, H.K., Boyer, J.L., Hartley, L.H., Loggie, J. 1976. Exploring the effects of exercise on hypertension. Physician Sportsmed 4(12):36–49.

25. Penpargkul, S., Scheuer, J. 1970. The effect of physical training upon the mechanical and metabolic performance of the rat heart. J Clin Invest 49:1859–1868.

26. Scheuer, J., Stezoski, S.W. 1972. Effect of physical training on the mechanical and metabolic response of the rat heart of hypoxia. Circ Res 30:418–429.

27. Bhan, A.K., Scheuer, J. 1972. Effects of physical training on cardiac actomycin adenosine triphosphate activity. Am J Physiol 223:1486–1490.

28. Currens, J.H., White, P.D. 1961. Half a century of running. N Engl J Med 265:988–993.

29. Tepperman, J., Pearlman, D. 1961. Effects of exercise and anemia on coronary arteries of small animals as revealed by the corrosion-cast technique. Circ Res 9:576–584.

30. Tomanek, R.J. 1969. Effects of age and exercise on the extent of the myocardial capillary bed. Anat Rec 167:55–62.

31. Eckstein, R.W. 1957. Effect of exercise and coronary artery narrowing on coronary collateral circulation. Circ Res 5:230–235.

32. Holloszy, J.O. 1973. Long-term metabolic adaptations in muscle to endurance exercise. In: Naughton J.P., Hellerstein H.K., (eds): Exercise Testing and Exercise Training in Coronary Heart Disease. Academic Press, New York, pp 211–222.

33. Blair, N.L., Youker, J.E., McDonald, I.G., Telford, R., Jelinek, Y.M. 1980. Echocardiographic assessment of cardiac chamber size and left ventricular function in aerobically trained athletes. Aust N Z J Med 10:540–547.

34. Sonnenblick, E.H., Ross, J. Jr., Braunwald, E. 1968. Oxygen consumption of the heart: Newer concepts of its multifactorial determination. Am J Cardiol 22:328–336.

35. Klocke, F.H., Braunwald, E., Ross, J. Jr. 1966. Oxygen cost of electrical activation of the heart. Circ Res 18:357–365.

36. Coleman, H.N., Sonnenblick, E.H., Braunwald, E. 1969. Myocardial oxygen consumption associated with external work: The Fenn effect. Am J Physiol 217:291–296.

37. Sonnenblick, E.H., Ross, J. Jr., Covell, J.W., Kaiser, G.A., Braunwald, E. 1965. Velocity of contraction as a determinate of myocardial oxygen consumption. Am J Physiol 309:919–927.

38. Hartley, L.H., Jones, L.G., Mason, J. 1973. The usefulness of exercise therapy in the management of coronary heart disease. Adv Cardiol 9:174–202.

39. Frick, M.H., Katila, M. 1968. Hemodynamic consequences of physical training after myocardial infarction. Circulation 37:192–202.

40. Lueker, R.D., Atterbom, H.A. Improved maximum work capacity in patients with coronary artery disease and decreased left ventricular function after aerobic training. In preparation.

41. Varnauskas, E., Bergman, H., Houk, P., Bjorntorp, P. 1966. Haemodynamic effect of physical training in coronary patients. Lancet 2:8–12.

42. Clausen, J.P., Trap-Jensen, J. 1970. Effects of training on the distribution of cardiac output in patients with coronary artery disease. Circulation 42:611–624.

43. Redwood, D.R., Rosing, D.R., Epstein, S.E. 1972. Circulation and symptomatic effects of physical training in patients with coronary artery disease and angina pectoris. N Engl J Med 286:959–965.

44. Detry, J.R., Rousseau, M., Vandenbrowcke, G., Kusumi, F., Brasseur, L.A., Bruce, R.A. 1971. Increased arteriovenous oxygen difference after physical training in coronary artery disease. Circulation 44:109–118.

45. Benge, W., Litchfield, R.L., Marcus, M.M. 1980. Exercise capacity in patients with severe left ventricular dysfunction. Circulation 61:955–959.

46. Kavanagh, T., Shephard, T.H., Pandit, V. 1974. Marathon running after myocardial infarction. JAMA 229:1602–1605.

47. Cantwell, J.D. 1977. Stress testing indicated in a variety of complaints. Physician Sportsmed 5(2):70–74.

48. Gertenblith, G., Lakatta, E.G., Weisfeldt, M.L. 1976. Age changes in myocardial function and exercise response. Prog Cardiovasc Dis 19:1–21.

49. Kavanagh, T., Shephard, R.J. 1977. The effects of continued training on the aging process. Ann NY Acad Sci 301:656–670.

50. Pollock, M.L. 1974. Physiological characteristics of older champion track athletes. Res Q 45:363–373.

51. Granath, A., Jonsson, B., Strandell, T. 1964. Circulation in healthy old men, studied by right heart catheterization at rest and during exercise in supine and sitting position. Acta Med Scand 176:425–446.

52. Tartulier, M., Bourret, M., Deyrieux, F. 1972. Pulmonary arterial pressures in normal subjects, effects of age and exercise. Bull Physiopathol Resp 8:1295–1321.

53. Port, S., Cobb, F.R., Colman, R.E., Jones, R.H. 1980. Effect of age on the response of the left ventricular ejection fraction to exercise. N Engl J Med 303:1133–1137.

54. Goodrick, C.L. 1980. Effects of long-term voluntary wheel exercise on male and female Wistar rats. I. Longevity, body weight, and metabolic rate. Gerontology 26:22–23.

55. Scaff, J.H. Jr. 1977. People Weekly 7(9):88.

56. Asano, K., Ogawa, S., Furuta, T. 1976. Aerobic work capacity in middle and old-aged runners. International Congress of Physical Activity Sciences, Quebec City, Canada.

57. Grimby, G., Saltin, B. 1966. Physiological analysis of physically well trained middle-aged and old athletes. Acta Med Scand 179:513–539.

# Chapter 13

# Sudden Cardiac Death in Sports

by Jerry E. Goss

## Introduction

Sudden death is death within 6 h (WHO [1]) to 24 h (Kuller et al. [2]) after onset of symptoms, but sports-associated sudden death usually occurs within 30 sec (Pickering [3]). Instant death suggests fatal arrhythmia, usually ventricular fibrillation, followed by immediate circulatory collapse (Doyle [4]). The clinical setting for this situation exists during long-distance running, since plasma norepinephrine, potassium, and lactic acid are high, and ventricular premature contractions are frequent (Pickering [3]). Although uncommon in sports, sudden death is a dramatic event that gains attention.

## General Survey

Approximately 450,000 people die suddenly each year in the United States (DeSilva and Lown [5]), but relatively few sudden deaths are sports-related (DeSilva and Lown [5]; Vuori et al. [6]). Of 2606 sudden deaths in Finland, only 22 were associated with sports—16 with skiing, 2 with jogging, and 4 with other activities, an incidence of 0.8% compared to 2.2% incidence of sudden death among Finnish sauna bathers. Eight sudden deaths occurred among 1,030,000 ski hikers during a 16-year period (Vuori et al. [6]). The hikes were vigorous, covered from 30 to 90 km and lasted 5–11 h. In a small number of skiers, ages 32–64 years, mean heart rates during the hikes were between 132 and 165 beats per minute, or 80%–90% of maximal rates.

Twenty-one sudden deaths among athletes were reported in South African newspapers over 18 months, and 19 of them were probably of cardiac causes. The sports involved were: rugby, 7; refereeing, 4; soccer and tennis, 2 each; golf, mountaineering, jogging, and yachting, 1 each. Ages ranged from 17 to 58 years. One sudden death per 50,000 player-hours of rugby occurred, and the average age of death was 26 years. Sudden death among rugby referees was one per 3000 hours of refereeing, and the average age was 56 years.

Seven subjects with pathologic diagnoses showed advanced coronary atherosclerosis. Two others had ischemic heart disease, according to electrocardiographic evidence of acute myocardial infarction in one and a history of myocardial infarction in the other. In 7 athletes, chest pain preceded death; histories of angina and positive findings in exercise tests in the 7 were thought to be strong indications of ischemic heart disease. In 2 remaining athletes, the clinical picture was "suggestive" of ischemic heart disease (Opie [7]). There have been several reports of myocardial infarction with classic electrocardiographic changes in athletes in whom the coronary arteries were found to be normal at autopsy (Green et al. [8]; Kimbiris et al. [9]; Maron et al. [10]). Chest pain may be a feature of other potentially lethal forms of heart disease such as hypertrophic cardiomyopathy, valvular aortic stenosis, coronary artery anomalies, and mitral valve prolapse. Therefore, chest pain alone cannot be the sole criterion for a diagnosis of ischemic heart disease.

Shephard [11] estimated one sudden death per 2500 gymnasium hours among middle-aged businessmen who attended unsupervised gymnasium programs. The estimate was based on reports reaching Ontario newspapers. Ventricular fibrillation occurred less often in supervised programs (Shephard [11]; Pyfer [12]). Pyfer [12] reported eight episodes of ventricular fibrillation occurring over a period of 50,000 gymnasium hours in Seattle, and at the Toronto Rehabilitation Center one episode occurred in over 100,000 man-hours of exercise (Shephard [11]).

Autopsy studies of 29 competitive athletes showed that death occurred during or shortly after strenuous exercise in 22 (Maron et al. [10]). Subjects included 26 men and 3 women, 20 whites and 9 blacks. Ages ranged from 13 to 30 years. Eleven athletes competed in basketball, 10 in football, 4 in track, 3 in wrestling, and 1 each in swimming, boxing, soccer, tennis, baseball, and gymnastics. Pathologic diagnoses included hypertrophic cardiomyopathy in 14, anomalous origin of the left coronary artery from the anterior sinus of Valsalva in 4, and coronary atherosclerosis in 3. Rupture of the aorta, due to Marfan's syndrome, occurred in 2. Five had idiopathic concentric left ventricular hypertrophy; 2 of these athletes also had narrowed atrioventricular node arteries. In 1 subject both leaflets of the mitral valve prolapsed. The only autopsy findings in 1 athlete were smaller-than-normal branches from the left circumflex and right coronary arteries to the posterior ventricular wall. The remaining subject had no discernible cardiac abnormality, but complete examination of the conduction system was not possible.

# Sudden Death Associated with Running

With the increase in the popularity of running as a recreational and competition sport for all ages, the occurrence of sudden death during or after a run has drawn attention (Pyfer [12]; Thompson et al. [13]; Noakes and Opie [14]; Noakes et al. [15]; Waller et al. [16]; Thompson et al. [17]). Autopsy findings in 18 persons who died while jogging or immediately afterward showed that 13 men died of coronary artery disease, and 4 men and 1 woman died of other causes (Thompson et al. [13]). One subject had myocardial lymphocytic infiltrate suggesting myocarditis, and another died of heat stroke. Three remaining subjects had no clear diagnosis although unexplained myocardial fibrosis was present in 2, suggesting that myocardial bridging was present but unnoticed. Morales et al. [18] report three cases of sudden death during exercise in which myocardial bridging was found at autopsy. During rapid heart rate, contraction of bridging muscle may constrict coronary arteries and narrow their lumens more than 75%. Bridging usually involves the left anterior descending coronary artery. The combination of arterial narrowing during systole plus short diastolic filling time can compromise blood supply to the septum. In such cases, focal scarring has been seen in septal areas.

Sudden death in marathon runners from advanced coronary atherosclerosis (Noakes and Opie [14]; Noakes et al. [15]; Waller et al. [16]) helps lay to rest the myth that marathon running provides complete immunity from this disorder (Bassler and Cardello [19]). One 44-year-old subject had completed eight marathons and two ultramarathons during the 14 months prior to his sudden death. He was a nonsmoker, but serum cholesterol was 298 mg/dl, high-density lipoprotein cholesterol was 43 mg/dl, and triglycerides were 145 mg/dl, unexpected values for a marathon runner. Sudden death occurred at 19 km in a 24-km road race.

Autopsy showed healed anteroseptal infarction with grade IV (75%–100%) atherosclerotic narrowing 5 mm from the origin of the left anterior descending artery, and at 15 mm from its origin, it was occluded by an organized thrombus in which recanalization had occurred. The left circumflex coronary artery showed grade IV eccentric atherosclerotic narrowing 3.5 cm from its origin. Special staining and chemical studies were consistent with acute infarction of the posterior wall (Noakes et al. [15]).

The second death was that of a 41-year-old athlete who had run marathons for 2 years prior to acute inferior myocardial infarction. Angiography confirmed inferior infarction and showed complete occlusion of the left circumflex coronary artery and 50% narrowing in the proximal right coronary, with minor irregularities of the lumen in the left anterior descending coronary artery. Cholesterol was 265 mg/dl, and triglycerides, 235 mg/dl. He had smoked pipes and up to three cigarettes per day for 20 years, but stopped after the infarction. He was advised to continue jogging but not to participate in marathon races. In the 28 months following infarction he logged 3624 km and completed five marathons.

Thirty-one months after infarction he was admitted to the hospital with unstable angina. Coronary angiography showed progression of the atherosclerotic narrowings. The left circumflex was unchanged, with total occlusion, but the right coronary had progressed from 50% narrowing to total occlusion, and the left anterior descending, from irregularities of the lumen to 80% narrowing. While in the hospital awaiting coronary bypass surgery, he developed acute anterolateral infarction followed by death within 1.5 h.

Autopsy revealed severe advanced coronary atherosclerosis, which included grade IV narrowing in the left anterior descending coronary artery and superimposed total occlusion by fresh thrombus. The left circumflex was totally occluded by long-standing organized thrombus, and the right coronary had grade IV narrowing, with total occlusion by recent organized thrombus (Noakes et al. [15]).

Waller [16] described five cases of sudden death in conditioned runners over 40 years of age, two of whom were marathoners. All five had severe three-vessel disease at autopsy. Both marathon runners had systemic hypertension and hypercholesterolemia with total cholesterol values of 310 mg/dl and 305 mg/dl. One year before death the more experienced marathoner had an HDL cholesterol of 41 mg/dl while running an average of 173 km per week. He had been running for 10 years and had completed six Boston marathons and seven 80-km JFK races. He had had angina pectoris with running for 2 years and positive treadmill stress tests without pain on two occasions.

In all four cases, advanced coronary atherosclerosis developed while the runners were actively engaged in marathoning. These case reports (Noakes and Opie [14]; Noakes et al. [15]; Waller et al. [16]) are important, for most runners and physicians believe in the Bassler hypothesis (Bassler and Cardello [19]), and distance runners may ignore important symptoms because of this unproven popular belief that promises immunity from atherosclerotic cardiovascular events. These reports should caution middle-aged distance runners. Serum lipids in the four cases were striking: All four men had high serum cholesterol, and high-density lipoprotein cholesterol was low in the two runners in whom it was measured (Hooper and Eaton [20]). The abnormal lipids are the most apparent reason these four marathoners developed advanced coronary atherosclerosis, and their demise might have been sooner if they had not been long-distance runners.

When a person dies during or immediately after running, it is assumed that the exercise caused the death. Koplan [21] estimated the number of cardiac deaths that might occur by chance alone during running. If runners live a marathoner's life style, four cardiac deaths while running are expected per year in the United States. If the runners' life-style is that of the average white American male, then 15 deaths per year are expected. If the running period includes 2 h after exercise, expected cardiac deaths are increased to 34 and 119, respectively. The average runner's risk of death during running is somewhere between these two extremes. Without an accurate method for recording deaths during running, it is impossible to say whether a given death was a chance occurrence or was directly related to the last run.

Using information from the Office of the Rhode Island State Medical Examiner and a random-digit telephone survey, it was estimated that one death per 7,620 joggers per year occurred in Rhode Island from 1975 to 1980 (Thompson et al. [17]). Although this estimated risk of death is higher than that of Koplan [21], both studies indicate that exercise risk is small, and suggest that routine pretraining exercise testing of asymptomatic adults, who are without significant risk factors for coronary artery disease, is not justified.

The more common causes of sudden death in sports are considered in detail below, with special consideration given to detection and prevention.

## Hypertrophic Cardiomyopathy

Hypertrophic cardiomyopathy, a genetically transmitted disease of cardiac muscle characterized by disproportionate thickening of the ventricular septum (Maron et al. [22]), has frequently been associated with sudden death (Shephard [11]; Maron et al. [22]; Lambert et al. [23]; Sturner and Spruill [24]; Evans et al. [25]). The hearts of 22 patients with this disorder showed multiple abnormalities in all parts of the conducting system, which could be responsible for electrical instability and ventricular fibrillation (James and Marshall [26]). Sudden death has been recognized in symptomatic patients, but most symptomatic patients do not compete in sports.

Maron et al. [22] studied 26 patients in whom sudden death was the first symptom of disease, and 13 of these persons died suddenly during or immediately after moderate to heavy physical exertion. Five were competitive athletes. This group had two characteristics: 1) an abnormal electrocardiogram, usually showing left ventricular hypertrophy, and 2) a moderately to severely thickened interventricular septum revealed at autopsy. Evans et al. [25] reported sudden death in two 17-year-old brothers while playing basketball, with pathologic changes of hypertrophic cardiomyopathy.

Symptoms associated with hypertrophic cardiomyopathy include chest pain, exertional dyspnea, palpitations, and syncope. Physicians frequently are not alert to the importance of these symptoms in young people. Asymptomatic patients with this disorder may have a systolic murmur at the lower left sternal border and apex. When a patient has the symptoms described and/or murmur, if the echocardiogram shows disproportional hypertrophy of the intraventricular septum, and the electrocardiogram indicates left ventricular hypertrophy, one should consider advising the patient to limit physical activity.

## Coronary Artery Anomalies

The incidence of aberrant origin of the coronary arteries is about 0.6% (Liberthson et al. [27]; Kimbiris et al. [28]). In most cases this is a benign condition. However, origin of the left coronary artery from the pulmonary artery is often associated with heart failure in early life and, if not discovered and treated, can result in death. This anomaly has rarely been associated with sudden death during sports (Jokl and Melzer [29]; McClelland and Jokl [30]). The coronary artery anomaly most often associated with exertional sudden death is at the origin of the left coronary from the anterior sinus of Valsalva. The vessel then passes obliquely between the aorta and the pulmonary artery (Shephard [11]; Liberthson et al. [27]; Kimbiris et al. [28]; McClellan and Jokl [30]; Tunstall-Pedoe [31]; Cheitlin et al. [32]; Schaumburg and Simonsen [33]).

The most plausible mechanism of exertional sudden death with this anomaly related to compromise of the lumen of the coronary artery by the angle formed as it arises from the anterior sinus of Valsalva (Cheitlin et al. [32]). The first part of the left main coronary artery may also be encased in the wall of the aorta (Kimbiris et al. [28]). With increased expansion of the aorta during exercise, the already slit-like opening of the left coronary artery may be further occluded (Cheitlin et al. [32]). Clinical recognition of this anomaly depends upon careful evaluation of young athletes with symptoms of exertional chest pain or syncope. Treadmill exercise testing and coronary angiography are used to make the diagnosis, and if established, enlargement of the slit-like ostia corrects the exertional ischemia (Cheitlin et al. [32]).

## Atherosclerotic Coronary Heart Disease

Atherosclerosis of the coronary arteries is a disease of all age groups (Opie [7]; Green et al. [8]; Shephard [11]; Noakes and Opie [14]; Noakes et al. [15]; Koskenvuo et al. [34]). Its occurrence in young athletes is always a surprise, and risk factors may be lacking. On the other hand, many middle-aged athletes smoke cigarettes, are hypertensive, have abnormal serum lipids, are diabetic, have a strong family history of atherosclerosis, or have stress-filled lives. Although exercise may modify many risk factors of coronary artery disease (CAD), (Wood et al. [35]; Cooper et al. [36]; Paolone et al. [37]), it cannot make an athlete immune to its development.

Many middle-aged athletes have well-developed CAD before starting to exercise, and symptoms develop with increased physical activity. Exercise in the presence of significant CAD can cause ischemia and transient angina pectoris, life-threatening myocardial infarction, or sudden death. Which condition occurs depends upon the extent of disease and the clinical setting. Those who might benefit the most from an exercise program also are most often at risk from exercise.

No large experience exists for successfully screening individuals before they start on an exercise program, and controversy prevails among those with limited experience (Vuori et al. [6]; Thompson et al. [13]). Persons with significant risk factors for development of CAD should have treadmill testing to identify exercise-induced ischemia or arrhythmia before they start physical fitness programs. Those with known CAD should be supervised in a coronary rehabilitation program to minimize risks (Green et al. [8]).

Prodromal symptoms before exercise-induced cardiac events are common (Opie [7]; Thompson et al. [13]; Waller et al. [16]), but denial by the patient is also common, and the exaggerated claims for the benefits of exercise may contribute to this denial (Noakes et al. [38]). Physicians are also vulnerable to the same claims and may underestimate the significance of new symptoms in athletes. Thompson et al. [13] and others (Opie [7]; Noakes et al. [15]) pointed out great variation in exercise capacity in subjects whose sudden death was associated with physical activity. The veteran superior athlete is at risk for exercise-induced sudden death, as well as the beginning or middle-aged exercise enthusiast.

This discussion is not meant to discourage sports in mid and later life but is intended to place the risks involved in perspective. Casualties will continue to occur no matter how careful the screening.

# Myocarditis

In a cooperative international study (Lambert et al. [23]) involving 20 pediatric cardiac centers in 10 countries, acute myocarditis accounted for 5% of sudden unexpected deaths, but none were associated with exertion. Sudden death associated with exercise and myocarditis has been reported (Thompson et al. [13]; Jokl and Melzer [29]; Jokl [39]), and several anecdotal reports exist of athletes dying during or shortly after a run to "sweat out" influenza or coryza (Tunstall-Pedoe [31]). Cardiac arrhythmias are common in myocarditis, and presumably death occurs from an arrhythmia potentiated by exercise (Tunstall-Pedoe [31]). Myocardial involvement may be detected during or shortly after even mild viral infections (Tunstall-Pedoe [31]; Barlow [40]; Burch [41]). Verel et al. [42] found that 43% of patients seen during an epidemic of A2 influenza had electrocardiographic changes. Other studies have reported electrocardiographic changes in 14%–76% of patients with influenza (Gibson et al. [43]; Walsh et al. [44]). Nonspecific ST segment and T-wave changes are the earliest and most common indicators of myocardial involvement, and when present should indicate temporary restriction of athletic activities. Severe exertion during or in early convalescence from an acute viral febrile illness is potentially dangerous and should be discouraged.

## Valvular Aortic Stenosis

With critical stenosis of the aortic valve, exercise produces marked elevation of left ventricular pressure, and normal cardiac output may not occur. When the stenosis is present, along with a thickened left ventricle, coronary perfusion may be inadequate for the muscle mass. This produces a relatively ischemic myocardium, which in turn may cause progressive electrical instability and ventricular fibrillation. In the international cooperative study reported by Lambert et al. [23] 38 children died suddenly as a result of valvular aortic stenosis, but only 5 of the deaths occurred during sports. To determine which patients with aortic stenosis were at risk for sudden death, Doyle et al. [45] reviewed the literature and found that most cases were associated with symptoms and/or severe electrocardiographic changes. Left ventricular hypertrophy with "strain pattern" was observed in 70% of reported cases of sudden death and only 9% of electrocardiograms were normal (Doyle et al. [45]). Most patients with mild to moderately severe aortic stenosis are asymptomatic, but in cases of sudden death one or more of the following symptoms were present: easy fatigability, chest pain, exertional dyspnea, or syncope.

All athletes with valvular aortic stenosis should undergo thorough history-taking, physical examination, and electrocardiogram. If these are consistent with mild stenosis, further studies and limitations are not indicated. If more significant stenosis is suspected, cardiac catheterization should be performed and the transvalvular gradient at rest and exercise should be assessed. The severity of the stenosis can be determined, and the patient can be counseled regarding participation in sports. Aortic stenosis is a progressive disease; therefore, continued observation for appearance of symptoms and electrocardiographic changes is necessary. Cardiac catheterization studies (Cohen et al. [46]; El-Said et al. [47]) may be repeated to identify progression and, it is hoped, prevent sudden death.

## Prolapsed Mitral Valve Leaflet

Mitral valve leaflet prolapse is characterized by valvular redundancy and myxomatous thickening of the mitral leaflets, with elongation of the chordae tendineae (Marshall and Shappell [48]). It is most commonly found in young women who complain of nonspecific chest pain, palpitations, and dizziness. On physical examination, a mid to late systolic click and/or a mid to late systolic murmur of mitral regurgitation can be heard. The electrocardiogram may show nonspecific ST–T wave changes in the inferior leads and borderline prolongation of the QT interval (Marshall and Shappell [48]). Echocardiogram and cineangiography will show prolapse of the posterior leaflet or of both leaflets of the mitral valve. The deformity is associated with arrhythmias and sudden death (Marshall and Shappell [48]; Swartz et al. [49]). In a literature review, 6.1% of patients had supraventricular tachycardia, 6.3% had ventricular tachycardia, and 1.4% (8 patients) died suddenly (Swartz et al. [49]).

Delayed repolarization arrhythmias have a prolonged QT interval with delayed recovery of parts of the myocardium. This is the essential ingredient to the occurrence of reentrant arrhythmias such as ventricular tachycardia (Han and Goel [50]). In 94 patients with mitral valve prolapse, 44 (47%) had prolonged QT interval during rest (Swartz et al. [49]). Prolonged QT interval has also been reported in patients with prolapsed mitral valve disease during exercise (Pocock and Barlow [51]).

Mitral valve prolapse has been reported in 6%–10% of asymptomatic young women (Brown et al. [52]; Markiewicz et al. [53]), a finding that could present a formidable problem in determining who should participate in sports. Restriction from sports should be advised only if the patient has paroxysmal ventricular tachycardia that is poorly controlled. Many women complain of postexercise palpitations that are not significant when evaluated by Holter and treadmill exercise testing. The threat of sudden death with this deformity, however, has been overemphasized and has caused undue anxiety and limitation for many patients (Jeresaty [54]).

# Activity Guidelines
# for Patients with Heart Disease

It is impossible to classify the energy requirements of sporting or recreational activities, as people pursue them with different degrees of vigor. For example, swimming may require energy expenditure of less than 5 cal/min or may require more than 20 cal/min, depending upon the individual intensity of performance (American Heart Association [55]). A person's skill also determines the amount of energy expenditure in a particular sport. Since many variables exist, a sports participation and skills history must be obtained so that more accurate prescriptions of activities can be outlined. Treadmill exercise testing with maximal oxygen consumption can be helpful in verifying the safety of the proposed exercise prescription.

Sports requiring isometric work, such as weight lifting, wrestling, and gymnastics, demand special consideration because of a disproportionate increase in systemic blood pressure relative to oxygen consumption (American Heart Association [55]). Although specific information is not available regarding the effects of transient systemic blood pressure elevation, it seems wise to discourage patients with left ventricular outflow obstruction, aortic insufficiency, significant coarctation of the aorta (American Heart Association [55]), and moderate or severe hypertension from participating in sports that require primarily isometric work.

Patients who have had repair of congenital defects and are without symptoms may be too casually evaluated. Special attention should be given to patients who have undergone total repair of tetralogy of Fallot. Trifascicular block and right bundle branch block with premature ventricular contractions have been associated with a high incidence of sudden death in this group (Quattlebaum et al. [56]), but none of these deaths were associated with sports. If a patient with repaired tetralogy of Fallot seeks advice regarding sports participation, the presence or absence of right bundle branch block or trifascicular block should be determined. If either is present, the patient should have Holter monitoring and treadmill exercise testing before a decision on sports participation is made. If significant ventricular arrhythmia is present, the patient should receive appropriate antiarrhythmic therapy and should be advised that moderate restriction be observed in choosing sports activities.

# References

1. World Health Organization. 1970. Report of the 4th working group with revised operating protocol. Working Group on Ischemic Heart Disease Registers, June 29–July 1, 1970, Copenhagen. Regional Office for Europe, World Health Organization, EURO 5010(4), Copenhagen.

2. Kuller, L., Lillienfeld, A., Fisher, R. 1967. An epidemiological study of sudden and unexpected death in adults. Medicine 46:341–361.

3. Pickering, T.G. 1979. Jogging, marathon running, and the heart. Am J Med 66:717–719.

4. Doyle, J.T. 1975. Profile of risk of sudden death in apparently healthy people. Circulation 52(suppl 3):176–179.

5. DeSilva, R.A., Lown, B. 1978. Ventricular premature beats, stress, and sudden death. Psychosomatics 19:649–661.

6. Vuori, I., Mäkäräinen, M., Jääskeläinen, A. 1978. Sudden death and physical activity. Cardiology 63:287–304.

7. Opie, L.H. 1975. Sudden death and sport. Lancet 1:263–266.

8. Green, L.H., Cohen, S.I., Kurland, G. 1976. Fatal myocardial infarction in marathon racing. Ann Intern Med 85:704–706.

9. Kimbiris, D., Segal, B.L., Munir, M., Katz, M., Likoff, W. 1972. Myocardial infarction in patients with normal patient coronary arteries as visualized by cineangiography. Am J Cardiol 29:724–728.

10. Maron, B.J., Roberts, W.C., McAllister, H.A., Rosing, D.R., Epstein, S.E. 1980. Sudden death in young athletes. Circulation. 62:218–229

11. Shephard, R.J. 1974. Sudden death—a significant hazard of exercise. Br J Sports Med 8:101–110.

12. Pyfer, H. 1974. Group exercise rehabilitation for cardiopulmonary patients. A five year study. 20th World Congress of Sports Medicine, Melbourne.

13. Thompson, P.D., Stern, M.P., Williams, P., Duncan, K., Haskell, W.L., Wood, P.D. 1979. Death during jogging or running, JAMA 242:1265–1267.

14. Noakes, T.D., Opie, L.H. 1979. Marathon running and heart: The South African experience. Am Heart J 98:669–671.

15. Noakes, T.D., Opie, L.H., Rose, A.G., Kleynhans, P.H.T. 1979. Autopsy proven coronary atherosclerosis in marathon runners. N Engl J Med 301:86–89.

16. Waller, B.F., Roberts, W.C. 1980. Sudden death while running in conditioned runners aged 40 years or over. Am J Cardiol 45:1292–1300.

17. Thompson, P.D., Funk, E.J., Carleton, R.A., Sturner, W.Q. 1982. Incidence of death during jogging in Rhode Island from 1975 through 1980. JAMA 247:2535–2538.

18. Morales, A.R., Romanelli, R., Boucek, R.J. 1980. The mural left anterior descending coronary artery, strenuous exercising, and sudden death. Circulation. 62:230–237.

19. Bassler, T.J., Cardello, F.P. 1976. Fiber feeding and atherosclerosis. JAMA 235:1841–1842.

20. Hooper, P.L., Eaton, R.P. 1978. Exercise, high density lipoprotein and coronary heart

disease. In: Appenzeller O., Atkinson R. (eds): Health Aspects of Endurance Training, Vol. 12, Medicine and Sport Series. Karger, Basel, pp 72–84.

21. Koplan, J.P. 1979. Cardiovascular deaths while running. JAMA 242:2578–2579.

22. Maron, B.J., Roberts, W.C., Edwards, J.E., McAllister, H.A., Foley, D.D., Epstein, S.E. 1978. Sudden death in patients with hypertrophic cardiomyopathy: Characterization of 26 patients without functional limitation. Am J Cardiol 41:803–810.

23. Lambert, E.C., Menon, V.A., Wagner, H.R., Vlad, P. 1974. Sudden expected death from cardiovascular disease in children. Am J Cardiol 34:89–96.

24. Sturner, W.Q., Spruill, F.G. 1974. Asymmetrical hypertrophy of the heart: Two sudden deaths in adolescents. J Forensic Sci 19:565–571.

25. Evans, A.T., Korndorffer, W.E., Boor, P.J. 1980. Sudden death of two brothers while playing basketball: Familial hypertrophic cardiomyopathy. Texas Med J 76:45–51.

26. James, T.N., Marshall, T.K. 1975. Asymmetrical hypertrophy of the heart. Circulation 51:1149–1166.

27. Liberthson, R.R., Dinsmore, R.E., Bharati, S., Rubenstein, J.J., Caulfield, J., Wheeler, E.O., Harthorne, J.W., Lev, M. 1974. Aberrant coronary artery origin from the aorta, Circulation 59:744–779.

28. Kimbiris, D., Iskandrian, A.S., Segal, B.L., Bemis, C.E. 1978. Anomalous aortic origin of coronary arteries. Circulation 58:606–615.

29. Jokl, E., Melzer, L. 1971. Acute fatal nontraumatic collapse during work and sport. In: Jokl, E., McClellan, J.T. (eds): Exercise and Cardiac Death, Vol. 5, Medicine and Sport Series. Karger, Basel, pp 5–18.

30. McClellan, J.T., Jokl, E. 1971. Congenital anomalies of coronary arteries as cause of sudden death associated with physical exertion. In: Jokl, E., McClellan, J.T. (eds): Exercise and Cardiac Death, Vol. 5, Medicine and Sport Series. Karger, Basel, pp 91–98.

31. Tunstall-Pedoe, D. 1979. Exercise and sudden death. Br J Sports Med 12:215–219.

32. Cheitlin, M.D., DeCastro, C.M., McAllister, H.A. 1974. Sudden death as a complication of anomalous left coronary origin from the anterior sinus of Valsalva. Circulation 50:780–787.

33. Schaumburg, H., Simonsen, J. 1978. Sudden death due to congenital malformation of the left coronary artery: A case report. Forensic Sci Int 12:83–85.

34. Koskenvuo, K., Karvonen, M.J., Rissanen, V. 1978. Death from ischemic heart disease in young Finns aged 15 to 24 years. Am J Cardiol 42:114–118.

35. Wood, P.D., Haskell, L., Stern, M.P., Lewis, S., Perry, C. 1977. Plasma lipoprotein distribution in male and female runners. Ann NY Acad Sci 301:748–763.

36. Cooper, K.H., Pollock, M.L., Martin, R.P., White, S.R., Linnerud, A.C., Jackson, A. 1976. Physical fitness levels vs. selected coronary risk factors. JAMA 236:166–169.

37. Paolone, A.M., Lewis, R.R., Lanigan, W.R., Goldstein, M.J. 1976. Results of two years' training in middle-aged men. Physician Sportsmed 4(12):72–77.

38. Noakes, T., Opie, L., Beck, W., McKechnie, J., Benchionol, A., Desser, K. 1977. Coronary heart disease in marathon runners. Ann NY Acad Sci 301:593–619.

39. Jokl, E. 1971. Sudden death after exercise due to myocarditis. In: Jokl, E., McClellan, J.T. (eds): Exercise and Cardiac Death, Vol. 5, Medicine and Sport Series. Karger, Basel, pp 99–101.

40. Barlow, J.B. 1976. Exercise, rugby, football and infection. S Afr Med J 50:1351.

41. Burch, G.E. 1976. Of URI and cardiomyopathy. Am Heart J 91:538.

42. Verel, D., Warrack, A.J.N., Potter, C.W., Ward, C., Richards, D.F. 1976. Observations on the A2 England influenza epidemic. Am Heart J 92:290–299.

43. Gibson, T.C., Arnold, J., Craige, E., Curnen, G.C. 1959. Electrocardiographic studies in Asian influenza. Am Heart J 57:661–668.

44. Walsh, J., Burch, G.E., White, A., Mogabgab, W., Digtlein, L. 1958. A study of the effects of type A (Asian strain) influenza on the cardiovascular system. Ann Intern Med 49:502–528.

45. Doyle, E.F., Arumugham, P., Lara, E., Rutkowski, M.R., Kiely, B. 1974. Sudden death in young patients with congenital aortic stenosis. Pediatrics 53:481–489.

46. Cohen, L.S., Friedman, W.F., Braunwald, E. 1972. Natural history of mild congenital aortic stenosis elucidated by serial hemodynamic studies. Am J Cardiol 30:1–5.

47. El-Said, G., Galioto, F.M., Mullins, C.E., McNamara, D.G. 1972. Natural hemodynamic history of congenital aortic stenosis in childhood. Am J Cardiol 30: 6–12.

48. Marshall, C.E., Shappell, S.D. 1974. Sudden death and the ballooning posterior leaflet syndrome. Arch Pathol 98:134–138.

49. Swartz, M.H., Terchholz, L.E., Donoso, E. 1977. Mitral valve prolapse. A review of associated arrhythmias. Am J Med 62:377–389.

50. Han, J., Goel, B.G. 1972. Electrophysiologic precursors of ventricular tachyarrhythmias. Arch Intern Med 129:749–755.

51. Pocock, W.A., Barlow, J.B. 1980. Post exercise arrhythmias in the billowing posterior mitral leaflet syndrome. Am Heart J 80:740–745.

52. Brown, O.R., Kloster, F.E., DeMots, H. 1975. Incidence of mitral valve prolapse in the asymptomatic normal. Circulation 51(suppl 2):77 (abstract).

53. Markiewicz, W., Stoner, J., London, E., Hunt, S.A., Popp, R.L. 1975. Mitral valve prolapse in one hundred presumably healthy females. Circulation 51(suppl 2):77 (abstract).

54. Jeresaty, R.M. 1976. Sudden death in the mitral valve prolapse-click syndrome. Am J Cardiol 37:317–318.

55. Ad Hoc Committee on Rehabilitation of the Young Cardiac, Council on Cardiovascular Disease in the Young, American Heart Association. 1976. Activity guidelines for young patients with heart disease. Physician Sportsmed 4(8):47–52.

56. Quattlebaum, T.G., Varghese, P.J., Neill, C.A., Donahoo, J.S. 1976. Sudden death among postoperative patients with tetralogy of Fallot. Circulation 54:289–293.

# Chapter 14

# Lipids and Sports: Protection from Coronary Artery Disease

by Philip L. Hooper and R. Philip Eaton

Coronary artery disease in the United States accounts for 650,000 deaths annually at a cost of over $28.5 billion per year (American Heart Association [1]). The magnitude of personal tragedy associated with these deaths is immeasurable. In spite of many scientific advances, the epidemic of coronary artery disease (CAD) continues. However, recent mortality statistics have shown a modest decline in CAD deaths (Gordon and Thom [2]). Increased exercise, better management of heart disease, prudent diets, and less cigarette smoking are factors thought to have contributed to this decline. The number of participants in endurance sports such as jogging, swimming, bicycling, and cross-country skiing is increasing. The enthusiasm for exercise is best evidenced by the increasing number of joggers and bicyclists on city streets. People exercise to reduce their waistlines, to heighten enjoyment of life, and to improve their well-being. Many people exercise because they believe that exercise reduces the risk of CAD.

## Exercise and Coronary Artery Disease

Epidemiologic studies have isolated physical activity as a protective factor against CAD. Morris [3] examined death certificates and occupations of 2 million middle-aged men in Great Britain. He found lower CAD mortality in those with higher levels of job-related physical activity. A study of 31,000 London transport employees compared sedentary bus drivers with more active bus conductors (Froelicher and Oberman [4]). The sedentary drivers had 1.5 times higher rate of CAD deaths and twice the incidence of sudden death after the first myocardial infarction. Both studies have been criticized because job selection created a natural bias.

Paffenbarger et al. [5] reported a 22-year follow-up of 3686 longshoremen in San Francisco. Work energy requirements were determined from measurements of oxygen consumption in each job assignment. When CAD risk factors such as cigarette smoking, blood pressure, and cholesterol were taken into account, the study revealed that workers having jobs with high energy output had one-third the incidence of fatal CAD, compared to workers with less active jobs.

In another study (Paffenbarger et al. [6]), physical activity as an index of CAD risk was studied in 16,936 Harvard male alumni. Those who had not been particularly athletic as students but who had a high level of physical activity in middle age were at lower risk of heart attack than were former athletes whose later exercise levels were low. Furthermore, they found that middle-aged men who exerted less than 2000 kcal in exercise per week had 64% higher risk of CAD than alumni who exerted more than 2000 kcal per week.

Other retrospective epidemiologic studies seem to support the concept that regular vigorous exercise reduces morbidity and mortality from CAD in middle-aged men. There are a few studies showing no benefit from long-term exercise, but none report that exercise aggravates CAD or hastens the development of clinical disease.

The mechanism by which exercise reduces risk of CAD probably comprises many factors. Improved cardiovascular function associated with exercise is reviewed elsewhere. The health-conscious life-style of the exercise enthusiast itself often reduces CAD risk (weight control, prudent dietary habits, abstinence from smoking, etc.). One recently identified benefit of exercise is an increase in the antiatherogenic fat transport substance, high-density lipoprotein (HDL, α-lipoprotein).

# High Density Lipoprotein

## Coronary Artery Disease

In 1951, Barr et al. [7] studied atherosclerosis and serum lipoproteins. They stated that "the outstanding fact in our observations is the relative and absolute reduction of α-lipoprotein (HDL) in atherosclerosis." They also observed that human babies and laboratory animals had elevated HDL and were resistant to CAD. Therefore, they proposed that HDL has a protective effect upon the heart. Unfortunately, the majority of lipid research since 1951 has focused on total serum cholesterol and its major lipoprotein carrier, low-density lipoprotein (LDL), rather than HDL. However, recent data from large prospective studies indicate that HDL is a better predictor of CAD risk than either serum cholesterol or LDL.

The highly publicized Framingham Heart Study (Gordon et al. [8]) gave evidence that HDL is an important CAD risk factor; it has shifted medical attention from serum cholesterol levels toward serum HDL levels. The Framingham Study was initiated in 1948 when the United States Public Health Service began a comprehensive study of factors associated with the development of atherosclerotic and hypertensive cardiovascular disease. A sample of the adult population of Framingham, Mass., was observed for 30 years. In 1968, 2815 of these men and women, aged 40–82 years, had lipids and lipoproteins

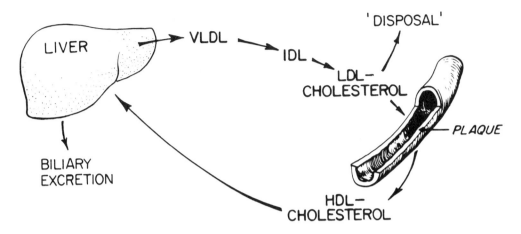

**14–1**   Schematic representation of the low density lipoprotein-generating system (*LDL*), and the high-density lipoprotein (*HDL*) cholesterol removal system. *IDL,* intermediate-density lipoproteins; *VLDL,* very-low-density lipoprotein. (From: Hooper P.L., Eaton R.P. 1978. Exercise, high density lipoprotein, and coronary artery disease. In: Appenzeller O., Atkinson R.A., (eds): Health Aspects of Endurance Training. Medicine and Sport Series, Vol. 12, S. Karger, Basel, p 77. Reprinted with permission from S. Karger AG, Basel.)

determined. Four years after the measurements, 142 subjects had developed CAD; their average cholesterol level was normal (244 mg/100 ml). Most people dying from CAD in the United States have normal serum cholesterol levels.

The Framingham study also showed that subjects with HDL-cholesterol levels below 35 mg/100 ml had eight times higher CAD incidence than those with HDL levels greater than 65 mg/100 ml. In addition, a study in Georgia (Castelli et al. [9]), the Tromso Heart Study in Norway (Miller and Miller [10]), the Hiroshima Study (Kajiyama et al. [11]), the Stockholm Prospective Study (Carlson [12]), and the Honolulu Heart Study (Rhoads et al. [13]) have all shown the same inverse relationship between HDL levels and CAD.

Further evidence that HDL protects the heart from atherosclerosis comes from studies of conditions associated with high or low HDL levels. Glueck et al (14) found 18 kindred with genetically elevated HDL levels. The average HDL-cholesterol in this group was 81 mg/100 ml compared to 53 mg/100 ml in controls. In kindreds with elevated HDL, life expectancy was longer and incidence of CAD was lower when compared to those in the general United States population.

Women have higher HDL levels than men (Gustafson et al. [15]). Under age 50, they also have one-fifth the number of CAD deaths compared to men (Statistical Bulletin [16]). Lower HDL values are seen with obesity (Wilson and Lees [17]), poorly controlled diabetes mellitus (Lopes-Virella et al. [18]), chronic renal failure (Brunzell et al. [19]), and smoking (Garrison et al. [20]). All these conditions significantly increase CAD risk. Therefore, the foregoing epidemiologic findings show that a high HDL level seems beneficial and, conversely, a low HDL level is detrimental.

Ethanol ingestion increases HDL levels. Belfrage et al. [21] gave nonintoxicating doses of alcohol to 9 healthy males for 5 weeks. Plasma HDL concentration steadily rose to 30% above control values over 5 weeks. Levels fell as soon as alcohol was discontinued. Johansson and Medhus [22] found elevated HDL levels in 60 of 69 alcoholic patients

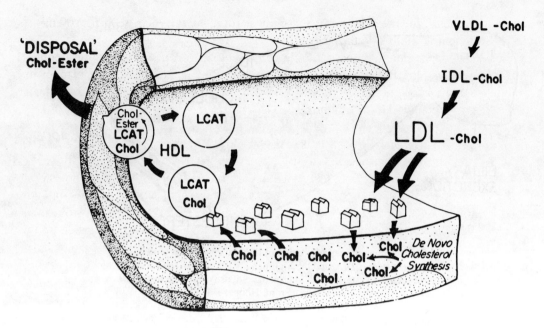

**14-2**   Cholesterol (*Chol*) accumulation in arterial smooth muscle cells: A net result of low-density lipoprotein (*LDL*) cholesterol deposition, *de novo* synthesis, and high-density lipoprotein (*HDL*) cholesterol removal. *IDL,* intermediate-density lipoproteins; *LCAT,* lecithin cholesterol acyltransferase; *VLDL,* very-low-density lipoproteins. (From: Hooper, P.L., Eaton R.P. 1978. Exercise, high density lipoprotein, and coronary artery disease. In: Appenzeller O., Atkinson R.A., (eds): Health Aspects of Endurance Training. Medicine and Sport Series, Vol. 12, S. Karger, Basel, p 77. Reprinted with permission from S. Karger AG, Basel.)

admitted to an alcohol withdrawal unit. After 2 weeks of abstinence, the patients' HDL values returned to normal. Yano et al. [23] studied the relationship of alcohol consumption to CAD in 7705 Japanese men living in Hawaii over 6 years. Those who drank 40 ml alcohol per day (equivalent to 3 bottles of beer, or 3 glasses of wine, or 2½ jiggers of hard liquor) had less than one-half the CAD events experienced by nondrinkers. They also found HDL levels higher in drinkers and lower in coronary-prone nondrinkers. These studies suggested that alcohol ingestion reduced CAD risk—perhaps by increasing HDL. However, the toxicity and abuse potential of alcohol decrease its therapeutic usefulness in CAD.

## Pathogenesis of Coronary Artery Disease

Research in coronary atherosclerosis has focused on cholesterol accumulation within proliferating smooth muscle cells of blood vessels. The accumulation of cholesterol in these cells is the result of three processes: synthesis, deposition, and removal.

Synthesis of cholesterol in the cell is thought to contribute little to cholesterol accumulation. Goldstein and Brown [24] have shown that cholesterol synthesis is blocked when its receptor is occupied by LDL. Since only 25 mg/100 ml LDL-cholesterol is required to suppress synthesis, the mean level of LDL-cholesterol in western man (120 mg/100 ml) is clearly sufficient to inhibit synthesis.

Cholesterol deposition in smooth muscle cells of blood vessels by circulating lipoproteins has received much attention. The cholesterol within atherosclerotic plaques is thought to come predominantly from LDL (Portman [25]). Low-density lipoprotein is derived from very-low-density lipoproteins (VLDL) by degradation (Fig. 14–1). Very-low-density lipoprotein is synthesized in the liver and is the major transport vehicle for triglycerides. The triglyceride fraction is hydrolyzed by lipoprotein lipase, and the VLDL particle is degraded to intermediate density lipoprotein (IDL), and then further to LDL. Low-density lipoprotein is left with the remaining cholesterol and is the major cholesterol carrier in the body (Eaton et al. [26]). Low-density lipoprotein is slowly cleared from the blood by a number of processes, including deposition into smooth muscle cells of blood vessels. The LDL binds to specific binding sites on cell membranes, and is taken up by pinocytosis to form intracellular vacuoles (Fig. 14–2). Cellular lysosomes then digest these lipoprotein vacuoles (Peters and DeDuve [27]). Accumulation of cholesterol occurs when LDL blood levels are high (Smith and Slater [28]) and when intracellular degradation is impaired (Peters and DeDuve [27]). Until recently, emphasis has been placed upon LDL influx as the major determinant of cholesterol accumulation within the cell.

Recent evidence suggests that cholesterol within smooth muscle cells can be removed by HDL. Moreover, a decrease in the removal of cholesterol from smooth muscle cells, due to a reduced plasma concentration from HDL, may be of greater importance in the accumulation of cholesterol than the deposition of cholesterol. High-density lipoprotein has the unique ability to bind to a cellular receptor (Miller et al. [29]), remove free cholesterol from the cell (Stein et al. [30]), esterify it (Glomset [31]), and transport the cholesterol ester to the bile (Sodhi and Kudchodkar [32]) (Fig. 14–2). This mechanism was first proposed by Glomset [31] in a detailed study of three sisters with a deficiency of the enzyme lecithin-cholesterol acyltransferase (LCAT). The LCAT enzyme catalyzes the esterification of cholesterol. Glomset [31] was fascinated by the cholesterol-burdened foam cells found in these patients' bone marrow and kidneys, and the similarity to the foam cells seen in familial HDL deficiency (Tangier disease). He postulated that HDL and the LCAT enzyme together estify the cholesterol load removed from tissues by HDL. The nonpolar cholesterol ester could rapidly be internalized into the core of the HDL (preventing reaccumulation in tissues) and be carried to the liver for excretion in the bile.

Recently, Stein et al. [30] have shown rapid cholesterol efflux from cells incubated with HDL apoproteins. Others (Miller et al. [33]) have studied the relationship between plasma lipoproteins and tissue pool size of cholesterol. Neither VLDL nor LDL concentrations correlated with total cholesterol pool size. However, HDL concentrations were inversely related to both rapidly and slowly exchanging pools of tissue cholesterol. These findings support the concept that the major determinant of net tissue cholesterol accumulation is the removal of cholesterol by HDL rather than deposition by LDL. Therefore, the mechanism by which HDL may confer a lower CAD risk is through a reduction in the cholesterol burden of the body.

Recent research into the pathogenesis of CAD has focused upon both cholesterol accumulation within smooth muscle cells and in the cells' rate of proliferation. Early atherosclerotic lesions are formed from rapidly proliferating smooth muscle cells. Serum factors such as lipoproteins (Fisher-Ozoga et al. [34]), platelet factors (Ross et al. [35]), and hormones (Stout et al. [36]) have been shown to stimulate proliferation. Low-density lipoprotein has been found to be a particularly potent stimulus for smooth muscle proliferation (Fisher-Ozoga et al. [34]), whereas HDL appears to inhibit proliferation of smooth muscle cells. A recent study in Finland (Tammi et al. [37]) revealed that sera from physically active lumberjacks (high in HDL) were more effective than sera from sedentary men in inhibiting the rate of smooth muscle DNA synthesis. Thus, HDL may also protect against CAD through inhibition of arterial smooth-muscle proliferation.

## What Is High-Density Lipoprotein?

High-density lipoprotein consists of spherical micelles, approximately 110 μm in diameter, with a hydrophobic inner core of esterified cholesterol and triglyceride and a hydrophilic outer shell of protein, free cholesterol, and phospholipid (Stoffel et al. [38]). The composition of HDL is approximately 50% protein, 25% phospholipid, 20% cholesterol, and 5% triglyceride (Jackson et al. [39]).

The protein fraction of the lipoprotein is termed *apoprotein*. A primary function of apoproteins is to solubilize plasma lipids for transport in the blood. The apoproteins of HDL are A-I, A-II, and C peptides. The A-I peptide, the major apoprotein of HDL, initiates binding to cellular surface receptors and may participate in the lecithin-cholesterol acyltransferase reaction (Fielding et al. [40]). The A-II peptide of HDL is present in about one-fourth the concentration of A-I peptide and has, as yet, no recognized metabolic function (Chenny and Albers [41]). At least four peptide units have been identified in the C-peptide group, with differing functions. The C-peptides dynamically shuttle between the HDL, VLDL, and IDL circulating in the plasma (Havel et al. [42]). The C-II peptide functions as a major activator of lipoprotein lipase, while C-I and C-III peptides inhibit human tissue lipoprotein lipase (Ekman and Nilsson-Ehle [43]). The activation of lipase activity, at the surface of VLDL and IDL, accelerates degration of VLDL into IDL, and IDL into LDL in the process of lipid clearance from the blood.

Total HDL levels are determined by sophisticated ultracentrifugation or electrophoretic procedures. With electrophoresis, the HDL migrates as the α-lipoprotein. Measurements of cholesterol within the HDL fraction are easily performed and correlate well with total HDL values (Albers et al. [44]). The determination of HDL-cholesterol is made by first adding phosphotungstate and magnesium, or manganese and heparin to either plasma or serum, which precipitates all lipoprotein fractions except for HDL. A simple cholesterol analysis of the remaining supernatant solution will result in an HDL-cholesterol determination (Lopes-Virella et al. [45]). The simplicity of the HDL-cholesterol determination has permitted its utilization in large epidemiologic studies of CAD.

## Exercise and High-Density Lipoprotein

Studies of exercise and lipid metabolism, like studies of coronary artery disease, have focused on total serum cholesterol. These have found that exercise has little or no effect on total serum cholesterol but reduces triglyceride levels. Recently it has been suggested (Simonelli and Eaton [46]) that one mechanism of exercise-induced triglyceride reduction

**Table 14.1**   Cross-Sectional Studies of Exercising and Nonexercising Populations and Their HDL-Cholesterol Levels.

| Subjects | | HDL-cholesterol | | Location of Study and Reference |
|---|---|---|---|---|
| Type of Exercise | Sex & No. | Mg/100 ml ± SD | p Value | |
| Runners, at least 15 miles/wk | M  41 | 64 ± 13 | | Stanford, CA (Wood et al. [55]) |
| | | | <0.05 | |
| Controls | M145 | 43 ± 10 | | |
| Runners | F  43 | 75 ± 14 | | |
| | | | <0.05 | |
| Controls | F 101 | 56 ± 14 | | |
| Lumberjacks | 12 | 67 ± 10 | | Finland (Lehtonen and Viikari [48]) |
| | | | <0.001 | |
| Electricians | 15 | 49 ± 11 | | |
| Runners & skiers | M  23 | 69 ± 15 | | Finland (Lehtonen and Viikari [49]) |
| | | | <0.01 | |
| Controls | M  15 | 54 ± 12 | | |
| Sprinters, 12–23 miles/wk | M   8 | 50 ±  6 | | |
| | | | <0.01 | |
| Long-distance runners, 62–82 miles/wk | M  12 | 66 ±  7 | | Finland (Nikkila et at. [50]) |
| | | | <0.01 | |
| Controls | M  10 | 47 ±  6 | | |
| Long-distance runners, 25–58 miles/wk | F   6 | 74 ± 19 | | |
| | | | <0.05 | |
| Controls | F  16 | 61 ±  3 | | |
| Boston Marathon runners | M  49 | 55 ± 14 | | |
| | F   1 | | | Massachusetts (Adner and Castelli [51]) |
| | | | <0.001 | |
| | M  42 | 45 ±  9 | | |
| Controls | | | | |
| | F   1 | | | |
| Ice hockey players (not endurance trained) | M  24 | 50 ±  7 | | |
| | | | <0.001 | Finland (Lehtonen and Viikari [52]) |
| Soccer team players (endurance trained) | M  21 | 64 ± 14 | | |
| | | | <0.001 | |
| Controls | M  61 | 53 ±  9 | | |
| Marathon runners, 40 miles/wk | M  59 | 65 ± 15 | | |
| | | | <0.001 | |
| Joggers, 6 miles/wk | M  85 | 58 ± 18 | | Houston, TX |
| | | | <0.001 | |
| Controls | M  74 | 43 ± 14 | | (Hartung et al. [53]) |

is through a reduction in VLDL production by the liver. This effect can be demonstrated in normal and Zucker rats, the animal model for type IV hyperlipoproteinemia. In patients with type IV hyperlipoproteinemia, only 30 min of treadmill walking a day for 4 days has a similar effect (Gyntelberg et al. [47]).

Both cross-sectional and longitudinal studies suggest that exercise increases HDL levels. The results of cross-sectional studies comparing HDL-cholesterol in exercising and nonexercising populations are presented in Table 14–1. All studies show significantly higher HDL-cholesterol levels in endurance athletes in comparison to sedentary controls. Furthermore, physically active lumberjacks have higher HDL levels than less active electricians (Lehtonen and Viikari [48, 49]).

The type of exercise appears important for a rise in HDL-cholesterol concentration. Anaerobically trained sprinters and ice-hockey players have no elevations of HDL-cholesterol concentration when compared to aerobically (endurance) trained long-distance runners and soccer players (Nikkila et al. [50]; Adner and Castelli [51]; Lehtonen and Viikari [52]). In the Houston Study, Hartung and co-workers [53] found that the distance run per week was the best predictor of HDL-cholesterol levels. In another study Schwane and Cundiff [54] found a statistically significant correlation between HDL-cholesterol and aerobic capacity, as determined by a treadmill test.

Investigators doing cross-sectional studies have all had difficulty controlling other factors that alter HDL-cholesterol. For instance, the Stanford runners consumed almost six times the amount of wine that controls had drunk (Wood et al. [55]). Similarly, runners smoke less, eat differently, and weigh less than do sedentary subjects. Hartung and co-workers [53] examined dietary, smoking, and alcohol habits in all subjects. Although differences were found among marathon runners, joggers, and sedentary subjects, the investigators could not attribute the different HDL levels to differences in life-style alone. Although a negative correlation has been observed between HDL-cholesterol concentration and body weight in a free-living population, no correlation has been found between adiposity and HDL-cholesterol concentration in runners (Hartung et al. [53]; Schwane and Cundiff [54]). All studies point to the fact that those who engage in endurance training have higher HDL-cholesterol concentrations than their sedentary counterparts.

Longitudinal exercise intervention studies have found that exercise elevates HDL-cholesterol concentrations. Altekruse and Wilmore [56] were early investigators to document this. Thirty-nine sedentary males, averaging age 33 years, were studied before and after 10 weeks of walking, jogging, or running 3 times a week. Subjects averaged 5.2 miles per week at 7.5 miles per hour. Mean weight loss was 1 kg. Diet, alcohol consumption, and cigarette smoking were not measured. Levels of HDL increased from 36.9% to 55.5% of total lipoprotein at the expense of VLDL and LDL.

Lopez et al. [57] studied 13 medical students who exercised 4 times a week for 7 weeks. Each exercise period consisted of 10–15 min of jogging, 5–10 min of bicycling, and 5–10 min of calisthenics. There was no weight loss. Diet, alcohol consumption, and cigarette smoking were not monitored. Total HDL rose 16%, from 57 mg/100 ml to 66.4 mg/100 ml ($p < 0.01$).

In 12 marathon runners who participated in a 20-day road race, HDL-cholesterol values rose 18% after 1 week of running 28 km/day. After 3 days of rest, the values returned to near baseline levels (Dressendorfer et al. [58]).

Two studies (Erkelens et al. [59]; Streja and Mymin [60]) have examined the effect of participation in a moderate exercise program after myocardial infarction. In both studies, exercise consisted of 30–45 min walking or jogging three times a week. In one study (Erkelens et al. [59]), a prompt rise in HDL-cholesterol concentration occurred (from 35 ± 8 mg/100 ml to 40 ± 8 mg/100 ml, $p < 0.001$) after only 1 week of exercise. Thereafter, the HDL-cholesterol remained unchanged for 6 months.

The effect of exercise on the apoproteins of HDL has been studied. Lehtonen et al. [61] examined HDL apoproteins in 23 athletes and found that the major apoprotein of HDL, A-

I, was 32% higher in the athletes than in controls. No difference was found in A-II levels. Similarly, the longitudinal study of Lopez and co-workers (57) reported a 37% rise in serum LCAT enzyme activity after 7 weeks of moderate exercise.

We conclude that 1) exercise increases HDL-cholesterol and HDL-apoprotein concentration; 2) a relatively low level of exercise is needed to raise HDL-cholesterol levels; and 3) aerobic endurance exercise appears to raise HDL-cholesterol better than anaerobic training. These observations are gratifying. To raise HDL-cholesterol, only moderate exercise within the reach of most of us is required. However, the exercise enthusiast, like the marathon runner, does benefit by a greater rise in HDL-cholesterol level. In other words, the extra mile is worth while.

The hypothesis that exercise elevates HDL-cholesterol levels, resulting in protection from CAD, is attractive and scientifically sound. The hypothesis, however, remains unproven. Well-controlled, long-term longitudinal studies of runners and nonrunners should help clarify the issue. In the meantime, we need encouragement to participate in endurance sports.

# References

1. American Heart Association. 1978. Heart Facts. American Heart Association, Dallas.
2. Gordon, T., Thom, T. 1975. The recent decrease in coronary heart disease mortality. Preventive Med 4:115–125.
3. Morris, J.N. 1960. Epidemiology and cardiovascular disease of middle age; I, II. Mod Concepts Cardiovasc Dis 29:625–631.
4. Froelicher, V.F., Oberman, A. 1972. Analysis of epidemiologic studies of physical inactivity as a risk for coronary artery disease. Prog Cardiovasc Dis 15:41–65.
5. Paffenbarger, R.S. Jr., Hale, W.E., Brand, R.J., Hyde, R.T. 1977. Work-energy level, personal characteristics and fatal heart attack: A birth cohort effect. Am J Epidemiol 105:200–213.
6. Paffenbarger, R.S. Jr., Wing, A.L., Hyde, R.T. 1978. Physical activity as an index of heart attack risk in college alumni. Am J Epidemiol 108:161–175.
7. Barr, D.P., Russ, E.M., Eder, H.A. 1951. Protein–lipid relationships in human plasma. Am J Med 11:480–495.
8. Gordon, T., Castelli, W.P., Hjortland, M.C., Kannel, W.B., Dawber, T.R. 1977. High density lipoprotein as a protective factor against coronary heart disease. Am J Med 62:707–714.
9. Castelli, W.P., Doyle, J.T., Gordon, T., Hames, C.E., Hjortland, M.C., Hulley, S.B., Kagan, A., Zukel, W.J. 1972. HDL-cholesterol and other lipids in coronary heart disease. The cooperative lipoprotein phenotyping study. Circulation 55:767–772.
10. Miller, G.J., Miller, N.E. 1975. Plasma high density lipoprotein concentrations and development of ischaemic heart disease. Lancet 1:16–19.
11. Kajiyama, G., Mizuno, T., Matsuura, C., Yamada, K., Suzukawa, M., Fujiyama, M., Miyoshi, A. 1974. The lowered serum phospholipids in alpha-lipoprotein in patients with atherosclerosis. Hiroshima J Med Sci 23:229–236.
12. Carlson, L.A. 1973. Lipoprotein fractionation. J Clin Pathol 26(suppl 15):32–37.
13. Rhoads, G.G., Gulbrandsen, C.L., Kagan, A. 1976. Serum lipoproteins and coronary heart disease in a population study of Hawaii Japanese men. N Engl J Med 294:293–298.

14. Glueck, C.J., Gartside, P., Fallat, R.N., Sielski, J., Steiner, P.M. 1976. Longevity syndromes: Familial hypobeta and familial hyperalpha-lipoproteinemia. J Lab Clin Med 88:941–957.

15. Gustafson, A., Lillienberg, L., Svanberg, A. 1974. Human plasma high-density lipoprotein composition during the menstrual cycle. Scand J Clin Lab Invest 137(suppl):63–70.

16. Statistical Bulletin. 1975. 56(June):1–6.

17. Wilson, D.E., Lees, R.S. 1972. Metabolic relationships among the plasma lipoproteins. J Clin Invest 51:1051–1057.

18. Lopes-Virella, M.F.L., Stone, P.G., Colwell, J.A. 1977. Serum high-density lipoprotein in diabetic patients. Diabetologia 13:285–291.

19. Brunzell, J.D., Albers, J.J., Haas, L.B. 1977. Prevalence of serum lipid abnormalities in chronic hemodialysis. Metabolism 26:903–910.

20. Garrison, R.J., Kannel, W.B., Manning, F., Castelli, W.P., McNamara, P.M., Padgett, S.J. 1977. Cigarette smoking and HDL-cholesterol: The Framingham Study. Circulation 55–56 (suppl III):44.

21. Belfrage, P., Berg, B., Hagerstrand, I., Nilsson-Ehle, P., Tonnquist, H., Wiebe, I. 1977. Alterations of lipid metabolism during long-term ethanol intake. Eur J Clin Invest 7:127–131.

22. Johansson, B.G., Medhus, A. 1974. Increase in plasma alpha-lipoproteins in chronic alcoholics after acute abuse. Acta Med Scand 195:273–277.

23. Yano, K., Rhoads, G.G., Kagan, A. 1977. Coffee, alcohol, and risk of coronary heart disease among Japanese men living in Hawaii. N Engl J Med 297:405–409.

24. Goldstein, J.L., Brown, M.S. 1977. The low-density lipoprotein pathway and its relation to atherosclerosis. Ann Rev Biochem 46:897–930.

25. Portman, O.W. 1970. Arterial composition and metabolism. Esterified fatty acids and cholesterol. Adv Lipid Res 8:41–114.

26. Eaton, R.P., Crespin, S., Kipnis, D.M. 1976. Incorporation of 75-seleno-methionine into human apoproteins. III. Kinetic behavior of isotopically labeled plasma apoprotein in man. Diabetes 25:679–690.

27. Peters, T.J., DeDuve, C. 1974. Lysosomes of the arterial wall. II. Subcellular fractionation of aortic cells from rabbits with experimental atheroma. Exp Mol Pathol 20:228–256.

28. Smith, E.B., Slater, R.S. 1972. Relationship between low-density lipoprotein in aortic intima and serum lipid levels. Lancet 1:463–469.

29. Miller, N.E., Weinstein, D.B., Canew, T.E. 1977. Interaction between high density and low density lipoproteins during uptake and degradation by cultured human fibroblasts. J Clin Invest 60:78–89.

30. Stein, Y., Glangeaud, M.C., Fainaru, N., Stein, O. 1975. The removal of cholesterol from aortic smooth muscle cells in culture and landschutz ascites cells by fractions of human high density apolipoproteins. Biochim Biophys Acta 380:106–118.

31. Glomset, A. 1978. The plasma lecithin: Cholesterol acyltransferase reaction. J Lipid Res 9:155–167.

32. Sodhi, H.S., Kudchodkar, B.J. 1973. Correlating metabolism of plasma and tissue cholesterol with that of plasma-lipoproteins. Lancet 1:513–519.

33. Miller, N.E., Nestel, P.J., Clifton-Bligh, P. 1976. Relationships between plasma lipoprotein cholesterol concentrations and the pool size and metabolism of cholesterol in man. Atherosclerosis 23:535–547.

34. Fisher-Ozoga, K., Chen, R., Wissler, R.W. 1974. Effects of serum lipoproteins on the morphology, growth, and metabolism of arterial smooth muscle cells. Adv Exp Med Biol 43:299–311.

35. Ross, R., Glomset, J., Kariya, B., Harker, L. 1974. A platelet-dependent serum factor that stimulates the proliferation of arterial smooth muscle cells in vitro. Proc Natl Acad Sci USA 71:1207–1210.

36. Stout, R.W., Bierman, E.L., Ross, R. 1975. Effect of insulin on the proliferation of cultured primate arterial smooth muscle cells. Circ Res 36:319–327.

37. Tammi, M., Ronnemaa, T., Vihersaari, T. 1979. High density lipoproteinemia due to vigorous physical work inhibits the incorporation of ($^3$H) thymidine and the synthesis of glycosaminoglycans by human aortic

smooth muscle cells in culture. Atherosclerosis 32:23–32.

38. Stoffel, W., Zierenberg, O., Tunggal, B., Schreiber, E. 1976. $^{13}$C nuclear magnetic resonance spectroscopic evidence for hydrophobic lipid-protein interactions in human high density lipoproteins. Proc Natl Acad Sci USA 71:3696–3700.

39. Jackson, R., Morrisett, J., Gotto, A.M. 1976. Lipoprotein structure and metabolism. Physiol Rev 56:259–316.

40. Fielding, C.J., Shore, V.G., Fielding, P.E. 1972. A protein cofactor of lecithin: Cholesterol acyltransferase. Biochem Biophys Res Commun 46:1463–1498.

41. Chenny, M.C., Albers, J.J. 1977. The measurement of apolipoprotein A-I and A-II levels in men and women by immunoassay. J Clin Invest 60:43–51.

42. Havel, R.J., Kane, J.P., Kashyap, M.L. 1973. Interchange of apoproteins between chylomicrons and high density lipoproteins during alimentary lipemia in man. J Clin Invest 52:32–38.

43. Ekman, R., Nilsson-Ehle, P. 1975. Effect of apolipoproteins on lipoprotein lipase activity of human adipose tissue. Clin Chim Acta 63:29–35.

44. Albers, J.J., Wahl, P.W., Cabana, V.G., Hazzard, W.R., Hoover, J.J. 1976. Quantitation of apolipoprotein A-I of human plasma high density lipoprotein. Metabolism 25:633–644.

45. Lopes-Virella, M.F., Stone, P., Ellis, S., Colwell, J.A. 1977. Cholesterol determinations in high-density lipoproteins separated by three different methods. Clin Chem 23:882–884.

46. Simonelli, C., Eaton, R.P. 1978. Reduced triglyceride secretion: A metabolic consequence of chronic exercise. Am J Physiol 234:221–227.

47. Gyntelberg, F., Brennan, R., Holloszy, J.O., Schonfeld, G., Rennie, M.J., Weidman, S.W. 1977. Plasma triglyceride lowering by exercise despite increased food intake in patients with type IV hyperlipoproteinemia. Am J Clin Nutr 30:716–720.

48. Lehtonen, A., Viikari, J. 1978. The effect of vigorous physical activity at work on serum lipids with a special reference to serum high-density lipoprotein cholesterol. Acta Physiol Scand 104:117–121.

49. Lehtonen, A., Viikari, J. 1978. Serum triglycerides and cholesterol and serum high-density lipoprotein cholesterol in highly physically active men. Acta Med Scand 204:111–114.

50. Nikkila, E.A., Taskinen, M.R., Rehunen, S., Harkonen, M. 1978. Lipoprotein lipase activity in adipose tissue and skeletal muscle of runners: Relation to serum lipoproteins. Metabolism 27:1661–1667.

51. Adner, M.M., Castelli, W.P. 1980. Elevated high-density lipoprotein levels in marathon runners. JAMA 243:534–536.

52. Lehtonen, A., Viikari, J. 1980. Serum lipids in soccer and ice-hockey players. Metabolism 29:36–39.

53. Hartung, G.H., Foreyt, J.P., Mitchell, R.E. 1980. Relation of diet to high-density lipoprotein cholesterol in middle-aged marathon runners, joggers, and inactive men. N Engl J Med 302:357–361.

54. Schwane, J.A., Cundiff, D.E. 1979. Relationships among cardiorespiratory fitness, regular physical activity, and plasma lipids in young adults. Metabolism 28:771–776.

55. Wood, P.D., Haskell, W.L., Stern, M.P., Lewis, S., Perry, C. 1977. Plasma lipoprotein distributions in male and female runners. Ann NY Acad Sci 301:748–763.

56. Altekruse, E.B., Wilmore, J.H. 1973. Changes in blood chemistries following a controlled exericse program. J Occup Med 15:110–113.

57. Lopez, A., Vial, R., Balart, L., Arroyave, G. 1974. Effect of exercise and physical fitness on serum lipids and lipoproteins. Atherosclerosis 20:1–9.

58. Dressendorfer, R.H., Wade, C.E., Hornick, C., Timmis, G.C. 1982. High-density lipoprotein-cholesterol in marathon runners during a 20-day road race. JAMA 247:1715–1717.

59. Erkelens, W.D., Albers, J.J., Hazzard, W.R. 1979. High density lipoprotein-cholesterol in survivors of myocardial infarction. JAMA 242:2185–2189.

60. Streja, D., Mymin, D. 1979. Moderate exercise and high density lipoprotein-cho-

lesterol. JAMA 242:2190–2192.

61. Lehtonen, A., Viikari, J., Ehnholm, C. 1979. The effect of exercise on high density (HDL) lipoprotein apoproteins. JAMA 106:487–488.

Chapter 15

# Exercise and the Lung

## by Jonathan M. Samet and Thomas W. Chick

The exercising athlete is merely performing work. Thus, his or her activities are appropriately described in terms borrowed from Newtonian physics (Table 15–1). The endurance athlete—the runner, swimmer, or cross-country skier—must work to accelerate and then maintain his or her pace. The isometric athlete—the weight lifter or football player—also performs work, even if no motion occurs. Power, the rate at which work is performed, is the usual measure of work capacity. The mechanical efficiency of work is the proportion of energy input that is transformed to external work.

Power demands in athletics vary with the type of activity and the rate at which it is performed (Fig. 15–1) (Astrand and Rodahl [1]). For example, an increase in running speed from 5.5 to 10 mph doubles the rate of work from 150 to 300 watts. This energy expenditure comprises not only the external work performed but the energy costs that accompany exercise of the body. The hyperpnea of exercise is paralleled by increased oxygen demand by the respiratory muscles themselves. In normal people, even with extreme exertion, the energy required by the respiratory system is never greater than approximately 10% of the total expended.

# Fuel Utilization During Exercise

Human work, including athletics, is always accomplished by muscle contraction, which is powered by the high-energy phosphate bonds of adenosine triphosphate (ATP). The ATP stored within muscle will meet energy requirements only transiently, for less than 1 sec (Astrand and Rodahl[2]; Wasserman and Whipp [3]). Regeneration of ATP by creatine phosphate is another short-term, limited ATP source (Astrand and Rodahl [2]). Sustained exercise with continued demand for ATP ultimately requires the utilization of body energy stores. Fuels available for exercise include fat and carbohydrate; protein utilization requires muscle and parenchymal tissue breakdown and does not occur with ordinary endurance exercise (Felig and Wahren [4]). Body stores are primarily in the form of fat.

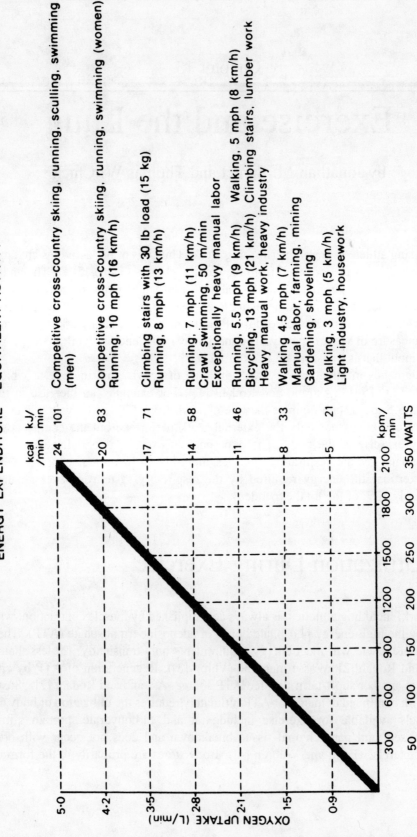

**Table 15-1**    Work Performed by the Exercising Athlete

| Term | Definition* | Measurement |
|------|------------|-------------|
| Force | Accelerates a mass | 1 newton = $1 \text{ kg} \times \text{m} \times \text{S}^{-2}$ |
| Work | Force acting through a distance | 1 joule = 1 newton × 1m |
| Efficiency | Work output per energy input | percent |
| Work load | Work demand of a task | watts |

*These units are in the International Standard (SI) system. In the previous system, work was measured in kilopond-meters (kpm). For conversion, 1 watt = $6.12 \text{ kpm} \times \text{min}^{-1}$

An untrained 70-kg man has approximately 140,000 kcal of fat and only 2000 kcal of carbohydrate. The carbohydrate is stored principally as muscle glycogen, 350 g, and hepatic glycogen, 40–90 g (Felig and Wahren [4]). These fuel supplies vary with diet and with exercise patterns.

Muscle cells convert fats and carbohydrates to ATP through both aerobic and anaerobic processes. The aerobic pathways require adequate numbers of mitochondria, adequate tricarboxylic acid (Krebs) cycle enzymes, and an adequate oxygen supply at the mitochondria (Wasserman and Whipp [3]). When these conditions are not met and aerobic metabolism becomes inadequate, ATP regeneration must occur by anaerobic processes.

During exercise, the muscles use muscle glycogen and blood-borne glucose as carbohydrate fuel. Under both aerobic and anaerobic conditions, the initial sequence of glucose metabolism is the same; the glycolytic enzymes convert glucose to pyruvate. When the requirements for aerobic metabolism are fulfilled, pyruvate then enters the mitochondria and undergoes oxidative decarboxylation by the tricarboxylic acid cycle enzymes to carbon dioxide and water. Under anaerobic conditions, pyruvate must accept hydrogen and is reduced to lactate. Fat is supplied to the muscle as blood-borne free fatty acids. These fatty acids are converted to acetyl coenzyme A, two carbon units, which are metabolized by the tricarboxylic acid cycle (Astrand and Rodahl [2]).

The ATP yield of aerobic metabolism markedly exceeds that of anaerobic metabolism. Aerobically, glucose supplies 37 molecules of ATP for each molecule of glucose, whereas anaerobically, 2 ATP molecules are generated for each glucose molecule. The actual efficiency of the two processes is remarkably similar: 53% for aerobic, and 55% for anaerobic. Fatty acids of composition similar to human adipose tissue are estimated to supply 138 moles of ATP per mole of fatty acid (Astrand and Rodahl [2]). For endurance athletics with a sustained demand for ATP, aerobic is clearly preferable to anaerobic metabolism.

Skeletal muscles are mixtures of two fiber types, which vary in their capacity to sustain aerobic metabolism (Gollnick and Sembrowich [5]). Type I, or slow-twitch fibers, have low myosin ATPase activity, high mitochondrial enzyme activity, and high myoglobin concentration. Type II, or fast-twitch fibers, have high myosin ATPase activity, low mitochondrial enzyme activity, and low myoglobin content. These contrasting metabolic capacities imply different roles for the two fiber types. The higher aerobic capacity of Type I fibers suggests their suitability for endurance activities. Type II fibers, with high ATPase activity, appear suited for the brief, high-power demands of isometric exercise.

◄——— **15-1** Ergometer work, equivalent physical activity, and oxygen uptake. (From Åstrand P. 1976. Quantification of Exercise Capability and Evaluation of Physical Capacity in Man. Prog Cardiovasc Dis 19:51–67. Reprinted with permission.)

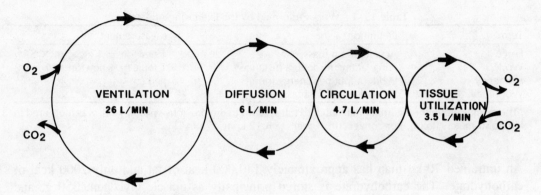

**15–2**   Schematic representation of $O_2$ and $CO_2$ transport. *Circles*, transport capacity of each step for $O_2$.

The fuels expended during exercise vary with the intensity and duration of the activity. Initially, before circulatory compensation occurs, stored ATP and ATP derived from creatine phosphate drive muscle contraction. Anaerobic glycolysis is also important initially but declines unless the work load is high. In the early phase of sustained exercise, muscle glycogen is the principal energy source. Subsequently, uptake of blood-borne glucose and free fatty acids increases. As muscle glycogen supplies are depleted during the first hour of exercise, blood-borne glucose becomes the major source of carbohydrate. With continued exercise, glucose utilization may decline while free fatty acid utilization continues to increase and becomes the predominant energy source. Heavy exercise increases the demand for muscle glycogen (Astrand and Rodahl [2]; Wasserman and Whipp [3]; Felig and Warren [4]). In fact, heavy and sustained exercise may result in hypoglycemia in some persons (Felig et al. [6]).

The performance of work requires a continuous supply of ATP to sustain muscle contraction. The ATP can be derived from either aerobic or anaerobic metabolism, but the latter yields less energy, more quickly depletes glycogen, and results in lactic acid accumulation. Endurance exercise requires prolonged muscle use, and must be accomplished primarily with aerobic metabolism.

# Maximal Oxygen Uptake

The maintenance of aerobic metabolism during exercise is critically dependent upon a continued availability of oxygen at the mitochondria. The respiratory and circulatory systems operate in series to deliver oxygen to the muscles and to remove the carbon dioxide generated by oxidative decarboxylation (Fig. 15–2). As work load increases, oxygen uptake $(\dot{V}O_2)$[1] must rise in compensation, or the proportion of ATP derived from anaerobic metabolism will increase. Because of the close correlation between work load

[1]Oxygen uptake per unit of time $(\dot{V}O_2)$ is expressed as milliliters per minute (ml/min) with the gas volume at standard conditions (STPD).

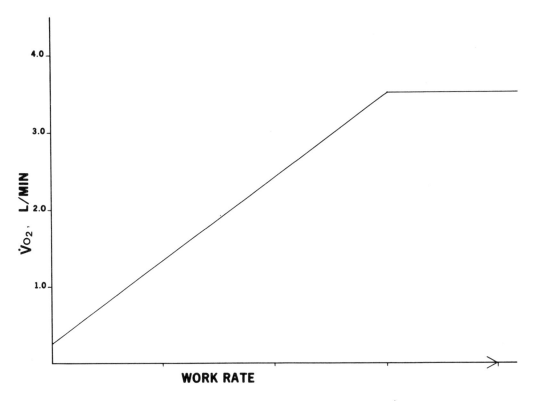

**15-3**   Relationship between work rate and oxygen uptake $\dot{V}O_2$.

and oxygen uptake, the energy requirements of specific activities can be expressed in terms of oxygen uptake (Fig. 15–1).

As work load increases, however, oxygen uptake will eventually attain a plateau and fail to increase further (Fig. 15–3). This level of oxygen utilization is termed the maximal oxygen uptake ($\dot{V}O_{2max}$), and this level of work is termed the maximal aerobic power. Further increases in work load may be achieved but only with reliance on anaerobic processes.

The transport of oxygen from atmospheric air to exercising muscles is performed by four distinct systems in series: pulmonary ventilation, diffusion, circulation, and tissue extraction (Fig. 15–2).

# Pulmonary Response to Exercise

## Gas Exchange at Rest

Pulmonary gas exchange is the transfer of oxygen from atmosphere to blood and of carbon dioxide from blood to atmosphere. In a steady state the quantity of carbon dioxide produced by tissue metabolism equals the quantity exhaled ($\dot{V}CO_2$, ml/min STPD). Similarly, oxygen uptake by the lungs matches oxygen utilization by tissues. The ratio of $\dot{V}_{CO_2}$ to $\dot{V}_{O_2}$ is the respiratory exchange ratio ($R$), which in a steady state equals the tissue ratio (R). R is determined by the type of substrate utilized by the tissues. The R for pure carbohydrate metabolism is 1; for fat, 0.7; and for protein, 0.9. The R for a normal individual at rest is 0.85 (Wasserman and Whipp [3]).

The components of gas exchange are ventilation, diffusion of gas across the alveolar-capillary membrane, and chemical reactions of $CO_2$ and $O_2$ in blood. Ventilation is accomplished by the respiratory muscles, which include primarily the intercostal muscles and the diaphragm. The exhaled minute ventilation ($\dot{V}_E$)[2] is the product of tidal volume ($V_T$) in liters BTPS, and the respiratory frequency (f). The $\dot{V}_E$ is also the sum of alveolar ventilation ($\dot{V}_A$) in liters/min BTPS and of dead space ventilation ($\dot{V}_D$, liters/min BTPS). The $V_A$ is the volume that reaches the alveolar surface and functions in gas exchange. The $\dot{V}_D$ is the ventilation distributed to the conducting airways and unperfused alveoli, and is ineffective in gas exchange. The ratio of dead space volume ($V_D$) to $V_T$ is normally 0.3.

Gas diffusion across the alveolar capillary membrane occurs along partial pressure gradients. The diffusing capacity of the lung is determined in part by the thickness and the surface area of the alveolar-capillary membrane. Blood within the pulmonary capillaries functions as a sink for oxygen, and thus pulmonary blood flow is the other principal determinant of diffusing capacity. Imperfect matching of ventilation with perfusion reduces the efficiency of gas exchange.

## Gas Exchange During Exercise

To meet the metabolic demands of exercise, each component of gas exchange increases. Ventilation rises in proportion to work load (Fig. 15–4) to maintain constant arterial blood gas tensions. The increase in ventilation is approximately 20–25 liters/min per liter of oxygen consumption with moderate work loads (Astrand and Rodahl [7]).

Initially, rising $V_T$ is principally responsible for the increase in $\dot{V}_E$; as work load increases, $V_T$ does not increase beyond approximately 50% of the vital capacity, and ventilation is increased by a more rapid respiration rate. In normal subjects the $V_D/V_T$ ratio declines with exercise, as $V_D$ remains constant and $V_T$ increases.

The increase in ventilation with exercise is immediate (Astrand and Rodahl [7]; Wasserman [8]). The stimuli and control mechanisms underlying the hyperpnea of exercise are not well understood. The coupling of ventilation to excess $CO_2$ delivery to the lungs suggests that $CO_2$ is the primary stimulus for the ventilatory response to exercise (Wasserman [8]). Other factors such as the carotid bodies, muscle mechanoreceptors, and psychogenic stimuli may also have a role (Wasserman [8]).

As work load increases and tissue $O_2$ supplies become inadequate, lactic acid production increases. The resulting rise in blood lactate decreases arterial pH and stimulates an increase in ventilation greater than needed for $CO_2$ elimination (Fig. 15–4) (Wasserman and Whipp [3]; Wasserman [8]). The work load at which this occurs defines the anaerobic threshold (AT). At higher work loads, $\dot{V}_E$ and $\dot{V}_{CO_2}$ increase more than does the $\dot{V}_{O_2}$. Consequently arterial $CO_2$ tension (Pa$_{CO_2}$) decreases.

---

[2]$\dot{V}_E$ is expressed as liters/min at body temperature, pressure, and saturation (BTPS).

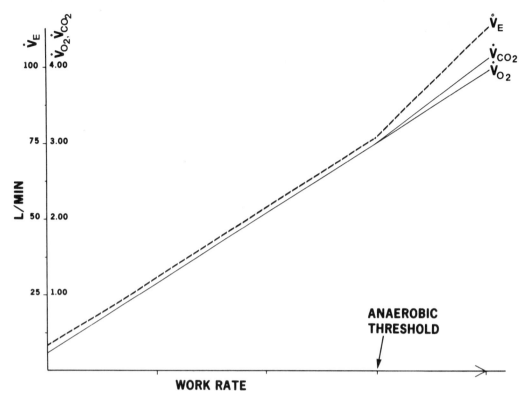

**15–4**   Relationship between work rate and $\dot{V}_{O_2}$, $\dot{V}_{CO_2}$, and $\dot{V}_E$.

Diffusion, the next step, increases primarily as a result of pulmonary capillary recruitment by the increased cardiac output. Attainment of $\dot{V}_{O_2max}$ is accompanied by a doubling of the diffusing capacity (Johnson [9]).

Gas exchange during exercise meets tissue metabolic demands remarkably well. Arterial carbon dioxide tension remains constant until the anaerobic threshold is reached; the arterial oxygen tension ($PaO_2$) also remains constant, and $CO_2$ production appears to be the principal stimulus for control of respiration during exercise.

## Oxygen Transport Capacity During Exercise

The respiratory and circulatory systems operate in series to deliver oxygen to exercising muscle. As described by the Fick equation, oxygen uptake is the product of the cardiac output and the arteriovenous oxygen difference:

$$\dot{V}_{O_2} = \dot{Q} \times (Ca_{O_2} - C\bar{v}_{O_2})$$

($\dot{Q}$ = cardiac output; $Ca_{O_2}$ = arterial $O_2$ content; $C\bar{v}_{O_2}$ = mixed venous $O_2$ content). The respiratory system serves to maintain $Ca_{O_2}$. The following analysis of oxygen transport capacity shows that normally $\dot{V}_{O_2max}$ is not limited by the respiratory system.

**Table 15–2**   Effects of Aging on the Components of the Oxygen Transport System

| Component | Effect |
|---|---|
| Ventilation | ↓ FEV$_1$* |
| | ↓ FVC† |
| | ↓ MVV‡ |
| | ↑ Closing volume |
| Gas Exchange | ↑ Ventilation-perfusion imbalance |
| | ↓ Diffusing capacity |
| Control of Respiration | ↓ Response to hypercapnia and to hypoxia |
| Cardiac Function | ↓ Maximal heart rate |
| | ↓ Stroke volume |
| | ↓ Maximal cardiac output |
| Peripheral Circulation | Importance not determined |
| Skeletal muscle | Importance not determined |

*Forced expiratory volume in 1 sec.
†Forced vital capacity.
‡Maximum voluntary ventilation.

An average size adult male can achieve a maximum $\dot{V}_A$ of 150 liters/min, which delivers 26 liters of oxygen. The oxygen transport capacity of the diffusion and chemical reaction steps of gas exchange are estimated to be 6 liters $O_2$ per minute (Johnson [9]). Circulation is the next step; maximum cardiac output is approximately 23 liters/min, which delivers oxygen at a rate of 4.7 liters/min. At most, 75% of this oxygen can be utilized during heavy exercise. Thus, as suggested by the Fick equation, cardiac output and muscle capacity to extract oxygen are the principal determinants of $\dot{V}_{O_{2max}}$.

# Factors Influencing Exercise Performance

## Aging

Cross-sectional and longitudinal studies demonstrate that $\dot{V}_{O_{2max}}$ declines progressively from the maximum value attained in an individual's early 20s. (Astrand and Rodahl [10]). The annual loss of aerobic power is approximately 0.5 ml/kg/min and is less for persons who remain fit. Performance in athletic events declines in parallel with $\dot{V}_{O_{2max}}$ (Shephard [11]).

Effects of aging on several components of the oxygen transport system result in the diminished maximal aerobic power (Table 15–2) (Murray [12]). The forced expiratory volume in 1 sec (FEV$_1$), forced vital capacity (FVC), and maximum voluntary ventilation (MVV) decline progressively from peak values attained in the mid-20s. In many cigarette smokers the rates of decline of these ventilatory parameters are increased. Deteriorating ventilation–perfusion relationships reduce the efficiency of gas exchange in the aging lung. Ventilatory responses to hypercapnia and to hypoxia also decline with aging. Decreased maximal heart rate and decreased stroke volume reduce the maximum cardiac output that can be achieved during exercise. Changes in the peripheral circulation and in skeletal muscle metabolism may contribute to the reduction in $\dot{V}O_{2max}$ related to aging, but their importance has not been determined. The observed decline in maximum arterio-venous oxygen difference may reflect changes in these two peripheral factors. Although the specific contribution of changes in each component of the oxygen transport system has not been experimentally assessed, theoretically the declining alveolar ventilation and cardiac output are principally responsible for reduced $\dot{V}O_{2max}$ with aging.

Middle-aged and elderly people respond to endurance training with increased $\dot{V}O_{2max}$ (Shephard [13]). Unlike the response in younger people, this increase results from increased cardiac output only and not from both increased cardiac output and increased arteriovenous oxygen difference. Nevertheless, elderly subjects can safely participate in endurance training (Shephard [13]).

# Training

Training is the regular performance of a work load that stresses the athlete and results in physiologic adaptation. Training activities may be loosely categorized as directed at increasing muscle strength and anaerobic processes or at increasing endurance and aerobic processes. The former type requires brief bursts of intense muscle activity, whereas the latter type requires more prolonged submaximal activity. Because the respiratory system has a limited role in adaptation to isometric exercise, the following discussion focuses on endurance training. Both human and animal data concerning the effects of training are available. The human investigations, however, are frequently flawed by inability to separate training effects from inherent constitutional capabilities.

Performance is determined by a complex interaction between psychological and phys-ical factors. Fatigue, the signal to stop exercising, is hypothesized to arise from lactic acid accumulation within muscle or from depletion of muscle and liver glycogen (Astrand and Rodahl [14]). Endurance training appears to postpone the development of fatigue by increasing $\dot{V}O_{2max}$. As aerobic power increases, the anaerobic threshold is reached at higher work loads; correspondingly, lactic acid accumulation begins at higher work loads and glycogen stores are less rapidly depleted. The development of dyspnea, the perception of breathlessness, also continues to the breaking point of exercise (Cotes [15]). During exercise, dyspnea occurs when the required ventilation is a large proportion of the MVV and high forces must be generated by the respiratory muscles (Cotes [15]). In normal subjects, dyspnea does not arise from limitation of oxygen transport capacity by the respiratory system.

The correlation between performance and $\dot{V}O_{2max}$ has been established by cross-sectional studies of athletes and by longitudinal studies of untrained subjects (Astrand and Rodahl [14]). The $\dot{V}O_{2max}$ of champion endurance athletes may exceed that of untrained persons by as much as 40 ml/kg/min. Similarly, the mean $\dot{V}O_{2max}$ for 8 elite marathon runners was 74.1 ml/kg/min, approximately 50% greater than predicted (Pollock [16]). Although a high $\dot{V}O_{2max}$ is requisite for champion endurance athletes, the level of $\dot{V}O_{2max}$ is a poor predictor of performance. These cross-sectional investigations of $\dot{V}O_{2max}$ also cannot determine the relative contributions of training and of genetic endowment to the increased aerobic power of elite endurance athletes. Longitudinal studies of both males and females have consistently shown that untrained persons increase their $\dot{V}O_{2max}$ in response to a training program. The magnitude of the increase varies with the training program from approximately 10% to 50%; those with the lowest $\dot{V}_{O_{2max}}$ sustain the greatest increments (Astrand and Rodahl [14]). Performance generally improves in parallel. Although the increase in $\dot{V}_{O_{2max}}$ appears to be the principal determinant of improved performance, other factors, such as improved technique and psychologic adaptation, are probably also important. The magnitude of the increase in $\dot{V}_{O_{2max}}$ is determined by the intensity, duration, and frequency of the training; the relative importance of these training program characteristics is currently controversial. Whether untrained athletes can be trained to the aerobic power levels attained by elite endurance athletes is unclear.

As anticipated from the Fick equation, training increases $\dot{V}_{O_{2max}}$ by increasing cardiac output and by increasing oxygen extraction by the muscles (Astrand and Rodahl [14]). Although training may affect some pulmonary function parameters and the pulmonary physiology of elite athletes may differ from that of normal individuals, alterations in the respiratory system do not contribute to increasing $\dot{V}_{O_{2max}}$ with training.

Increased cardiac output and increased tissue oxygen extraction contribute equally to the increase of $\dot{V}_{O_{2max}}$ (Rowell [17]) as follows:

**Heart**
1. Increased stroke volume, decreased rate at submaximal loads
2. Increased maximal cardiac output

**Skeletal Muscle**
1. Increased myoglobin content
2. Increased size and number of mitochondria
3. Increased enzymes involved in fatty acid metabolism
4. Increased glycogen synthetase activity and elevated skeletal muscle glycogen
5. Increased muscle capillary density

Training increases stroke volume, reduces heart rate at submaximal levels, and increases maximal cardiac output (Astrand and Rodahl [14]). Although specific relationships between skeletal muscle adaptations and increased $\dot{V}_{O_{2max}}$ are not well defined, each appears to increase the capacity for aerobic metabolism (Gollnick and Sembrowich [5]). In fact, the enzyme adaptations are remarkably specific. For example, mitochondrial enzymes that are not involved in aerobic pathways do not increase, nor do glycolytic enzymes. Whether these adaptations occur differentially in the two human muscle fiber types is uncertain (Gollnick and Sembrowich [5]). Similarly, we do not know the relative importance of training and of genetic endowment in producing the increased percentage of Type I fibers found in endurance athletes. Short-term studies suggest that the usual training does not convert a fiber of one type to the other.

These adaptations are linked to improved performance primarily through increased aerobic power (Astrand and Rodahl [14]). The increased cardiac reserve, increased capillary density (Gollnick and Sembrowich [5]; Anderson and Henriksson [18]), and increased myoglobin concentration facilitate oxygen delivery to exercising muscles. The trained muscle appears adapted for aerobic metabolism. The increases in oxidative enzymes may allow the muscle to function effectively at lower tissue $P_{O_2}$, anticipated as oxygen extraction rises. Known consequences of muscle enzyme changes include increased glycogen stores, increased reliance on fat metabolism during exercise, and increased capacity to oxidize carbohydrates (Gollnick and Sembrowich [5]; Astrand and Rodahl [14]). Thus, for the trained endurance athlete, submaximal exercise results in lower lactate levels and slower glycogen depletion; fatigue is delayed and performance improved.

Current knowledge of training effects on the respiratory system is limited and derived largely from cross-sectional studies of athletes. The data have not conclusively established that pulmonary function of trained-endurance athletes is superior to that of untrained normal persons; published reports provide conflicting observations concerning the total lung capacity, forced vital capacity, and diffusing capacity (Astrand and Rodahl [14]). Interesting recent cross-sectional studies of endurance athletes have demonstrated decreased ventilatory responsiveness to hypoxia and to hypercapnia (Bryne-Quinn et al. [19]; Scoggins et al. [20]). Family members of these athletes displayed similar reduction of ventilatory responsiveness (Scoggins et al. [20]). This implies that ventilatory response patterns of endurance athletes may be the consequence of familial factors rather than training. Mechanisms by which decreased responsiveness might be linked to improved performance are currently speculative.

The respiratory muscles, including the diaphragm, are skeletal muscles; thus, training should increase their aerobic power, although this has not been documented in human subjects. In guinea pigs, training increases the proportion of Type I fibers in the diaphragm (Lieberman et al. [21]). Longitudinal studies of training effects have not consistently found a resulting increase in the maximal voluntary ventilation (MVV); an increase in the proportion of the MVV that can be utilized without dyspnea has been demonstrated (Leith and Bradley [22]). Recently, Leith and Bradley [22] found that the endurance of the respiratory muscles could be specifically trained. Four subjects trained with voluntary hyperventilation. Their MVV increased by 14% and the proportion of the MVV at which they could sustain hyperventilation increased from 81% to 96%. These training-related changes in the respiratory muscles may contribute to improved performance by reducing the sensation of dyspnea.

# Hypertransfusion

Exercise performance may also be enhanced by hypertransfusion or "blood doping." This technique involves phlebotomy and subsequent storage of the blood until the hematocrit has returned to normal. Reinfusion of the whole blood or packed erythrocytes increases the hematocrit and hence oxygen-carrying capacity. Buick and co-workers (Buick et al. [23]) showed that this technique increases $\dot{V}O_{2max}$ and running time to exhaustion. The enhancement of performance lasted 16 weeks even though the hematocrit returned to normal. We speculate that the ability to train at higher intensity may explain the persistence of the effect. Buick's and other studies of hypertransfusion confirm the relationship between oxygen-carrying capacity and performance (Buick et al. [23]; Ekblom et al. [24]).

# Pulmonary Response to Exercise in Lung Disease

## Clinical Exercise Testing

Exercise testing is usually performed either with a progressively increasing work load or with a constant work load. The work load is applied either by a bicycle ergometer or by treadmill. During an exercise test, collection, measurement, and analysis of exhaled air allows the determination of tidal volume ($V_T$), volume of expired gas ($\dot{V}_E$), oxygen consumption ($\dot{V}_{O_2}$), carbon dioxide production ($\dot{V}_{CO_2}$), anaerobic threshold (AT), and respiratory exchange ratio (R). If arterial blood gases are measured, alveolar ventilation ($\dot{V}_A$), dead space ventilation ($\dot{V}_D$), and the alveolar-arterial oxygen gradient can also be determined. Heart rate and respiratory frequency are usually monitored (Jones [25]).

## Chronic Airflow Obstruction

Dyspnea on exertion is the most common symptom in patients with chronic airflow obstruction. In this syndrome, loss of elastic recoil in pulmonary tissue as a result of emphysema, and increased airway resistance because of airway narrowing and obliteration, reduce expiratory flow (Thurlbeck [26]). Consequently, the work of breathing is increased and dyspnea occurs because the ventilatory demands of a given work load are met with difficulty. Additionally, in some patients, decrease of the arterial oxygen tension contributes to dyspnea on exertion (Jones [25]). Dyspnea usually occurs when the $FEV_1$ is less than 2.0 liters, a reduction of approximately 50%. Ventilation limits performance with exercise testing. At the maximum work load, voluntary ventilation reaches the maximum (MVV); at that point, heart rate is submaximal and the $\dot{V}_{O_2max}$ is below the predicted level.

Although the exercise performance of patients with chronic airflow obstruction is limited, they may exercise and participate in physical training programs. A properly designed exercise program should result in improved exercise tolerance (Chester et al. [27]; Belman and Kendregan [28]). However, the mechanisms underlying the improved performance are uncertain and may differ from those important in normals (Chester et al. [27]; Belman and Kendregan [28]; Degre et al. [29]). Specific training of the respiratory muscles may be accomplished by repetitive breathing against a resistance device (Belman and Mittman [30]). The physician should use both routine pulmonary function tests and measurement of exercise capacity in designing realistic activity programs for such patients.

# Asthma

The exercise performance of patients with asthma is limited as a result of the same mechanisms discussed in the foregoing section on chronic airflow obstruction. Moreover, some asthmatic patients have exercise-induced bronchospasm (EIB), an increase in airway resistance that usually occurs 5–10 min after cessation of an exercise challenge. McFadden and Ingram [31] have postulated that EIB results from increased respiratory heat exchange as minute ventilation rises. The exact mechanism by which heat flux triggers release of mediators of bronchospasm is unclear. Only certain types of exercise are associated with EIB—characteristically, activities such as bicycling and running, in which there is high aerobic demand. The severity of EIB is directly proportional to the intensity of the exercise (McFadden and Ingram [31]).

Clinically, EIB may be manifest as wheezing, dyspnea, or coughing during or after physical activity (Shephard [32]). Symptoms may be increased by exercise in cold, dry air (McFadden and Ingram [31]). The physician should consider EIB in patients whose wheezing, cough, or dyspnea is primarily associated with exercise—for example, the runner who complains of cough after his morning workout. The diagnosis should be confirmed with exercise testing. Characteristically, ventilatory measurements, such as $FEV_1$, and airway resistance begin to worsen during the exercise stimulus and show the maximum effect 5–10 min after cessation of exercise. Inhalation of sympathomimetic aerosols before exercise is the treatment of choice for EIB. These agents may improve basal pulmonary function, and in most patients they abolish post-exercise bronchoconstriction (Anderson et al. [33]; Eggleston et al. [34]). Oral sympathomimetics and theophylline compounds are less effective (Anderson et al. [33]; Eggleston et al. [34]). Cromolyn sodium may also be utilized, but it does not improve basal pulmonary function.

# Restrictive Lung Disease

Restrictive lung diseases limit vital capacity by reducing the volume of air that can be inhaled. Diseases of the pulmonary interstitium are the most common example. Exercise limitation parallels the reduction of vital capacity. With exercise testing, these patients characteristically increase $\dot{V}_E$ primarily through a marked increase in respiratory frequency. As with chronic airflow obstruction, $\dot{V}_{O_2}$ and heart rate fail to reach predicted values. In patients suffering interstitial lung disease or other diseases that stiffen the lung parenchyma, the loss of compliance is the cause of the increased work of breathing (Jones [25]).

# Exercise under Special Conditions

## Cigarette Smoking

Tobacco smoke is a complex mixture containing several thousand distinct chemical compounds. The physiological consequences of smoking are myriad, and only those relevant to the endurance athlete will be briefly discussed. Acute inhalation of cigarette smoke may increase airway resistance and elevate blood carboxyhemoglobin because of the high concentration of carbon monoxide in cigarette smoke. Chronic cigarette smoking may result in permanent reduction of ventilatory and gas exchange capacity. The effects on the circulatory system range from acute blood pressure and pulse rate elevation to promotion of degenerative cardiovascular disease. Thus, the empirical observation that cigarette smokers have reduced $Vo_{2max}$ is not surprising (Ingemann-Hansen and Halkjaer-Kristensen [35]), nor are the investigators' personal observations that endurance athletes do not smoke.

## Air Pollution

Both popular literature and scientific reports have hypothesized that ambient air pollution may limit exercise performance and that the high minute ventilation of the endurance athlete may place him or her at risk for pollution effects. Air pollution is a mixture of atmospheric contaminants that can be categorized into two major types. The sulfur oxide and particulate complex produced by the combustion of fossil fuels affects the industrialized urban areas of the eastern and central United States. Photochemical pollution, or smog, results principally from motor vehicle emissions and predominates in metropolitan areas of the western United States.

Few data are available to support the hypothesized effects of air pollution on the endurance athlete. In Los Angeles, Wayne et al. [36] found that performance of high school cross-country track teams was adversely affected by photochemical pollution. In Tucson, Arizona, which also has photochemical pollution, Lebowitz et al. [37] demonstrated that exercise on high pollution days decreased lung function. Similar studies of populations exposed to sulfur oxide and particulate-matter pollution have not been performed. Experimental chamber exposures of exercising human subjects generally support the cited studies. Effects of pollutants, however, are usually observed only at levels several-fold higher than those normally encountered in ambient air. Certain people, such as those suffering from asthma, may be more sensitive to pollution.

Carbon monoxide is of particular importance for the endurance athlete because of its effects on oxygen transport and the exposure of urban athletes to motor vehicle exhaust. Carbon monoxide limits oxygen transport by combining with hemoglobin to form nonfunctional carboxyhemoglobin and by limiting tissue oxygen availability by increasing hemoglobin affinity for oxygen. Exercise increases the rate at which hemoglobin achieves equilibrium with inhaled carbon monoxide. In young, healthy men, $Vo_{2max}$ declines linearly as carboxyhemoglobin increases from 5% to 35%. Effects on oxygen transport have not been demonstrated at levels below 4% in healthy subjects. Patients with coronary artery disease or with peripheral vascular disease, however, appear to be affected by levels as low as 2.5%–3% carboxyhemoglobin. Carbon monoxide pollution severe enough to limit the maximal performance of normal individuals rarely occurs. In certain western cities of the United States the combined effects of exercise, carbon monoxide, and altitude might limit oxygen transport under unusual circumstances (National Research Council [38]).

# Altitude

The partial pressure of oxygen in ambient air declines linearly with increasing altitude (Frisancho [39]). As a result, the alveolar partial pressure of oxygen is reduced at high altitude and the oxygen transport system delivers less oxygen to tissue than at sea level (Fig. 2). Each step of oxygen transport is affected by altitude (Frisancho [39]; Lenfant and Sullivan [40]). As a result, above 5000 feet, $\dot{V}_{O_{2}max}$ declines by approximately 3% per 1000 feet ascent. In both sojourners and natives at high altitude, a subnormal cardiac output with exercise causes the reduction of $\dot{V}_{O_{2}max}$ (Frisancho [39]; Lenfant and Sullivan [40]).

Acute exposure to high altitude results in increased ventilation with respiratory alkalosis, and resting tachycardia with increased cardiac output (Frisancho [39]; Lenfant and Sullivan [40]). With acclimatization, hyperventilation persists but at a lower level than initially; pulmonary diffusing capacity does not appear to increase; resting cardiac output declines; red cell mass increases and the oxygen hemoglobin dissociation curve shifts to the right; and tissue capillarization and enzymes related to oxidative metabolism increase. These adaptations result in a partial reversal of the altitude-related reduction of $\dot{V}_{O_{2}max}$. Reduced maximal cardiac output, however, continues to limit $\dot{V}_{O_{2}max}$.

Highland natives also have polycythemia and reduced maximal cardiac output (Frisancho [39]). Their level of ventilation at high altitude is less than that of sojourners, primarily because of reduced response to hypoxia. Compared with lowlanders, highland natives have increased lung volumes and pulmonary diffusing capacity (Frisancho [39]; Lenfant and Sullivan [40]). The $\dot{V}_{O_{2}max}$ (as milliliters per minute per kilogram of body weight) of the high altitude native exceeds that of the acclimatized lowlander, unless the latter moved to high altitude during childhood.

The physician may be asked to advise athletes about training at high altitude. Frequently asked questions relate to the potential advantages of training and exercise at high altitude and to the potential hazards of such training. Whether training at high altitude is advantageous is unclear from current reports. Several studies have been conducted in which performance and $\dot{V}_{O_{2}max}$ at sea level were measured after training at high altitude (Faulkner et al. [41]; Dill and Adams [42]). The conflicting results of these studies suggest that training at high altitude probably does not provide marked benefits.

Physicians should be aware of the syndrome of acute mountain sickness (Hacket et al. [43]; Hecht [44]). Both lowlanders acutely ascending to high altitude and highlanders returning to high altitude are at risk. Exercise, particularly by untrained individuals, increases the risk of acute mountain sickness. The incidence of this syndrome increases with altitude and is highest above 10,000 feet. Manifestations include headache, personality changes, lassitude, dyspnea, anorexia, nausea, and vomiting (Hackett et al. [43]). Acute pulmonary edema may occur and acute cerebral edema may result in coma, convulsions, and death. Normal individuals manifest a large range of susceptibility to acute mountain sickness. The pathophysiology of acute mountain sickness is unclear; the occurrence of widespread capillary leakage appears to have a crucial role in its development. Acetazolamide, a carbonic anhydrase inhibitor, is of proven prophylactic value (Hecht [44]; Forwand et al. [45]).

# References

1. Åstrand, P., Rodahl, K. 1977. Textbook of Work Physiology. McGraw-Hill Book Co., New York, pp 449–480.
2. Åstrand, P., Rodahl, K. 1977. Textbook of Work Physiology. McGraw-Hill Book Co., New York, pp 11–34.
3. Wasserman, K., Whipp, B.J. 1975. Exercise physiology in health and disease. Am Rev Respir Dis 112:219–249.
4. Felig, P., Wahren, J. 1975. Fuel homeostasis in exercise. N Engl J Med 293:1078–1084.
5. Gollnick, P.D., Sembrowich, W.L. 1977. Adaptations in human skeletal muscle as a result of training. In: Amsterdam E.A., Wilmore J.H., DeMaria A.N., (eds): Exercise in Cardiovascular Health and Disease. Yorke Medical Books, New York, pp 70–94.
6. Felig, P., Cherif, A., Minagawa, A. et al. 1982. Hypoglycemia during prolonged exercise in normal man. N Eng J Med 306:895–900.
7. Åstrand, P., Rodahl, K. 1977. Textbook of Work Physiology. McGraw-Hill Book Co., New York, pp 207–266.
8. Wasserman, K. 1978. Breathing during exercise. N Engl J Med 298:780–785.
9. Johnson, R.L. 1973. The lung as an organ of oxygen transport. Basics Resp Dis 2(1):1–6.
10. Åstrand, P., Rodahl, K. 1977. Textbook of Work Physiology. McGraw-Hill Book Co., New York, pp 291–329.
11. Shephard, R.J. 1978. Physical Activity and Aging. Year Book Medical Publishers, Inc, Chicago, pp 204–224.
12. Murray, J.F. 1976. The Normal Lung. The Basis for Diagnosis and Treatment of Pulmonary Disease. W.B. Saunders Co., Philadelphia, pp 307–324.
13. Shephard, R.J. 1978. Physical Activity and Aging. Year Book Medical Publishers, Inc, Chicago, pp 176–203.
14. Åstrand, P., Rodahl, K. 1977. Textbook of Work Physiology. McGraw-Hill Book Co., New York, pp 291–329, 391–445, 449–480.
15. Cotes, J.E. 1975. Lung Function. Assessment and Application in Medicine, 3rd Ed. Blackwell Scientific Publications, Oxford, pp 275–295.
16. Pollock, M.L. 1977. Submaximal and maximal working capacity of elite distance runners. I. Cardiorespiratory Aspects. Ann NY Acad Sci 301:310–322.
17. Rowell, L.B. 1974. Human cardiovascular adjustments to exercise and thermal stress. Physiol Rev 54:75–179.
18. Anderson, P., Henriksson, J. 1977. Capillary supply of the quadriceps femoris muscle of man: Adaptive response to exercise. J Physiol 270:677–690.
19. Bryne-Quinn, E., Weil, J.V., Sodal, I.E. et al. 1971. Ventilatory control in the athlete. J Appl Physiol 30:91–98.
20. Scoggins, C.H., Doekel, R.D., Kryger, M.H. et al. 1978. Familial aspects of decreased hypoxic drive in endurance athletes. J Appl Physiol 44:464–468.
21. Lieberman, D.A., Maxwell, L.C., Faulkner, J.A. 1972. Adaptation of guinea pig diaphragm muscle to aging and endurance training. Am J Physiol 222:556–560.

22. Leith, D.E., Bradley, M. 1976. Ventilatory muscle strength and endurance training. J Appl Physiol 41:508–516.

23. Buick, F.J., Gledhill N, Froese, A.B. et al. 1980. Effect of induced erythrocythemia on aerobic work capacity. J Appl Physiol 48:636–642.

24. Ekblom, B., Goldbarg, A.N., Gullbring, B. 1972. Response to exercise after blood loss and reinfusion. J Appl Physiol 33:175–180.

25. Jones, N.L. 1975. Exercise in pulmonary evaluation. Rationale, methods and the normal respiratory response to exercise. Clinical applications. N Engl J Med 293:541–544, 647–650.

26. Thurlbeck, W.M. 1977. Aspects of chronic airflow obstruction. Chest 72:341–349.

27. Chester, E.H., Belman, M.J., Bahler, R.C. et al. 1977. Multidisciplinary treatment of chronic pulmonary insufficiency. Chest 72:695–702.

28. Belman, M.J., Kendregan, B.A. 1981. Exercise training fails to increase skeletal muscle enzymes in patients with chronic obstructive pulmonary disease. Am Rev Respir Dis 123:256–261.

29. Degre, S., Sergysels, R., Messin, R. et al. 1974. Hemodynamic responses to physical training in patients with chronic lung disease. Am Rev Respir Dis 110:395–402.

30. Belman, M.J., Mittman, C. 1980. Ventilatory muscle training improves exercise capacity in chronic obstructive pulmonary disease patients. Am Rev Respir Dis 121:273–280.

31. McFadden, E.R. Jr., Ingram, R.H., Jr. 1979. Exercise-induced asthma: Observations on the initiating stimulus. N Engl J Med 301:763–769.

32. Shephard, R.J. 1977. Exercise-induced bronchospasm—a review. Med Sci Sports 9:1–10.

33. Anderson, S.D., Seale, J.P., Rosea, P. et al. 1976. Inhaled and oral salbutamol in exercise-induced asthma. Am Rev Respir Dis 114:493–500.

34. Eggleston, P.A., Beasley, P.P., Kindley, R.T. 1981. The effects of oral doses of theophylline and fenoterol on exercise-induced asthma. Chest 79:399–405.

35. Ingemann-Hansen, T., Halkjaer-Kristensen, J. 1977. Cigarette smoking and maximal oxygen consumption in humans. Scand J Clin Lab Invest 37:143–148.

36. Wayne, W.S., Wehrle, P.F., Carroll, R.E. 1967. Oxidant air pollution and athletic performance. JAMA 199:901–904.

37. Lebowitz, M.D., Bendheim, P., Cristea, G. et al. 1974. The effect of air pollution and weather on the lung function in exercising children and adolescents. Am Rev Respir Dis 109:262–273.

38. National Research Council, Committee on Medical and Biological Effects of Environmental Pollutants. 1977. Carbon Monoxide. National Academy of Sciences, Washington D.C.

39. Frisancho, A.R. 1975. Functional adaptation to high altitude hypoxia. Science 187:313–319.

40. Lenfant, C., Sullivan, K. 1971. Adaptation to high altitude. N Engl J Med 284:1298–1309.

41. Faulkner, J.A., Daniels, J.T., Balke, B. 1967. Effects of training at moderate altitude on physical performance capacity. J Appl Physiol 23:85–89.

42. Dill, D.B., Adams, W.C. 1971. Maximal oxygen uptake at sea level and at 3,090-m altitude in high school champion runners. J Appl Physiol 30:854–859.

43. Hackett, P.H., Dennie, D., Levine, H.D. 1976. The incidence, importance, and prophylaxis of acute mountain sickness. Lancet 2:1149–1155.

44. Hecht, H.H. 1971. A sea level view of altitude problems. Am J Med 50:703–708.

45. Forwand, S.A., Landowne, M., Follansbee, J.N. et al. 1968. Effect of acetazolamide on acute mountain sickness. N Engl J Med 279:839–845.

# Chapter 16

# Oxygen Transport During Exercise at Sea Level and High Altitude[1]

by Stephen C. Wood

## General Aspects of Oxygen Transport

For healthy persons at rest, the acquisition and transport of oxygen are subliminal processes. However, three situations bring the importance of oxygen transport, and the discomfort of hypoxia, to conscious levels. These are cardiopulmonary disease, exposure to high altitude, and vigorous exercise. These situations involve 1) an inadequate transfer (cardiopulmonary disease), 2) an inadequate supply (exposure to altitude) and 3) an inordinate consumption of oxygen (vigorous exercise). How the oxygen transport system adapts to altitude and exercise is the topic of this chapter.

## The Oxygen ''Cascade''

The transport of oxygen from the environment to tissue (muscles, especially) and of carbon dioxide ($CO_2$) in the reverse direction involves four processes, each of which has a variable rate. The components of $O_2$ supply to muscle are illustrated in Figure 16–1. They are as follows:

1. Ventilation
2. Diffusion from alveolar gas to pulmonary capillaries
3. Circulation
4. Diffusion from tissue capillaries to the cellular site of utilization (mitochondria)

[1]Supported by NSF Grant PCM-7724246.

## STEPS IN $O_2$ UPTAKE

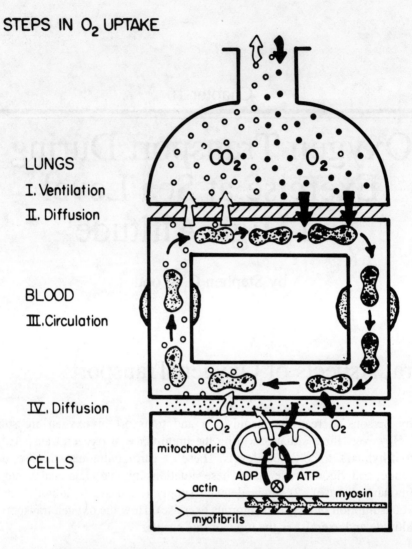

**16–1**   Respiratory system, indicating the four steps in $O_2$ uptake. (Adapted from Weibel, E. 1979. The scaling of oxygen transport in mammals. In Wood, S.C., and Lenfant, C., (eds): Evolution of Respiratory Processes: A Comparative Approach. Marcel Dekker, Inc., New York.)

The two active steps, ventilation and circulation, have variable rates and play major roles in compensation for exercise or disease. The $O_2$ stores (lung, hemoglobin, myoglobin) are of limited value in exercise, amounting to a total of only about 2 liters in a 70-kg person (Cherniak and Longobardo [1]).

The rate of $O_2$ transfer at each step is presented quantitatively in Figure 16–2. The first equation shows the measures actually used to assess $O_2$ uptake in the laboratory—i.e., ventilation of air and concentration of $O_2$ in exhaled air. Because these steps are in series, all equations give identical values of $\dot{M}_{O_2}$. Furthermore, the maximum $O_2$ uptake is obviously limited by the step that has the lowest capacity to increase during exercise. It is generally accepted that for sea level- or low altitude-exercise, the final two steps are limiting, with some investigators favoring a circulatory limitation, whereas others favor a

STEPS IN $O_2$ UPTAKE

EQUATIONS FOR
$O_2$ TRANSFER

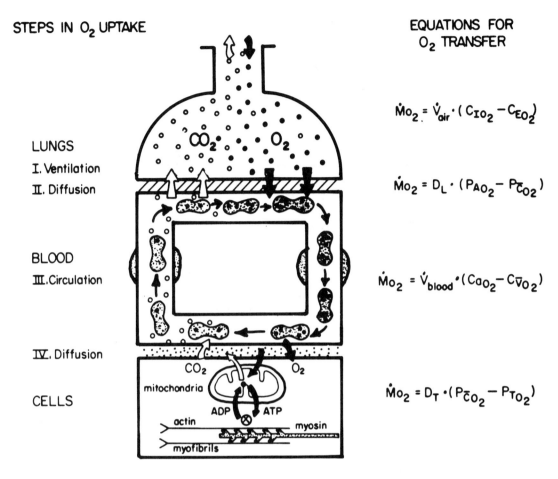

LUNGS

I. Ventilation

II. Diffusion

BLOOD

III. Circulation

IV. Diffusion

CELLS

$$\dot{M}_{O_2} = \dot{V}_{air} \cdot (C_{IO_2} - C_{EO_2})$$

$$\dot{M}_{O_2} = D_L \cdot (P_{AO_2} - P_{\bar{c}O_2})$$

$$\dot{M}_{O_2} = \dot{V}_{blood} \cdot (C_{aO_2} - C_{\bar{v}O_2})$$

$$\dot{M}_{O_2} = D_T \cdot (P_{\bar{c}O_2} - P_{TO_2})$$

**16–2** Quantification of steps in $O_2$ transport for convective and diffusive transfer of $O_2$. See text for discussion.

tissue or metabolic limitation. At high altitude, diffusive limitations for lung $O_2$ transfer become an important limitation, (see section on Oxygen Transport and Delivery at High Altitude later in this chapter).

Variables associated with each step in $O_2$ transfer are presented in Figure 16–3. Each variable is also potentially adaptive to exercise-induced increases in $O_2$ demand or altitude-dependent decreases in $O_2$ supply.

## Oxygen Uptake

Skeletal muscle cells account for most of the $O_2$ uptake during rest and exercise (Hill [8]). In these and other cells, the mitochondria are the primary sites of $O_2$ utilization. An adequate supply of $O_2$ to muscle ensures that metabolic fuels are combusted to $CO_2$ and $H_2O$ (Fig. 16–4). This oxidative metabolism produces 12 times as much adenosine triphosphate (ATP) per mole of glucose as anaerobic metabolism. Adenosine triphosphate, in turn, provides energy for muscle contraction and relaxation.

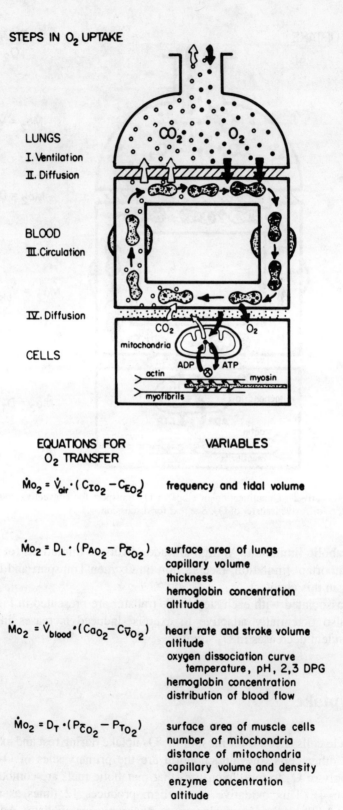

## STEPS IN $O_2$ UPTAKE

LUNGS
I. Ventilation
II. Diffusion

BLOOD
III. Circulation

IV. Diffusion

CELLS

$CO_2$    $O_2$

mitochondria

ADP    ATP

actin                    myosin
myofibrils

EQUATIONS FOR                 VARIABLES
$O_2$ TRANSFER

$\dot{M}_{O_2} = \dot{V}_{air} \cdot (C_{I_{O_2}} - C_{E_{O_2}})$     frequency and tidal volume

$\dot{M}_{O_2} = D_L \cdot (P_{A_{O_2}} - P_{\bar{c}_{O_2}})$     surface area of lungs
capillary volume
thickness
hemoglobin concentration
altitude

$\dot{M}_{O_2} = \dot{V}_{blood} \cdot (C_{a_{O_2}} - C_{\bar{v}_{O_2}})$     heart rate and stroke volume
altitude
oxygen dissociation curve
    temperature, pH, 2,3 DPG
hemoglobin concentration
distribution of blood flow

$\dot{M}_{O_2} = D_T \cdot (P_{\bar{c}_{O_2}} - P_{T_{O_2}})$     surface area of muscle cells
number of mitochondria
distance of mitochondria
capillary volume and density
enzyme concentration
altitude

**16–3**   Main variables at each step of $O_2$ transfer. Each variable is a potential limit to maximum $O_2$ uptake.

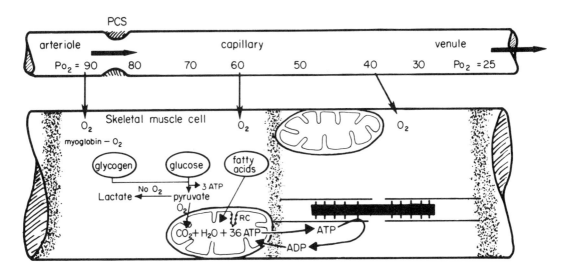

**16–4** General scheme of $O_2$ uptake by muscle cells. Precapillary sphincters (*PCS*) vary rate of muscle capillary blood flow. See text for discussion.

With increased physical activity, $O_2$ consumption increases as a result of increased ATP utilization by skeletal muscles. For adults weighing about 70 kg, the $O_2$ uptake at rest is approximately 250 ml/min, irrespective of their athletic prowess. For untrained adults, $O_2$ uptake may increase 16-fold (4000 ml/min) at maximum effort; trained adults may increase up to 25-fold (6250 ml/min) or more. There are, however, large differences between the sexes, among different types of athletes, and at various altitudes. The ability of athletes to increase their maximum $O_2$ uptake by training depends on variables shown in Figure 16–3.

The relative importance of these variables will be discussed, but it is useful first to consider how important a high maximum $O_2$ uptake is to athletic performance. The best available data apply to distance runners. The oxygen "cost" of running is independent of running speed; i.e., $O_2$ uptake increases linearly with running speed and is the same for male and female runners (Fig. 16–5a). Thus, the cost of running is about 5 ml $O_2 \times kg^{-1} \times min^{-1} \times mph^{-1}$, and this is a constant.

However, it should be noted that $O_2$ cost for improving performance in terms of time per unit distance is not a constant because time is the reciprocal of speed, and the $O_2$ cost of improving running time is not linear (Fig. 16–5b). For example, to decrease running time from 10 to 8 min/mile requires an increase in $O_2$ uptake of about 8 ml $\times kg^{-1} \times min^{-1}$ (from 30 to 38), but the same 2-min improvement from 7 to 5 min/mile requires an increase of about 25 ml $\times kg^{-1} \times min^{-1}$ (from 40 to 65).

Note also (Fig. 16–5) that a running speed slightly faster than 12 mph is necessary to complete a marathon in world class time. This, in turn, requires an $O_2$ uptake in excess of 70 ml $\times kg^{-1} \times min^{-1}$, or 20–30 ml $\times kg^{-1} \times min^{-1}$ greater than the maximum $O_2$ uptake of untrained adults.

The importance of a high maximum $O_2$ uptake for competitive performance depends largely on the length of the race. In sprints and other short-distance races, the value of maximum $O_2$ uptake is less important, as "oxygen debts" are easily tolerated for short

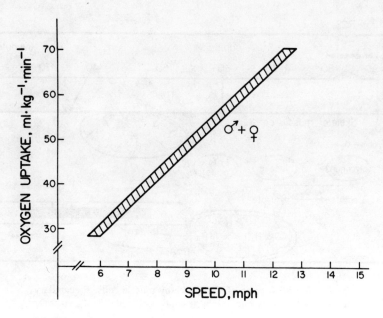

**16–5a**  Oxygen uptake as function of running speed in men and women. (Redrawn from Davies, C.T.M., Thompson, M.W. 1979. Aerobic performance of female marathon and male ultra marathon athletes. Eur J Appl Physiol 41:233–245.)

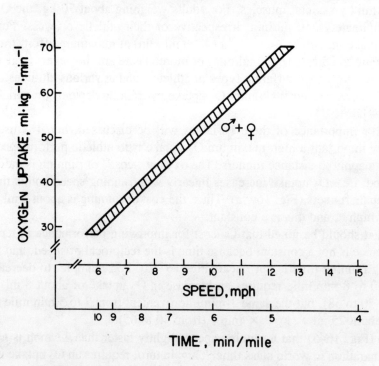

**16–5b**  Same as Figure 5a with time in minutes per mile shown on the x axis. (Redrawn from Davies, C.T.M., Thompson, M.W. 1979. Aerobic performance of female marathon and male ultra marathon athletes. Eur J Appl Physiol 41:233–245.) See text for discussion.

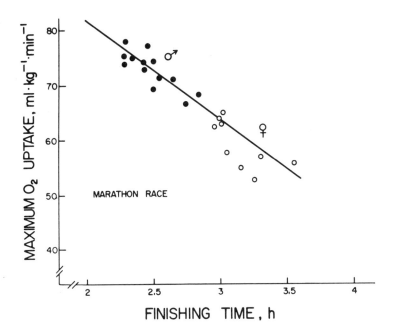

**16–6**  Finishing time in marathon race as function of maximum $O_2$ uptake for male and female runners. (Redrawn from Davies, C.T.M., Thompson, M.W. 1979. Aerobic performance of female marathon and male ultra marathon athletes. Eur J Appl Physiol 41:233–245.)

durations. In longer races, e.g., marathons, there is generally little or no lactic acid accumulation in trained competitors—i.e., the race is run under steady-state, aerobic metabolism. Under these conditions, there is a significant correlation between maximum $O_2$ uptake and finishing times for both male and female runners (Fig. 16–6). In a longer "ultramarathon" race, however, there is a much weaker correlation, indicating, perhaps, the importance of psychologic factors. For the marathon, measurement of maximum $O_2$ uptake on a treadmill will predict finishing time fairly well (Fig. 16–6). Of course, numerous other factors are also important. Chief among these is the fraction of maximum $O_2$ uptake at which a runner can perform. For most people, lactate accumulation begins at about 70% of maximum $O_2$ uptake, but in highly trained distance runners the so-called "anaerobic threshold" is not reached until $O_2$ uptake reaches 90% of maximum.

## Distribution of Blood Flow

The primary cardiovascular adaptations to exercise are an increase in total cardiac output and redistribution of blood flow to favor skeletal muscles. The change from rest to heavy work alters the proportion of cardiac output going to skeletal muscle from 15%–20% to 80%–85%. This redistribution of blood flow to exercising muscles is essential in assuring the increased $O_2$ supply during work. The $O_2$ uptake of muscles at $\dot{V}_{O_2max}$ is about 100 times their resting $O_2$ uptake. With an arteriovenous $O_2$ difference of twice normal, this requires a 50-fold increase in blood flow (Asmussen [2]).

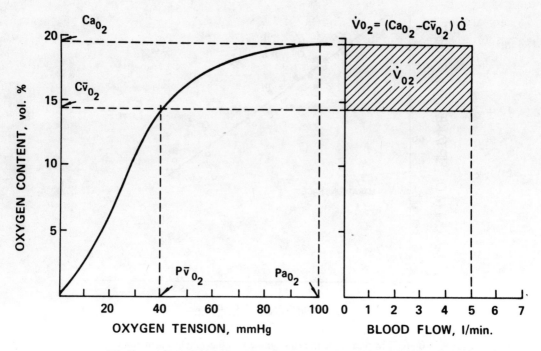

**16-7** Graphic representation of the Fick principle, $\dot{V}_{O_2} = \dot{Q} \times (Ca_{O_2} - C\bar{v}_{O_2})$, showing the oxygen dissociation curve for blood. See text for discussion.

The mechanism of this adaptive response to exercise has been attributed to: 1) stimulation of sympathetic vasodilator fibers resulting in an initial, even anticipatory decrease in resistance; and 2) local (auto) regulation, whereby low $O_2$ levels cause decreased resistance, either directly or via release of some vasodilator metabolite. More recent evidence indicates that intrinsic nerves act to maintain maximum vasodilation during muscle contraction. Intrinsic sympathetic fibers *initiate* vasodilation before contraction, assuring maximum flow at onset of contraction (avoiding early $O_2$ debt), and maintain maximum vasodilation during contraction. Moreover, local metabolites result in vasodilation, which persists after contraction ceases, allowing repayment of an $O_2$ debt (Honig [3]). In addition to vasodilation, the increase in flow is enhanced by the recruitment of capillaries that are usually closed at rest. For example, the number of open capillaries in guinea-pig muscle increases from about 30 per mm$^2$ at rest to 2500 per mm$^2$ during exercise (Krogh [4, 5]).

# Oxygen Transport vs. Oxygen Delivery

## The Fick Principle

The amount of oxygen made available to any tissue (per minute) is readily calculable as the product of blood flow and arterial $O_2$ content—e.g., $O_2$ transport (ml $O_2$/min) = $\dot{Q}$

(liters of blood/min) $\times$ $CaO_2$ (ml $O_2$/liter of blood). For a normal person at rest, $O_2$ transport to all tissues is about 1000 ml $O_2$/min (5 liters/min $\times$ 200 ml $O_2$/liter of blood). If arterial saturation is reduced (at constant hemoglobin content) to 50%, $O_2$ transport is halved.

The $O_2$ *transported* determines the maximum $O_2$ available. However, the $O_2$ *delivered* (or utilized) is a more important measure. Once $O_2$ is transported to tissue capillaries, its utilization and uptake depend on the rate of diffusion (passive or facilitated by myoglobin).

At this point it is helpful to use the Fick principle (Fig. 16–7), which relates the variables that determine $O_2$ delivery, i.e., $O_2$ delivered = ($O_2$ transported in − $O_2$ transported out), or:

$$\dot{V}_{O_2} = (\dot{Q} \times CaO_2) - (\dot{Q} \times C\bar{v}_{O_2})$$
$$\text{or}$$
$$\dot{V}_{O_2} = \dot{Q} \times (CaO_2 - C\bar{v}_{O_2})$$

## Role of the Oxyhemoglobin Dissociation Curve in Exercise

The relationship between blood $O_2$ content and partial pressure is described by the oxyhemoglobin dissociation curve (ODC) (Fig. 16–7). For a given ODC, the arterial ($CaO_2$) and venous ($C\bar{v}_{O_2}$) oxygen contents correspond to a unique $P_{O_2}$. The ultimate physiologic role of the ODC is to insure that capillary $P_{O_2}$ is high enough for an adequate $O_2$ diffusion into tissues. Any adaptation of the shape or position of the ODC must be one that minimizes a decrease in $P\bar{v}_{O_2}$.

**Influence of the Hematocrit**    One way of increasing capillary $P_{O_2}$ (as reflected by $P\bar{v}_{O_2}$) is to have an increased hematocrit causing an increased $O_2$ capacity (and increased $CaO_2$). If $O_2$ extraction ($CaO_2 - C\bar{v}_{O_2}$) is constant, an increase in $O_2$ capacity (hematocrit) will result in an increased $P\bar{v}_{O_2}$. This is a major component of acclimatization to mountaineering at high altitude but does not seem to play a role in adaptation to exercise at sea level and is not seen in endurance runners who train at moderate altitudes (up to 7000 ft).

**Influence of the Position of the ODC**    The relation of the ODC to the x axis, i.e., the oxygen affinity of blood, is usually quantified as the $P_{50}$. The $P_{50}$ is influenced by the ODC, as in Figure 16–8, in which the $P_{50}$'s (i.e., the $P_{O_2}$ of 50% saturated blood) are approximately 20, 27, and 30 mm Hg. The traditional view is that any factor that shifts the ODC to the left and lowers $P_{50}$ (Curve III, Fig. 16–8) will decrease $O_2$ delivery, whereas a shift of the ODC to the right (Curve II, Fig. 16–8) increases $O_2$ delivery, and a higher $P_{50}$ is always advantageous. However, this generalization must be qualified, particularly if arterial hypoxemia exists. (Lahiri [18]). Although an increase in $O_2$ capacity improves $O_2$ delivery, an increase in $P_{50}$ is advantageous only if arterial $P_{O_2}$ exceeds a certain value and $O_2$ "loading" in the lung is not significantly impaired. Consequently, a high $P_{50}$ may be detrimental during arterial hypoxemia if $O_2$ extraction is increased as a result of exercise or reduced cardiac output. Also, as $O_2$ extraction varies among different organs, so does the advantage or disadvantage of a given $P_{50}$.

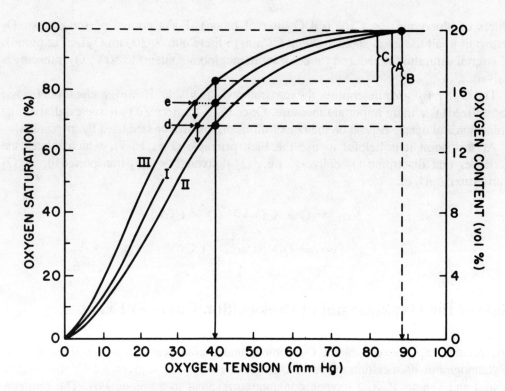

**16–8**  Influence of position of oxyhemoglobin dissociation curve (ODC) on $O_2$ extraction at normal sea level values of arterial and mixed-venous $P_{O_2}$. Curve I represents normal ODC in human subjects. Curve II, shift of ODC to right, increases $O_2$ delivery. Curve III decreases $O_2$ delivery (from bracket A to bracket C). (From Shappell, S.D., Lenfant, C. 1975. Physiological role of the oxyhemoglobin dissociation curve. In: Surgenor D.M., (ed): The Red Blood Cell, Vol 2. Academic Press, New York. Reprinted with permission of the publisher.)

Humoral factors that alter the position of the ODC during exercise are $P_{CO_2}$, and most potently, pH and temperature. (Most of the $CO_2$ effect is indirect—i.e., a pH effect.) These have an exponential effect on $P_{50}$ (Fig. 16–9). Thus, all humoral changes accompanying exercise act in concert to shift the ODC to the right, which, at sea level in healthy people, increases $O_2$ delivery to working muscles. Any accumulation of carboxyhemoglobin due, for instance, to air pollution and/or cigarette smoking will offset this increase in $P_{50}$ and decrease the $O_2$ capacity of blood.

In addition to humoral factors and elevated temperature and acidosis, a right-shifted ODC may result from an increase in the amount of 2,3 diphosphoglycerate (2,3 DPG) in red cells. The role of 2,3 DPG in adaptation to exercise is controversial. The results of studies at sea level on the effects of exercise on red cell 2,3 DPG levels are equivocal. The studies showing increased 2,3 DPG with exercise are almost evenly matched by those showing no change or a decrease in 2,3 DPG. At present, the best evidence indicates an insignificant effect of a shift mediated by 2,3 DPG in the ODC on $O_2$ delivery during exercise (see section on Oxygen Transport and Delivery at High Altitude later in this chapter). For example, men (and rats) whose ODCs were left-shifted (by 2,3 DPG depletion) showed no decrease in maximum $\dot{V}_{O_2}$ or endurance (Wranne et al. [6]).

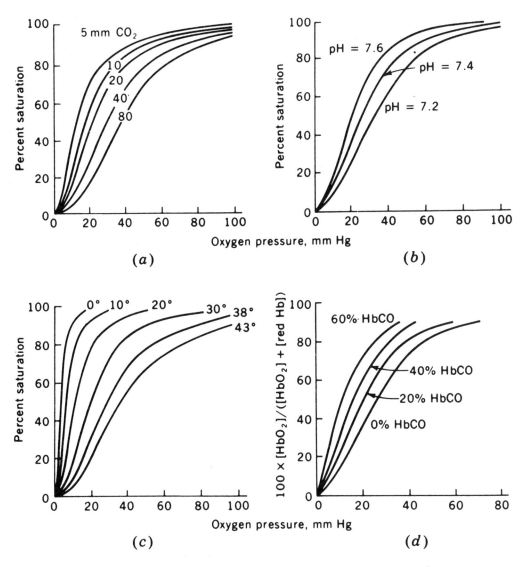

**16–9**   Effects of $P_{CO_2}$, pH, temperature, and carbon monoxide binding on $O_2$ affinity of hemoglobin. (From Astrand, P.O., Rodahl, K. 1977. Textbook of Work Physiology, 2nd Ed. McGraw-Hill Book Co., New York. Reprinted with permission of the publisher.)

The equivocal nature of the studies on 2,3 DPG and exercise probably reflects differences in experimental protocols and work levels. For example, a primary factor controlling red-cell DPG concentration is pH. Lactic acidosis would deplete 2,3 DPG, and the work levels needed to produce acidosis would depend on physical conditioning (see section on The Limits of Maximum Oxygen Uptake). Furthermore, a relatively small effect of 2,3 DPG-induced change in $P_{50}$ is expected because of the very large changes in $P_{50}$ from temperature and pH and the high $O_2$ extraction of muscle.

A graphic representation of the Fick principle (Fig. 16–10) illustrates the essentials of the foregoing discussion.

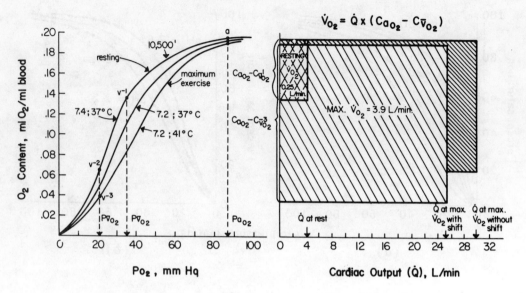

**16–10**   Graphic representation of Fick principle at rest and during maximum exercise. Shift of oxyhemoglobin dissociation curve to right occurs as a result of decreased blood pH (if lactic acid accumulates) and increased blood temperature. Values for flow, $O_2$ contents, and partial pressures represent normal values for a healthy man at rest. $O_2$ uptake of 5 liters/min $\times$ 50 ml $O_2$/liter = 250 ml $O_2$/min. *Arrow*, approximate $Pa_{O_2}$ at altitude of 10,500 ft.

What happens during exercise? In this example, $O_2$ uptake increases to a maximum; in untrained persons the increase is about 16-fold (to 3.9 liters/min). The ODC shifts to the right as a result of a decrease in pH (lactic acidosis) from 7.4 to 7.2 (middle ODC) and even farther to the right when there is an elevation in blood temperature from 37°C to 41°C. The combined factors increase $P_{50}$ from approximately 27 to 42 mm Hg. An important concept is illustrated by the vertical lines for mixed venous $P_{O_2}$ (Fig. 16–10). If the $P\bar{v}_{O_2}$ remained at resting value of 36 mm Hg, the increase in $P_{50}$ would almost double the $O_2$ extraction. However, actual extraction exceeds this, and actual $P\dot{v}_{O_2}$ decreases to about 20 mm Hg. At this value the ODCs converge and the effect of the large change in $P_{50}$ on extraction is greatly reduced.

Although the shift in the curve has a more limited effect on $C\dot{v}_{O_2}$ at low values of $P\dot{v}_{O_2}$, the adaptiveness of the increased $P_{50}$ is clear when the effect on cardiac output is considered. The actual cardiac output at max $\dot{V}_{O_2}$ is approximately 25 liters/min (Fig. 16–10), but without a shift in the ODC the required cardiac output would be approximately 30 liters/min, beyond the capacity of most people. A portion of the 1979 and 1980 endurance runs (28.5 miles) along the crest trail of the Sandia Mountains (near Albuquerque, New Mexico) was held at the altitude of 10,500 ft (Fig. 16–10, arrow), and most of the course is at about 9000 feet. At this level of hypoxemia ($Pa_{O_2} \approx 58$ mm Hg), the right-shifted ODC loses its advantage because "loading" of $O_2$ in the lungs is impaired more than the "unloading" of $O_2$ in muscle is increased.

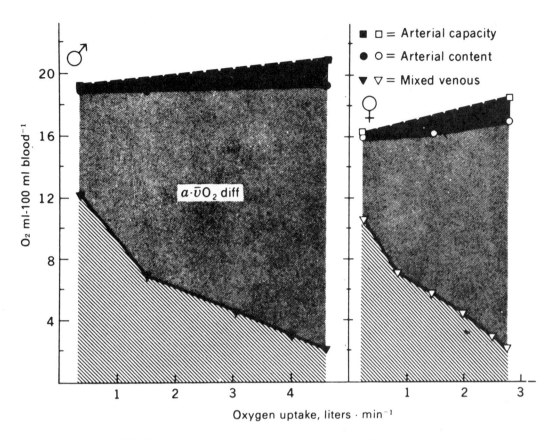

**16–11**  Sexual differences in $O_2$ capacity, arteriovenous $O_2$ difference at rest and during exercise up to maximum. (From Astrand, P.O., Rodahl, K. 1977. Textbook of Work Physiology, 2nd Ed. McGraw-Hill Book Co., New York. Reprinted with permission of the publisher.)

**Table 16–1**   Maximum Ventilation and Maximum Oxygen Uptake in Trained and Untrained Men and Women at Sea Level and Altitude

| Age | Sex | Condition* | Body Weight (kg) | $\dot{V}_E$MAX (L/min) | $\dot{V}_{O_2}$MAX Liters/min | $\dot{V}_{O_2}$MAX Ml/min/kg | Reference |
|-----|-----|-----------|------------------|------------------------|-------------------------------|------------------------------|-----------|
| 33 | M | UT | 80.7 | 100 | 4.15 | 50.8 | 20 |
| 33 | M | WCR | 63.5 | 162 | 4.64 | 72.5 | 9 |
| 30 | F | WCR | 52.3 | 115 | 3.04 | 58.2 | 9 |
| 25 | M | XCS | — | — | 6.20 | 85.0 | 7 |
| 25 | F | XCS | — | — | 3.80 | 73.0 | 7 |
| 26 | M | MC-SL | 73.0 | 97 | 3.21 | 45.3 | 14 |
| 26 | M | MC-5305m | 73.0 | 145 | 2.26 | 34.4 | 14 |

*UT, untrained; WCR, world class runners; XCS, cross-country skiers; MC-SL, mountain climbers at sea level; MC-5305m, mountain climbers at altitude of 5305 meters (17,400 ft)

**Sexual Differences**   The smaller $\dot{V}_{O_{2max}}$ of women athletes in comparison with men in the same sport persists when corrected for body size (Table 16–1). Part of the reason for this difference (Fig. 16–11) is that women athletes begin with a lower $O_2$ capacity (less hemoglobin) and lower arterial $O_2$ content. Thus, although the relative $O_2$ extraction increases with $\dot{V}_{O_2}$ almost equally in women and men, the amount of $O_2$ delivered and the

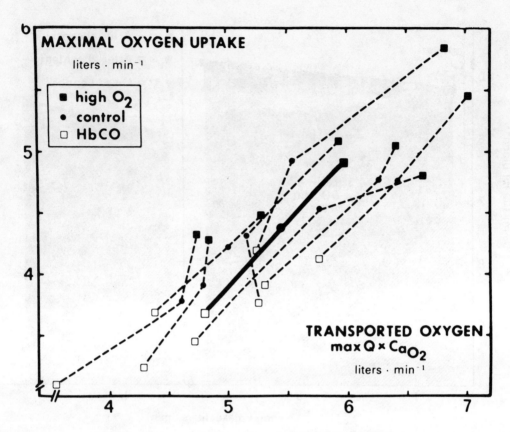

**16–12a**   Effect of transported $O_2$ on maximum $O_2$ uptake during maximum running of 8 subjects (top). Transported $O_2$ was lowered by inducing 15% carboxyhemoglobin and raised by adding 50% $O_2$ to inspired air.

arteriovenous $O_2$ difference is much higher in men. Consequently, assuming a lower limit of mixed venous $O_2$ content of 2 vol percent, men have an $O_2$ uptake of approximately 4.5 liters/min compared with 2.8 liters/min for women. The role of this relative anemia in accounting for sexual difference in $\dot{V}_{O_{2max}}$ has not been determined. However, data from experiments on blood removal and re-infusion (''doping'') suggest that the quantity of $O_2$ transported to tissues *is* a main factor limiting $\dot{V}_{O_{2max}}$.

## The Limits of Maximum Oxygen Uptake

Maximum $O_2$ uptake is unquestionably important to athletic performance. The question remains as to whether training increases maximum $O_2$ uptake and, if so, how.

Most evidence suggests that circulatory or metabolic factors limit maximum aerobic capacity. The principal circulatory limitation is the maximum transported $O_2$—i.e., $\dot{Q}_{max} \times Ca_{O_2}$. The foregoing discussion on women athletes and the evidence presented in Figure 16–12 support this argument. Figure 16–12a shows the effects of hypoxia (HbCO) and hyperoxia (high $O_2$) on transported $O_2$ during maximum running and the resulting

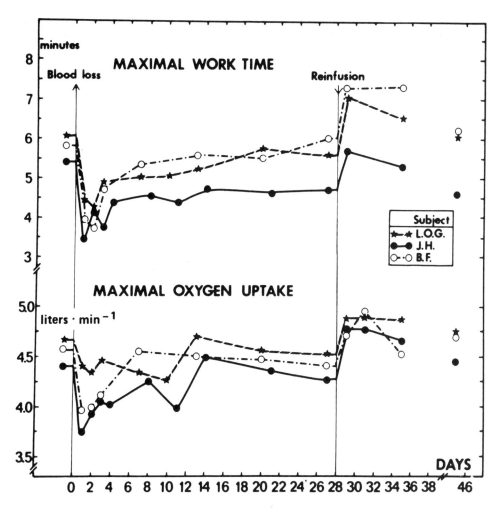

**16–12b**  Effects of 800 ml blood loss and reinfusion of packed cells in maximal work time (time to exhaustion during maximal running) and maximal $O_2$ uptake (bottom). (From Ekblom, B., Goldbarg, A.N., Gullbring, B. 1972. Response to exercise after blood loss and re-infusion. J Appl Physiol 33:175–180. Reprinted with permission of the publisher.)

effect on maximum $O_2$ uptake. The effect on breathing high $O_2$ (50% $O_2$) is attributed to an increase in dissolved $O_2$ delivered to tissues and not to an enhanced $O_2$ diffusion rate in the lungs. For example, inhalation of 25% $O_2$ enhances diffusion by increasing the alveolar to capillary $P_{O_2}$ gradient, but there is no increase in maximum $O_2$ uptake. However, diffusion limitation may be an important factor at altitude. Related evidence is shown in Figure 16–12b. Acute blood loss (lowering $O_2$ capacity) causes a sharp drop in both maximal work time (time to exhaustion during a standardized maximal run) and maximum $O_2$ uptake. Conversely, re-infusion of the packed red cells after 28 days (when $O_2$ capacity had returned to control values) caused a sharp increase (to supernormal values) in both measures. It is curious that analogous, but longer-term, increases in hematocrit due to altitude acclimation do not have the same effect in improving maximum $O_2$ uptake after return to sea level (Åstrand and Rodahl [7]; Cerretelli [14]).

**Table 16–2**  Summary of Responses of Oxygen Transport System to Endurance Training

| Transport System | Type of Response | | |
| --- | --- | --- | --- |
| | Increased | Unchanged | Decreased |
| $O_2$ uptake | Maximum $\dot{M}_{O_2}$ | Resting $\dot{M}_{O_2}$ | |
| Lungs | Maximum $\dot{V}_E$ | | Ventilation at sub-maximal loads |
| | | Diffusing capacity | $V_D/V_T$ ("dead space") |
| Blood | Maximum $\dot{Q}$ | Maximum HR | HR at submaximal loads |
| | Maximum SV | Hemoglobin | Blood lactate at submaximal loads |
| | $O_2$ delivery (2,3 DPG) | | Blood flow per unit muscle |
| Muscles | Capillary density Oxidative enzymes Mitochondria | Efficiency of fibers | |

Training does increase maximum $O_2$ uptake, and the most obvious effect of training is an increase in cardiac output. This, in turn, is due primarily to an increase in stroke volume. Training is also known to increase muscle capillary density and the concentration of oxidative enzymes (Saltin and Rowell [7]). Other responses of the $O_2$ transport system to endurance training are presented in Table 16–2.

# Anaerobic Work

If delivery of $O_2$ to working muscles is inadequate, there is increased lactate formation from anaerobic metabolism and generation of an "oxygen debt." Most runners associate "exhaustion" with excessive lactic acid, although a study by Hill and Lupton [10] clearly showed that subjective "exhaustion" could occur without lactate accumulation.

The level of blood lactate during muscular work depends on 1) the rate of lactate formation; 2) the rate of lactate utilization in cells; and 3) the rate of diffusion of lactate into blood. The intensity of work required for lactate accumulation is variable, but it is an excellent index of fitness (Fig. 16–13). Lactate accumulation occurs with moderate work in heart patients. In sedentary but otherwise normal people, lactate accumulates when $O_2$ uptake reaches approximately 1.2 liters/min. For an 80-kg person, this corresponds to a jogging speed of 5.7 km/hr or 17.5 min/mile. In contrast, a trained person may show no lactate accumulation until $O_2$ uptake reaches 2.5 liters/min, equivalent to a jogging speed of approximately 9 min/mile. The speeds at which lactate accumulates are more impressive for trained runners. Many marathon racers had little or no blood lactate at the finish; the highly trained distance runners could utilize up to 90% of $\dot{V}_{O_{2max}}$ for 30 min with only moderate lactate accumulation (Costill [11]). For most people, lactate accumulation begins at approximately 70% of $\dot{V}_{O_2}$.

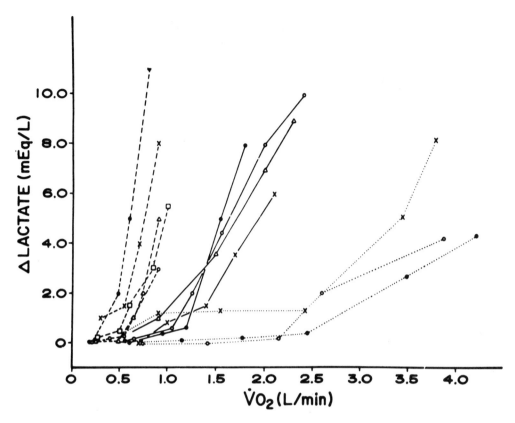

**16–13** Lactate accumulation in blood at different levels of work in heart disease patients (*dashed lines*), sedentary normals (*solid lines*), and trained athletes (*dotted lines*). (From Wasserman, K., Whipp, B.J. 1979. Exercise physiology in health and disease. Am Rev Resp Dis 112:219–249. Reprinted with permission of the publisher.)

# Oxygen Transport and Delivery at High Altitude

## Oxygen Availability

One factor that brings the need for oxygen from being subliminal to consciousness is high altitude. At moderate altitudes hypoxia-induced hyperventilation usually remains subliminal. For example, normal $Pa_{CO_2}$ at an altitude of 5000 ft is about 36 mm Hg compared to approximately 40 mm Hg at sea level. Most people become aware of a hypoxic drive to breathe at an altitude of 9000–11,000 feet. Although the fraction of oxygen is constant at about 21%, the inspired $Po_2$ ($Pi_{O_2}$) falls with falling barometric pressure (PB) according to the equation:

$$Pi_{O_2} = (PB - 47) \times 0.21$$

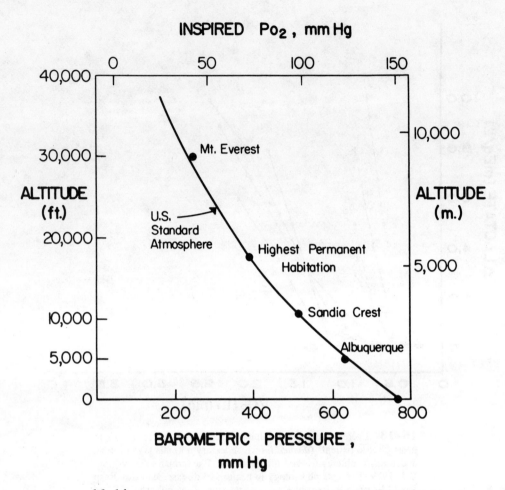

**16–14**  Relationship of altitude to barometric pressure ($P_B$) and inspired oxygen pressure ($P_{IO2} = (P_B - 47) \times 0.21$).

where 47 is the vapor pressure of water at normal body temperature. The effect of altitude on $P_B$ and $P_{IO_2}$ is illustrated in Figure 16–14. Alveolar $Po_2$ ($P_{AO_2}$) is determined by $P_{IO_2}$, $P_{ACO_2}$, and the respiratory exchange ratio (R) according to the equation:

$$P_{AO_2} \approx P_{IO_2} - \frac{P_{ACO_2}}{R}$$

The importance of hyperventilation in altitude adaptation is emphasized when $P_{AO_2}$ is calculated for the summit of Mt. Everest in climbers without supplemental $O_2$ in May 1978. Barometric pressure at this altitude ~ 29,200 feet) is approximately 250 mm Hg. Thus, inspired $Po_2$ would be $P_{IO_2}$ ~ $(250 - 47) \times 0.21 = 43$. If $P_{ACO_2}$ and R remained at sea level values (i.e., no hyperventilation), alveolar $Po_2$ would be:

$$P_{AO_2} = 43 - \frac{40}{0.8} = -7 \text{ mm Hg (!)}$$

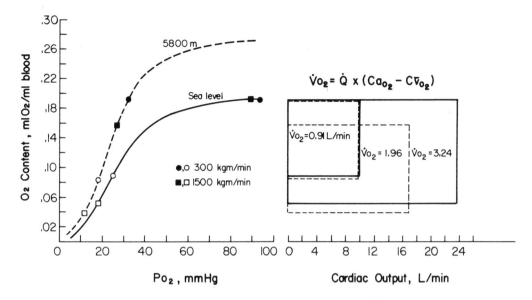

**16–15**  Graphic representation of Fick principle during light (300 kg/min), moderate (900 kg/min) $\dot{V}_{O_2} = 1.96$ liters/min, and heavy (1500 kg/min) work at sea level and at 5800 m altitude. The $\dot{V}_{O_2}$ of 1.96 liters/min corresponds to a work level of 900 kg/min at 5800 m. See text for discussion. (Based on data in Pugh, L.G.C.E. 1964. Cardiac outut in muscular exercise at 5,800 m (19,000 ft). J Appl Physiol 19:441–447.)

The observed survival of men breathing air at this altitude is due to a reduction of alveolar $P_{CO_2}$ by hyperventilation to about 10 mm Hg, which provides an alveolar $P_{O_2}$ of about 30 mm Hg. This, however, is not enough since, without a long period of acclimatization, an alveolar $P_{O_2}$ of 30 would render normal people unconscious.

## The Oxygen "Cascade"

The drop in $P_{O_2}$ at each step of $O_2$ transport becomes much less as altitude increases. The decrease in the first drop ($P_{I_{O_2}} - P_{A_{O_2}}$) reflects the increasing degree of hyperventilation as altitude increases. The second drop in $P_{O_2}$ ($P_{A_{O_2}} - P_{a_{O_2}}$) also decreases as arterial oxygenation begins to occur on the steeper portion of the ODC. However, because the driving pressure for diffusion ($P_{A_{O_2}} - P_{\bar{c}_{O_2}}$) is vastly reduced (from a $\Delta P_{O_2}$ of approximately 60 mm Hg at sea level to approximately 11 mm Hg at 29,000 feet), there is a substantial diffusion limitation on Mt. Everest, even at rest. Similarly, the reduced drop in blood $P_{O_2}$ ($P_{a_{O_2}} - P_{\bar{v}_{O_2}}$) reflects the fact that tissue $O_2$ delivery is occurring on the steep portion of the ODC.

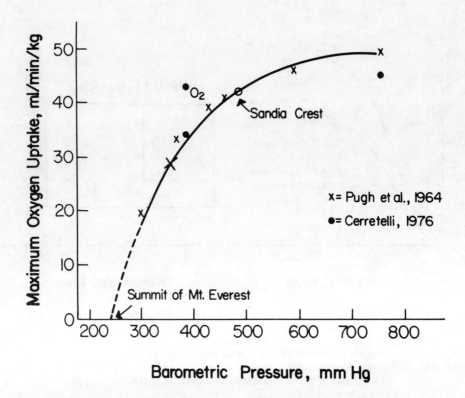

**16–16** Relationship between maximum $O_2$ uptake and barometric pressure. See text for discussion. (Based on data from Pugh, L.G.C.E. et al. 1964. Muscular exercise at great altitudes. J Appl Physiol 19:431–440; and Cerretelli, P. 1976. Limiting factors to oxygen transport on Mt. Everest. J Appl Physiol 40:658–667.)

## The Fick Principle at High Altitude

The graphic representation of the Fick principle in Figure 16–15 presents data (Pugh [12]; Pugh et al. [13]) on $O_2$ transport at high altitude and emphasizes the crucial importance of increased $O_2$ capacity in adaptation to altitude. Indeed, after acclimation to an altitude of 5800 m (19,000 feet), the arterial $O_2$ content at rest and during light work (300 kg/min) is (at 70% saturation) the same as or slightly higher than the preacclimation sea level value (97% saturation). For the $O_2$ uptake of 0.91 at this work rate, the $O_2$ delivery and cardiac output is the same at sea level and 5800 m.

At the higher work rate of 900 kg/min (equivalent to running about 5.5 mph), $\dot{V}O_2$ was 1.96 liters/min and the effects of altitude are pronounced. Arterial saturation decreases, presumably as a result of diffusion limitation, causing a smaller $O_2$ extraction than at sea level. This was the highest work rate for which adequate data were available. Maximum heart rate decreases at altitude, apparently as a result of increased parasympathetic tone and direct effects of hypoxia on the sinoatrial node (Cerretelli [14]). This accounts for the reduction in maximum cardiac output since maximum stroke volume is not affected by altitude.

Most of the evidence points to a circulatory limit of $\dot{V}O_{2max}$, i.e., the maximum $O_2$ transport ($\dot{Q}_{max} \times Ca_{O2}$). Studies in which subjects breathing $O_2$-enriched air show an increase in $\dot{V}o_{2max}$ indicate that the oxidative capacity of muscles exceeds the $O_2$ transport capacity of blood. At high altitude, diffusion limitation may also play a role in limiting $\dot{V}o_{2max}$ because arterial saturation and $Ca_{O_2}$ decrease as work rate increases. This would result from both a decrease in transit time of red cells in pulmonary capillaries and a decrease in the (alveolar-capillary) $\Delta Po_2$.

The decrease in $\dot{V}o_{2max}$ at high altitude is usually due to a decrease in both $Q_{max}$ and $Ca_{O_2}$. The upper portion of a curve illustrating $\dot{V}o_{2max}$ at different barometric pressures (Fig. 16–16) is relatively flat, but there are significant diminutions of athletic performance at moderate altitudes. For example, there were no world records established in endurance events in the Olympic games held in Mexico City ($P_B \approx 580$ mm Hg). The predicted $\dot{V}o_{2max}$ on Sandia Crest would be only 80% of the sea level value. Extrapolation of this curve suggests that $\dot{V}o_{2max}$ would be zero at $P_B$ of approximately 240 mm Hg. On the summit of Mt. Everest ($P_B = 250$ mm Hg) the $\dot{V}o_{2max}$ would be only 3–4 ml $O_2$/min/kg, roughly the basal $\dot{V}o_2$. Cerretelli [14] made an interesting observation (Fig. 16) in his study on factors limiting $O_2$ transport on Mt. Everest. He found that even when subjects were breathing 100% $O_2$ at $P_B$ of 390 mm Hg, they were unable to attain the preexisting sea level $\dot{V}o_{2max}$ in spite of a 40% increase in hematocrit and a limited reduction in maximum cardiac output ($\dot{Q}_{max}$). He speculated that changes in peripheral microcirculation—i.e., bypass of resistance blood vessels in muscle—could account for this.

## The Oxygen Dissociation Curve During High Altitude Exercise

For a given work rate, more lactic acid is produced at high altitude than at sea level. On the other hand, acute altitude-induced hyperventilation will produce respiratory alkalosis. Thus, the role of acid-base balance in $O_2$ transport is complex. In addition, the advantage or disadvantage of a left or right shift of the ODC depends on altitude and arterial $Po_2$. Therefore, the familiar and advantageous right shift of the ODC during exercise at sea level could be maladaptive at high altitude. Whether or not a right shift of the ODC occurs as a result of increased 2,3 DPG depends primarily on blood pH. A decrease in pH inhibits overall glycolytic rate and 2,3 DPG phosphatase, causing a depletion of 2,3 DPG. Alkalosis has the opposite effect by activating 2,3 DPG mutase, causing accumulation of 2,3 DPG. The redox potential of the red cell, reflected by the ratio of lactate to pyruvate (L/P), is also a key factor. In hypoxia, as L/P increases, 2,3 DPG levels decrease.

There is little agreement on the role of 2,3 DPG-induced shifts in the ODC as an adaptation to exercise at sea level (Thomson [20]). The picture is equally cloudy at high altitude. In a recent study of marathon racing at 1600 m altitude, 2,3 DPG and $P_{50}$ were found to increase in the slower finishers, but not in the runners with times under 3:20 (Wood et al. [15]). In two endurance runs along the crest of the Sandia Mountains (altitude 7000–10,650 feet) all runners (n = 40) who did not become acidotic had an increase in $P_{50}$, whereas those who were acidotic at the finish (n = 7) had a decrease in $P_{50}$. The changes in $P_{50}$ were related to the degree of acidosis and the consequent changes in red cell 2,3 DPG (Wood and Hoyt, unpublished observations). Because of the low $Pa_{O_2}$ during much of the run, it is not certain that runners with increased 2,3 DPG benefited by the right-shifted ODC, although the right shift in ODC offsets the effect of alkalosis, which has an opposite effect. Clearly, much work is needed to elucidate the role of ODC and its modulators in the adaptation to exercise at sea level and high altitude.

# Glossary and Index of Terms

**ATP**     Adenosine triphosphate, high energy molecule that provides the energy for muscle contraction

**Carboxy-hemoglobin**     Nonfunctional form of hemoglobin in which carbon monoxide is bound to the heme group

**$Ca_{O_2}$**     Oxygen content of arterial blood, e.g., ml $O_2$/100 ml blood

**$Cv_{\bar{O}_2}$**     Oxygen content of mixed venous blood

**2,3 DPG**     2,3 diphosphoglycerate, a compound found in red cells that has a strong influence on the affinity of hemoglobin for oxygen

**HbCO**     Carboxyhemoglobin

**ODC**     Oxyhemoglobin dissociation curve

**$P_{50}$**     Partial pressure of oxygen required for 50% saturation hemoglobin

**$PA_{O_2}$**     Partial pressure of oxygen in alveolar gas

**$Pa_{O_2}$**     Partial pressure of oxygen in arterial blood

**$PA_{CO_2}$**     Partial pressure of carbon dioxide in alveolar gas

**$Pa_{CO_2}$**     Partial pressure of carbon dioxide in arterial blood

**$P_B$**     Barometric pressure, e.g., 760 mm Hg at sea level, 630 mm Hg at 5500 feet

**$P\bar{c}_{O_2}$**     Partial pressure of oxygen in mixed capillary blood

**$PI_{O_2}$**     Partial pressure of oxygen in inspired (moist, tracheal) air

**$P\bar{v}_{O_2}$**     Partial pressure of oxygen in venous blood

**$\dot{Q}$**     Cardiac output or quantity of blood pumped per unit time, e.g., liters $\times$ min$^{-1}$

**R**     Respiratory exchange ratio, $\dot{V}_{CO_{O2}}/\dot{V}_{O_2}$. Depends (at steady state) on composition of metabolized foods, e.g., R = 1 for carbohydrates, 0.7 for fats, and about 0.8 for proteins.

**$\dot{V}_{O_2}$**     Oxygen uptake in volume of oxygen consumed per unit time. May also be given as $M_{O_2}$ or moles of oxygen consumed per unit time.

# References

1. Cherniak, N.S., Longobardo, G.S. 1970. Oxygen and carbon dioxide stores of the body. Physiol Rev 50:196–243.
2. Asmussen, E. 1965. Muscular exercise. In: Fenn, W.O., Rahn, H., (eds): Handbook of Physiology, Sec 3, Respiration, Vol 2. American Physiological Society, Washington, D.C., p 943.
3. Honig, C.R. 1976. Mechanisms of circulation metabolism coupling in skeletal muscle. In: Grote, J., Reneau, D., Thews G. (eds): Oxygen Transport to Tissue, Vol. 2, Plenum Publishing Corp., New York, pp 623–639.
4. Krogh, A. 1919. The supply of oxygen to the tissues and the regulation of the capillary circulation. J Physiol 52:457–474.
5. Krogh, A. 1936. The Anatomy and Physiology of Capillaries. Yale University Press, New Haven.
6. Wranne, B., Nordgren, L., Woodson, R.D. 1974. Increased blood oxygen affinity and physical work capacity in man. Scand J Clin Lab Invest 33:347–352.
7. Åstrand, P.O., Rodahl, K. 1977. Textbook of Work Physiology, 2nd Ed. McGraw-Hill Book Co., New York.
8. Hill, A.V. 1922. The maximal work and mechanical efficiency of human muscles and their most economical speed. Am J Physiol 56:19–26.
9. Davies, C.T.M., Thompson, M.W. 1979. Aerobic performance of female marathon and male ultramarathon athletes. Eur J Appl Physiol 41:233–245.
10. Hill, A.V., Lupton, H. 1923. Muscular exercise, lactic acid and the supply and utilization of oxygen. Quart J Med 16:135–171.
11. Costhill, D.L. 1970. Metabolic responses during distance running. J Appl Physiol 28:251–255.
12. Pugh, L.G.C.E. 1964. Cardiac output in muscular exercise at 5,800 m (19,000 ft). J Appl Physiol 19:441–447.
13. Pugh, L.G.C.E., Gill, M.B., Lahiri, S., Milledge, J.S., Ward, M.P., West, J.B. 1964. Muscular exeircse at great altitudes. J Appl Physiol 19:431–440.
14. Cerretelli, P. 1976. Limiting factors to oxygen transport on Mt. Everest. J Appl Physiol 40:658–667.
15. Wood, S.C., Schade, D.S., Hoyt, R.W. 1979. Marathon racing at 1600 m altitude: Effects on red cell 2,3 DPG and hemoglobin-oxygen affinity. Fed Proc 38:1050.
16. Wasserman, K., Whipp, B.J. 1979. Exercise physiology in health and disease. Am Rev Resp Dis 112:219–249.
17. Shappell, S.D., Lenfant, C. 1975. Physiological role of the oxyhemoglobin dissociation curve. In: Surgenor, D.M., (ed): The Red Blood Cell, Vol. 2. Academic Press, New York, Ch 20.
18. Lahiri, S. 1975. Blood oxygen affinity and alveolar ventilation in relation to body weight in animals. Am J Physiol 229:529–536.
19. Ekblom, B., Goldbarg, A.N., Gullbring, B. 1972. Response to exercise after blood loss and re-infusion. J Appl Physiol 33:175–180.
20. Thomson, J.M., Dempsey, J.A., Chosey, L.W., Shahidi, N.T., Reddan, W.G. 1974. Oxygen transport and oxyhemoglobin dissociation during prolonged muscular work. J Appl Physiol 37:658–664.
21. Saltin, B., Rowell, L.B. 1980. Functional adaptations to physical activity and inactivity. Fed Proc 39:1506–1513.

# Section 5
# Locomotion and Sports

# Chapter 17

# Ocular Injuries
# in Athletic Activities

by William Selezinka

## Introduction

Increasing emphasis on athletics in schools and in communications media, and the resulting surge in the numbers of persons engaging in exercise and body conditioning has led to an increased number of ocular injuries. Eye safety in athletics through preventive measures, public education, and design of protective eye devices has been emphasized, but eye injuries still occur (Pashby [1]). Some of these are unavoidable, others are due to carelessness or refusal to wear protective devices; nevertheless, three out of four people fear blindness more than any other illness except cancer (Research to Prevent Blindness, Inc. [2]). This is significant when one considers that 75% of sensory input is through the eye. Ophthalmologists treating ocular trauma see a substantial number of cases that result from recreational activities.

Eye injuries should not be ignored, because, initially, they may appear deceptively mild (irritation and some tearing, slightly blurred vision, or transient double vision). If associated with head injury, however, the symptoms may be attributed to central disturbances of the visual system when both central and peripheral injuries coexist. A superficial injury of the eye or surrounding structures may be the outward sign of a more severe contusion of the eye itself. An obvious severe injury of the lids or globe should be managed by an ophthalmologist. In other, less severe injuries, the examining physician should perform a thorough eye examination (Wilkinson [3]). Practical knowledge of management of ocular injuries is important for early correct diagnosis and treatment. This may prevent worsening of the injury and possible subsequent blindness (Morin [4]).

Between 2% and 4% of the population have unilateral amblyopia, so among 1 million sports participants, 20,000–40,000 can be expected to have varying degrees of unilaterally impaired vision (Pashby et al. [5]). In these people, injury of the normal eye may be tragic. A survey of eye injuries in ice hockey participants indicates that 15% became legally blind, and the highest number occurred in 11- to 15-year-olds (Pashby [6]).

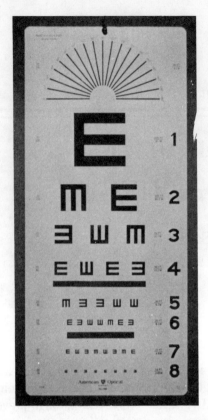 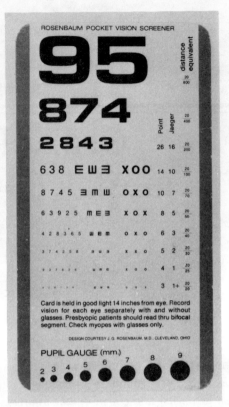

**17–1**   Visual acuity charts (Rosenbaum Vision Screener).

Another study showed that 16 of 38 eye injuries required hospitalization of the victims, 12 of whom needed follow-up care for late complications from angle recession, subluxated lens, traumatic cataract, and retinal detachment. Some even required enucleation (Vinger [7]). One-half of traumatic retinal detachments were legally blind even after successful surgery (Antaki et al. [8]), and 31%–44% had less than 20/40 vision. In racketball, tennis, and squash, up to one-half the injuries required hospitalization, mostly due to hyphema (Easterbrook [9]). Many eye injuries have peripheral retinal tears and detachments. Some of these can be repaired if treated early. Others have central retinal damage. In squash the likelihood of eye injury is not reduced even in an experienced player (Seelenfreund and Freilich [10]). Thorough ophthalmologic examination is urgent for all sports-injured eyes.

# Management of Ocular Trauma

Good records are essential. Notes are made of how the eye was injured, whether glasses, contact lenses, or a protective device was worn. Previous eye injury, disorder, or systemic disease (e.g., bleeding disorder) that might affect management or outcome should be noted (Levin and Bell [11]). Signs and symptoms such as decreased vision, diplopia, and pain should be recorded.

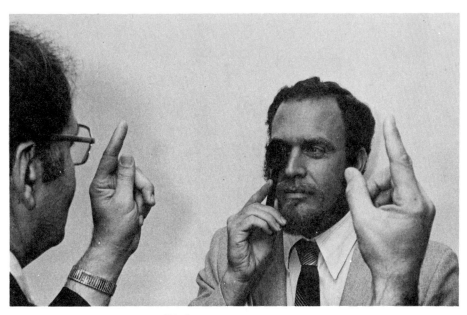

**17–2**   Confrontation field.

It is always important to check visual acuity. This can be done with a Snellen chart or a Rosenbaum near-vision card (Fig. 17–1) held 14 inches from the eyes, which should be individually tested. In a presbyope, near vision is tested with bifocals or reading glasses. If only finger-counting or hand-movement vision exists, the distance at which this is possible is noted. Care is taken to indicate whether the patient has light perception (LP). If he or she also detects the direction from which the light is coming (light projection—LP), then it is recorded as LP & LP, as light perception is required to detect light direction. No light perception (NLP) is recorded when the eye is totally blind, which may be the case in an optic nerve avulsion or in a fracture of the optic nerve canal in which the nerve is severed. Vision should be measured with spectacle correction or, if the glasses are broken, with a pinhole and a Snellen chart. Visual fields should be examined by confrontation (Fig. 17–2).

The extent of ecchymosis, chemosis, and conjunctival hemorrhages is recorded (Fig. 17–3), and preceding infection of the periorbital skin, lids, conjunctiva, or tear sac is noted. Ocular motility is checked in all directions of gaze and diplopia is looked for with a red glass. Restricted eye movements may indicate extraocular muscle entrapment in a bony orbital fracture. The orbital rim is palpated, and cutaneous sensation below the eye is tested. One should feel for lid crepitus from subcutaneous emphysema, usually originating from a fractured paranasal sinus. Displacement of the globe should be noted and measured if an exophthalmometer is available. Auscultation for orbitocranial bruit should also be done.

Depth and location of lid lacerations, especially if they involve the nasolacrimal system or the canthal tendons, should be noted. If present, they require the attention of an ophthalmic surgeon to reconstruct proper tear drainage, equal-sized eye apertures, and a good cosmetic result by a three-layer closure.

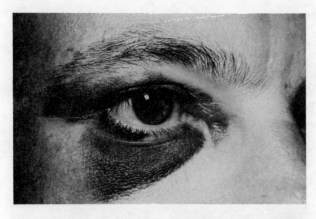

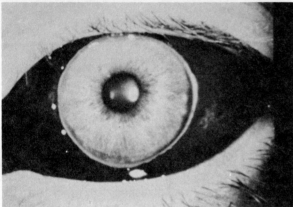

**17–3**    Ecchymosis (a) and subconjunctival hemorrhage (b). (Courtesy of University of Michigan)

Pupil size, shape, and equality, and reactions, including the results of the swinging penlight test for a possible Marcus Gunn pupil (usually from an optic nerve injury), are recorded.

The swinging penlight test is useful in the detection of pupillary afferent fiber defects. It consists of shifting a light back and forth from pupil to pupil, allowing approximately 5 sec at each eye to observe for dilatation of the pupil. In a normal eye, the illuminated pupil may redilate slightly. In the affected eye, however, pupillary redilatation during illumination is proportional to the severity of the conduction defect in the injured optic nerve (Paton and Goldberg [12]).

Actual pupillary size may be measured in millimeters with a pupil scale on a Rosenbaum chart. It is especially important to note a pupil dilated from trauma to the sphincter or ciliary ganglion, or a constricted pupil from traumatic iritis or Horner's syndrome, secondary to accompanying neck or brachial plexus injury. A "teardrop" pupil usually indicates iris entrapment in a corneal or scleral laceration.

One notes if a hyphema is present and if there is an iridodialysis or iridodonesis (a tremulous iris because of loss of support from a subluxated or dislocated lens).

Finally, a loupe or slit lamp (which many hospital emergency rooms now have) should be used to check for corneal abrasions, foreign bodies, and hyphema. The slit lamp helps in assessing the anterior chamber for microscopic hyphema, traumatic iritis, and the state of the lens—i.e., its location, and whether or not there is a traumatic cataract. The anterior vitreous can also be examined for red blood cells, which may be present from a peripheral retinal tear. At the same time, the intraocular pressure can be measured if the cornea is intact.

Systematic ophthalmoscopic examination after athletic injuries should include the optic nerve, retinal vessels, choroid, macula, and peripheral retina. An indirect ophthalmoscope is best for visualizing peripheral retinal dialysis or tears, hemorrhages, or retinal edema through a dilated pupil. This should be done soon after injury, as vitreous blood may later spread and obscure the retina. Central retinal edema (commotio retinae) is very common in contused eyes, and it can best be seen with the red-free light of the ophthalmoscope. It should be noted that more mistakes are made by not looking than by not knowing. Many eye injuries receive delayed, inadequate, or misguided treatment. Therefore, a methodical, thorough examination and proper treatment are essential.

*All extraocular injuries must have an intraocular examination.*

X-ray examinations of the orbits, facial bones, and, when indicated, skull and optic nerve canals should be made in contusion injuries or if an intraocular or intraorbital foreign body is suspected. In some cases, a CAT scan may be useful, and documentation by photography is also often helpful. The clinical evaluation of an injured eye may be difficult because of the patient's tendency to squeeze the eye shut and to blink vigorously as a result of photophobia and intense lacrimation. The examination should, therefore, be performed in subdued light. Some of the blepharospasm may be overcome by the use of local anesthetic. This should not be used indiscriminately, nor should it be given for self-medication at home, as a severe (chemical) keratitis may result from its overuse. After the lids are relaxed and open, one can measure visual acuity. If the lids are still closed, they can be retracted gently by hand or with a small lid retractor. At the same time, the cornea should be inspected for abrasions, lacerations, and foreign bodies. If examination cannot be done, one should gently apply an eye patch and send the patient to an ophthalmologist or hospital as soon as possible.

# Decreased Vision in Injured Eyes

Decreased vision after eye injury may result from trauma to various ocular structures. In severe lid injury resulting in massive swelling and/or blood on the cornea, vision is impaired. A hyphema, dislocated lens, or traumatic cataract may also be responsible. Commotio retinae (macular edema) or hemorrhages of the retina resulting from a direct blow may decrease vision, and choroidal rupture in the macular area or between the macula and the optic nerve also impairs vision. A central retinal artery or vein occlusion from direct compression of these vessels by orbital hemorrhage may decrease vision or cause total visual loss. Retinal detachment and vitreous hemorrhage are other causes. Lastly, cortical blindness (patient may be unaware of blindness) may result from a blow, usually to the back of the head, such as occurs in contact sports. Various causes of visual loss must, therefore, be considered in evaluating the injured eye.

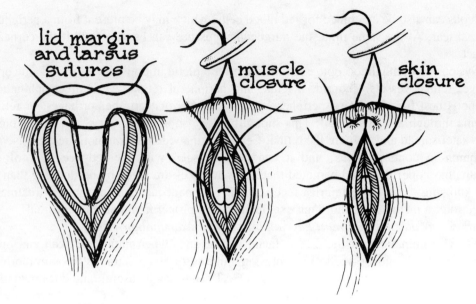

**17–4** Three-layer closure of full-thickness lid laceration.

# Lid Injuries

The extent of lid injuries should be ascertained. At the same time, the eye itself must also be examined. Tetanus prophylaxis should be given if indicated, as for lacerations and avulsions of other body parts. Simple lid lacerations need meticulous primary repair. Many oculoplastic ophthalmic surgeons recommend the use of a microscope for better approximation of the various layers and for removal of microscopic foreign bodies within the wound. Each anatomic lid layer (skin, orbicularis muscle, and tarsus-palpebral conjunctiva) should be repaired separately (Fig. 17–4). Because of the abundance of skin in the lid vicinity, large skin defects can be closed by undermining and sliding skin over the more fixed, deeper layers. Skin grafts may be obtained, if needed, from the area behind the ear.

Fat in the laceration, orbital septum perforation, and a deep injury in the eyelid could involve the eyeball (Fig. 17–5). An absent lid fold (in non-Orientals) or blepharoptosis may point to traumatic dehiscence of the levator palpebrae muscle, which requires repair by an ophthalmologist. However, soreness or photophobia can cause partial ''protective ptosis,'' which disappears when the irritation subsides.

Medial and, particularly, lateral canthal tendon damage is frequent in trauma and should be identified and repaired. Lacerated lid margins require proper reapposition at the gray line and the use of 7-0 or 9-0 silk for suturing. A continuous strip of tarsus at least 3 mm wide should be left at the margin. These injuries should be treated by an ophthalmologist.

The lacrimal duct canaliculus may be transected in lacerations near the medial canthus. This also requires meticulous repair with fine silicone tubing (Fig. 17–6). Dental malocclusion and facial bone fractures may be associated with a nasolacrimal duct tear between the tear sac and nose.

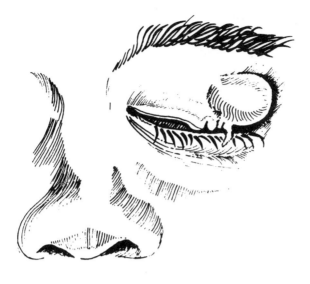

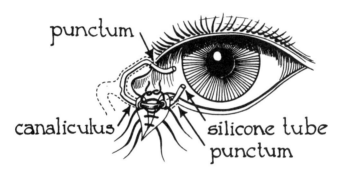

**17–5**   Orbital fat protruding through lid laceration.

Marked lid ecchymosis from a direct blow often results because of good blood supply to the area. Orbital or subconjunctival hemorrhage and even proptosis may also be present. Hemorrhage may spread subcutaneously across the midline from one eye to the other or may extend to the cheek and jaw over 24–48 hours. The spread is of no consequence, except that it may indicate coexisting serious orbital injury. For example, ringlike periorbital blood may indicate skull fracture. An orbital floor fracture is often associated with inferior orbital and lower lid ecchymosis and anesthesia of lateral skin of the lower lid, side of the nose, and cheekbone because of involvement of the infraorbital branch of the trigeminal nerve. Orbital roof fracture may present as ecchymosis of the upper lid and subconjunctival hemorrhage, the blood spreading along the levator muscle, and downward under the conjunctiva.

The treatment of lid ecchymosis is similar to that of contusions elsewhere. At first, cold compresses are used for 24–48 hours. This may be changed to warm compresses later. Sunglasses are worn for cosmetic reasons.

Enlarged submaxillary and preauricular nodes may indicate infection. The lymphatic drainage from the temporal third of the lids is to the preauricular nodes and the nasal two-thirds drains to the submaxillary lymph nodes.

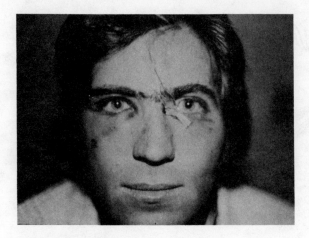

**17–6**   Canaliculus repair.

# Orbit Injuries

The orbital rim protects the eye from blows by objects larger than the rim circumference. An anterior orbit blow causes serum and blood release into the lids and surrounding tissues, forcing eyelid closure. Mild to severe proptosis and even ophthalmoplegia may result from orbital hemorrhage. Anesthesia of skin served by the supraorbital and infraorbital nerves occurs if they are involved in fracture margins. Diplopia and impaired upward gaze often result from inferior rectus and inferior oblique muscle entrapment in an orbital floor fracture (Fig. 17–7). Subcutaneous emphysema, which may be seen on X-ray, can cause lid crepitus and indicates medial orbital wall (ethmoid sinus) fracture. Systemic antibiotics should be given to these patients because of the possibility of orbital cellulitis due to organisms entering from the paranasal sinus. When orbital fractures are present, straining (heavy lifting) and nose-blowing should be avoided. Orbital roof fractures may cause cerebrospinal fluid rhinorrhea. Plain X-ray films of the skull, orbits, and sinuses miss many fractures of this type. Tomography or computerized axial tomography correlated with clinical findings is often required for identification of orbital fractures (Fig. 17–8).

The timing of surgery is important. Delay of up to 10 days may be required for edema to subside, but surgery should be done before fibrosis begins. Early repair may be justified if there is obvious enophthalmos, X-ray proof of the fracture, and the patient is undergoing surgery for another facial injury. Postoperative complications can occur. Many cases do not require surgery. Postoperative complications include enophthalmos, limitation of vertical gaze, lower lid ectropion, trichiasis, postoperative cellulitis, dacryocystitis, extrusion of implant, and even postoperative visual loss from surgical trauma to the optic nerve or from orbital hemorrhage.

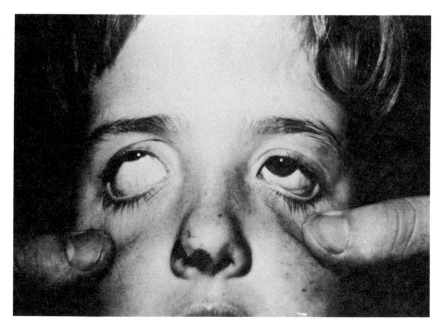

**17–7**   Blowout fracture, left orbit. (Courtesy of University of Michigan)

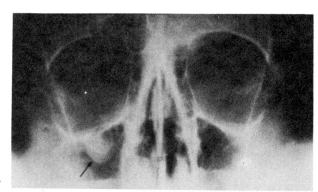

**17–8**   Plain X-ray film of blowout fracture (left) and tomography (right) for comparison. (Courtesy of Dr. Hanafee, University of California, Los Angeles.)

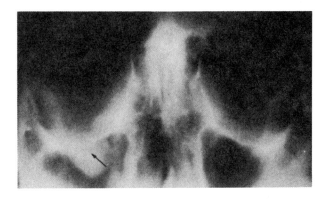

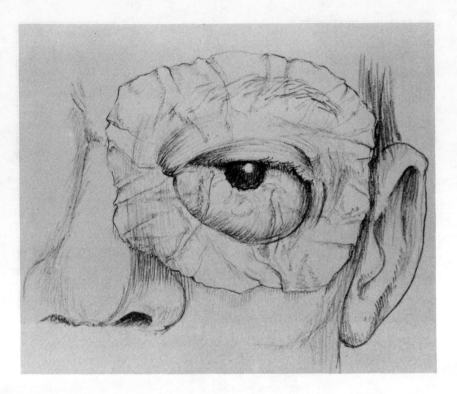

**17–9**   Adhesive transparent kitchen wrap protects excessive chemosis.

# Conjunctival and Corneal Injuries

Commonly seen conjunctival trauma leads to subconjunctival hemorrhage. Most of the time, specific treatment is not indicated. If the hemorrhage is severe, with chemosis, eye closure may not be possible. When this occurs, application of an ointment to the eye, and coverage with adhesive transparent kitchen wrap protects the cornea until the lids can be closed again (Fig. 17–9). An ice pack may help to reduce swelling. Associated injuries are of more concern. Severe chemosis may indicate an intraorbital foreign body, scleral rupture, and invisible conjunctival perforation—associated with an invisible scleral perforation, an orbital fracture, or a carotid-cavernous fistula. Therefore, careful avoidance of pressure on the eye during examination is essential to prevent prolapse of the intraocular contents through a possible hidden scleral wound. Foreign bodies removed from *perforating* conjunctival injuries should be cultured for bacteria and fungus even though perforations seldom become infected and usually heal rapidly. Conjunctival lacerations longer than 1 cm are repaired, or if they are contaminated and extensive, they require débridement. Traction on the plica semilunaris by sutures should be avoided, and Tenon's fascia should not be caught in wound edges, nor should conjunctival epithelium be trapped subconjunctivally.

Corneal abrasions are painful. Because of tearing, severe pain, and lid spasm, clinical examination is difficult and can be assisted by use of topical anesthetic and an oblique

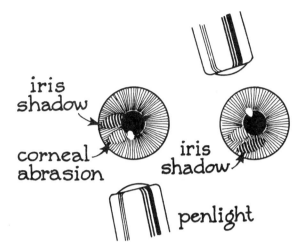

**17–10**   Shadow cast on iris by corneal abrasion.

light. A sterile fluorescein paper strip stains areas of corneal epithelial loss. If a fluorescein strip is not available (avoid aqueous fluorescein solutions, which may harbor *Pseudomonas* after the bottle has been opened), a light directed at suspected damage may reveal corneal abrasions. When the light is moved parallel to the iris, the corneal defect may be seen as a shadow on the iris opposite to the light (Fig. 17–10). The upper lid is everted to check for foreign bodies that may be responsible for the abrasion (Selezinka, [13]) (Fig. 17–11). Dry cotton swabs should not be used on the eye. However, a saline-moistened cotton swab may be used to remove foreign bodies from the corneal surface. Corneal abrasions are managed by the instillation of antibiotic and mydriatic drops, followed by snug application of two pads to the injured eye. The cul-de-sac accommodates only one drop of medication, therefore, the time of application of the two medications is spaced and the punctum occluded with tissue or cotton ball for 30 sec before patching. If healing is slow or there is doubt, an ophthalmology consultation should be obtained. Steroid-containing medications are not indicated for corneal abrasions because an occult herpetic infection of the cornea could spread.

Hard contact lenses should be removed soon after severe facial injury if this can be done easily before the lids swell (Selezinka [13]). Corneal and corneoscleral lacerations are the domain of the experienced ophthalmic surgeon. These may be present with iris prolapse and give the pupil a teardrop shape. Surgery should be performed as soon as possible.

# Contusive Injuries

In contusion, the anterior segment may be involved, causing a hyphema (Fig. 17–12). The hyphema may layer inferiorly or fill the entire chamber. Approximately 20% rebleed. Between 25% and 50% eventually result in 20/40 vision or less. Therefore, an ophthalmologist's care is essential (Paton and Goldberg [12]). Patients require hospitalization, biomicroscopy, and applanation tonometry for daily intraocular tensions, to record deterioration resulting from multiple areas of eye damage. In addition, approximately 7% of patients develop glaucoma in later years because of angle recession produced by the

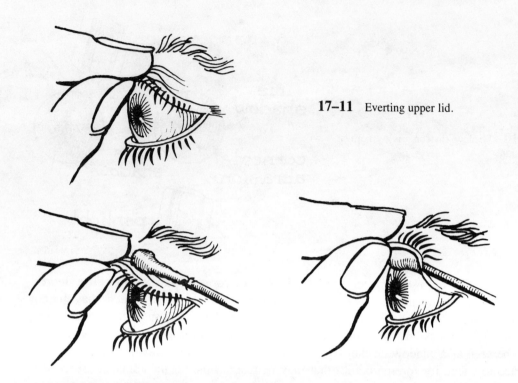

**17–11**   Everting upper lid.

trauma (Fig. 17–13). Somnolence is the hallmark of hyphemas, particularly in young people; the possibility of coexisting head injury must be excluded.

Traumatic **mydriasis** from rupture of the iris sphincter results in permanent pupillary deformity. The lens may be dislocated and produce visual changes or develop a cataract.

Scleral rupture with intact conjunctiva commonly occurs at the limbus and may not be easily visible. The rupture is usually arc-like and opposite the impact site but near the rectus muscle insertion on the nasal side (Fig. 17–14). Marked localized hemorrhagic chemosis and a hyphema are always present. The lens may be dislocated subconjunctivally through the rupture site. Surgical intervention is necessary.

The presence of a vitreous hemorrhage should be considered when the "red reflex" is lost and an ophthalmoscopic view is hazy or bloody. It signifies damage to the retina,

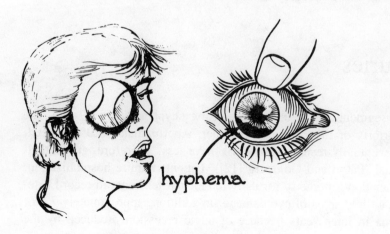

**17–12**   Hyphema.

hyphema

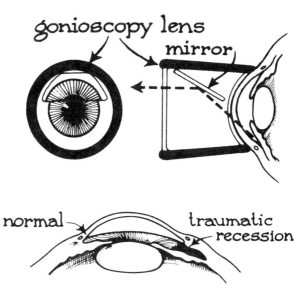

**17–13**   Angle recession.

choroid, or ciliary body. **Treatment** consists of bed rest. An old vitreous hemorrhage may eventually need vitrectomy.

Central retinal edema (**commotio retinae**) is common after direct blows. Initially, vision decreases as edema increases, and then it gradually improves. Return to normal depends upon the extent of the injury. Perimacular pigmentary changes eventually occur. In boxers, recurrent contusive injury may cause persistent edema, with macular cyst or hole formation and loss of central vision (Fig. 17–15). Chronic edema after a single injury may produce the same bad results. Central retinal edema appears as a whitish, cloudy discoloration. Comparison with the uninvolved eye using a red-free ophthalmoscope light aids in diagnosis. An Amsler grid shows irregular lines.

Retinal **hemorrhages**, edema, and exudates may result from a direct blow to the eye, a blow to the **back of the head**, or from contrecoup injury. Retinal detachment may occur as

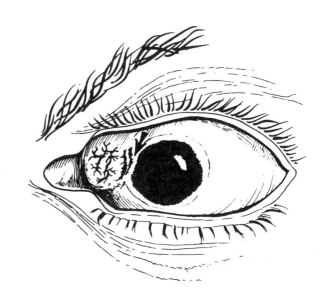

**17–14**   Scleral rupture at limbus.

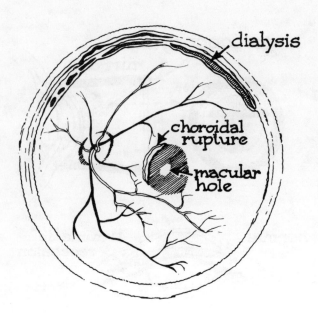

**17–15**  Schematic of traumatic retinopathy.

a result of a tear in the extreme peripheral retina (Cox et al. [14]; Weidenthal and Schepens [15]). It is estimated that 15% of all detachments result from trauma. Retinal dialysis may occur immediately after trauma (Fig. 17–16). About 80% of retinal detachments become symptomatic within 2 years of trauma, although the detachments usually occur soon after injury. Floating black specks, a persistent cobweb in the peripheral visual field, and light flashes are symptoms that make one suspicious of detachment. Ophthalmoscopy shows a billowy grayish retina that may shift as the patient moves the eye. Traumatic detachments occur near the ora serrata in 59.4% of cases, and 9.1% are of the posterior type (Cox et al. [14]). The ora serrata type progresses insidiously until the macula is involved, and is seen primarily in young people after sports accidents. Surgical

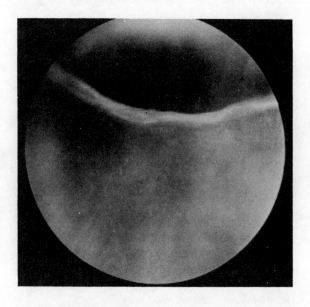

**17–16**  Retinal dialysis.

intervention is indicated. *All* orbital contusive injuries need careful indirect ophthalmoscopy to prevent eventual visual loss.

In sports the frequency of ocular injuries can be summarized as follows (adapted from Rousseau [16]):

| | |
|---|---|
| Hockey | 31.0% |
| Sporting equipment (BB, darts, etc.) | 19.3% |
| Transport (bicycle, snowmobile, etc.) | 16.5% |
| Racket sports | 10.3% |
| Baseball, etc. | 8.2% |
| Golf, fishing, boxing, skiing, basketball | 14.3% |

Sports cause significant eye injuries. Physicians need to impress sports participants of the need to prevent eye injury by the use of protective devices or by game rule changes. Recognition of a variety of eye injuries in athletics and subsequent proper management by the primary physician is important. Thorough examination and good records aid in treatment. The risk of visual loss from an unrecognized serious eye injury is high.

# References

1. Pashby, T.J. 1977. Eye injuries in Canadian hockey. Phase II. Can Med Assoc J 117:671–678.
2. Research to Prevent Blindness, Inc. Annual Report. 1977. New York.
3. Wilkinson, C.P. 1976. Injury in the vicinity of the eye. In: O'Donoghue, D.H., (ed): Treatment of Injuries to Athletes, 3rd Ed. W.B. Saunders Co., Philadelphia, pp 130–132.
4. Morin, D.J. 1978. Primary management of ocular trauma. Can Med Assoc J 118:305–307.
5. Pashby, T.J. et al. 1975. Eye injuries in Canadian hockey. Can Med Assoc J 113:663–674.
6. Pashby, T.J. 1979. Eye injuries in Canadian hockey. Phase III. Can Med Assoc J 121:643–644.
7. Vinger, P.F. 1976. Ocular injuries in hockey. Arch Ophthalmol 94:74–76.
8. Antaki, S., Labelle, P., Dumas, J. 1977. Retinal detachment following hockey injury. Can Med Assoc J 117:245–246.
9. Easterbrook, M. 1978. Eye injuries in squash. Can Med Assoc J 118:298–305.
10. Seelenfreund, M.H., Freilich, D.B. 1976. Rushing the net and retinal detachment. JAMA 235:2723–2776.
11. Levin, D.B., Bell, D.K. 1977. Traumatic retinal hemorrhages with angioid streaks. Arch Ophthalmol 95:1072–1073.
12. Paton, D., Goldberg, M.F. 1976. Management of Ocular Injuries. W.B. Saunders Co., Philadelphia.
13. Selezinka, W. 1979. Eye injuries. In Ryder, S.M., (ed): To Help You Save Lives. Rescue Publications, Scottsdale, pp 33–34.
14. Cox, M.S., Schepens, C.L., Freeman, H.M. 1966. Retinal detachment due to ocular contusion. Arch Ophthalmol 76:678–685.
15. Weidenthal, D.T., Schepens, C.L. 1966. Peripheral fundus changes associated with ocular contusion. Am J Ophthalmol 62:465–477.
16. Rousseau, A.P. 1979. Ocular trauma in sports. In: Freeman, H. MacK., (ed): Ocular Trauma. Appleton-Century-Crofts, New York, pp 353–361.

# Chapter 18

# General Surgery and Sports Medicine

### by William R. Schiller

## Introduction

Many athletic injuries are primarily orthopaedic in nature, but minor problems may be referred to a general surgeon. These include not only soft-tissue injuries, but also those involving thoracic and abdominal viscera. In addition, general surgeons may be asked to diagnose and manage surgical illnesses unrelated to injuries in athletes. The most common injuries of athletes are lacerations and contusions. Blisters, abrasions, and calluses also cause discomfort and loss of competitive edge in many sports.

## Soft-Tissue Injuries

### Contusion

Injury from being struck by another participant or by a piece of equipment is inevitable in a variety of contact sports. Although abrasion or laceration of overlying skin may occur, the common denominator of contusions is bleeding into soft tissues; the severity of this is directly proportional to the force applied. Blood from small vessels dissects into tissue planes, causing the appearance of diffuse bruising rather than presenting a localized hematoma. Bleeding usually does not result from injury to larger vessels. Much morbidity of bruises results from the large quantity of blood that extravasates and dissects tissue planes. Painless function is regained faster when extravasation is minimized. Measures that limit the effects of bruising include cold pack application—usually a dry, protected ice bag—to the injured part. This produces vasoconstriction and minimizes bleeding into the injured site. Though rebound vasodilatation may occur after cold application, it can be postponed by continued use of the cold pack until the injury is stable, usually up to 24 hours following injury. Thereafter, when further bleeding is less likely, warmth applied locally tends to decrease discomfort. Localized cutaneous injury from the cold application can be prevented by placing a layer of material such as pant leg between the ice bag and the skin. Moreover, keeping the area dry decreases the likelihood of cold injury. Compression of the injured area with a woven elastic bandage over the ice bag to hold it in place further limits bleeding. Finally, elevation of the injured part minimizes swelling.

Rest for the acutely injured part is beneficial, but athletes should be encouraged to maintain general conditioning by exercising uninjured body parts. Graded activity may be resumed when pain and swelling are gone. The use of a contused area should be regulated so that pain and/or swelling does not occur. If either of these occurs, the athlete is using the injured part too soon or too vigorously and should limit its use. This general program should allow a return to full athletic capability over the ensuing week.

## Hematomas

Subcutaneous hematomas are common in participants of contact sports. Small hematomas resorb with appropriate padding and should be allowed to do so. Larger, more localized hematomas resolve more quickly if aspirated one or more times. Diffuse hematomas within muscle bundles are difficult to aspirate, but localized hematomas are usually removed easily with a syringe fitted with a large-bore needle. Drainage of hematomas by incision should be resisted unless they are infected. Incising hematomas converts a trivial wound into a serious open wound that takes a long time to heal, causing loss of active participation in sports. Needle aspiration of hematomas should be preceded by proper antiseptic skin preparation to prevent introduction of pathogens into the wound.

## Lacerations

Small lacerations are frequent on the athletic field, and those that penetrate the skin should be sutured, since primarily closed wounds heal more rapidly and with less scarring than those that are allowed to heal secondarily. Minor lacerations not involving deeper structures can be sutured in the locker room, but larger ones should be cared for in the emergency department. After the wound has been cleansed thoroughly with soap and water, sterile drapes are applied. Many athletes feel that they are obliged to accept sutures without local anesthetic. However, a better and more meticulous repair can be done with local anesthetic use, and players will appreciate the afforded comfort. It is unpleasant, ineffective, and unnecessary to suture a writhing, grimacing athlete for purely "macho" reasons. If activity is resumed, a protective dressing, often including a splint, should be used over the healing laceration until a mature scar has formed. In lacerations of the hands, this is especially important since repeated trauma causes inflammation in the healing wound.

Lacerations in certain areas of the body require special attention.

**Eye**    When lacerations occur around the eye, the eye itself should also be examined. When facial lacerations are being treated, the eyebrow should never be shaved. The likelihood of infection is not increased if eyebrows are left, and the risk that they will not regenerate to a normal configuration is eliminated. The possibility of a facial fracture underlying a laceration should be kept in mind.

**Ear**    Ear lacerations must be treated with care if the cartilage, which is especially susceptible to infection, is involved. Cartilage infection may cause loss of substance and induce ear deformity. Aseptic techniques and thorough cleansing must be meticulously performed prior to wound closure with fine sutures. The cartilage should be reapproximated to its anatomic position with fine, soluble suture. Overlying skin can then be closed in a separate layer, using 6-0 nylon sutures. A splinting dressing will then support and maintain the normal shape of the ear during healing. The ear should be padded, inside a protective headgear, until healing is complete.

Hematoma formation between the skin and auricular cartilage, causing a painful "cauliflower ear," is a frequent injury in wrestlers. The clinical setting for this injury is as follows: The victim is held tightly around the head and either attemps to, or does, in fact, withdraw from the grip of the opponent, causing contusion and shearing of the ear. The hematoma must be drained, for maximal restoration of contour, through a small skin incision under local anesthesia. The underlying cartilage should be avoided, and several incisions may be necessary to completely evacuate the clot. The ear must then be encased in a splinting dressing. One should warn athletes with this injury that residual deformity may occur. More attention should be paid to preventing the injury through use of proper headgear.

**Tongue or Lip**    A bitten tongue or lip is another common injury that may be either self-induced or result from a blow to the mouth by an opponent. Tongue lacerations are best closed with absorbable sutures in layers, under local anesthesia. If the tongue is not sutured, a nodule of tissue, frequently bitten accidentally by the patient, will result. Prompt healing can be expected. Lip lacerations are common in many sports and should be closed in layers so that the orbicularis oris is reapproximated, as well as the overlying mucous membrane and skin. Careful attention must be paid to realigning the vermilion lip border so that normal contour is restored. Careless suturing of the vermilion border, with resultant offset after recovery, is not acceptable.

# Hand Injuries

Hand injuries are relatively frequent and include superficial abrasions, lacerations, and injury of underlying tendons and bones. Fingernails are commonly avulsed, partially or totally, or a blow to the finger may cause a subungual hematoma. If the avulsed fingernail is partially attached, it is best replaced on the nailbed. A proper dressing over the repositioned nail is needed and the finger should be protected until the nail regrows. Only completely avulsed nails should be discarded, and the nailbed in this case should be covered with a sterile dressing. Occasionally a laceration involves the nail without avulsion. This should be treated as any other laceration, with reapproximation of tissue planes and a sterile dressing.

Subungual hematomas are painful because of increased pressure caused by blood between the nail and nailbed. The throbbing pain can be incapacitating even to a stoic athlete. Treatment is drainage through a hole drilled into the nail. A hot paper clip may be used to melt a small hole in the nail to allow the underlying blood to escape. In most cases, this can be done painlessly without local anesthetic. Drainage provides instantaneous relief of pain. A fracture of the underlying distal phalanx is commonly present with subungual hematomas; therefore X-ray examination of the finger is recommended. This injury is not usually a cause of prolonged disability, and most athletes promptly return to full activity, especially if damage has not occurred to the underlying phalanx.

Hand injuries may involve more than the overlying skin. Therefore, examination of nerve and tendon function is necessary when lacerations are deep. If these structures are clinically involved, the injury should be treated by a surgeon with a special expertise in hand injuries. A final good result is often related to proper early management, so the team physician must be alert to the possibility of complicated hand injury.

Fractures of hand bones may occur either from direct involvement in athletic events or from an altercation, commonly seen in hockey games. Fifth metacarpal fracture from such incidents may cause residual hand and finger deformity if not cared for properly. With metacarpal fracture, the hand must be carefully examined for teeth marks, for the human bite is prone to infection. Careful cleaning of the laceration is, therefore, important. Consideration should be given to primary or subsequent closure of human bite wounds, and most surgeons give antibiotics to victims of human bites.

# Neck Injuries

Neck injuries may involve associated damage to the cervical vertebrae and underlying spinal cord. Those who complain of neck pain after an injury should be carefully evaluated for contusion of cervical musculature or more serious injuries, such as vertebral fractures. If the diagnosis is not clear, the athlete must have cervical spine X-rays and neurologic evaluation. Poorly conditioned athletes who take unexpected falls are especially prone to cervical vertebral injuries. Indications of injury to these vital structures require neurosurgical consultation. Less devastating is neck contusion, which may produce a hematoma in the cervical musculature. This can be managed as for any other contusion, but attention should be given to assuring an adequate airway, since a large hematoma may produce tracheal compression. Injuries to the larynx must also be considered. An athlete who is struck in the neck and then has hemoptysis should be suspected of sustaining airway injury, which requires prompt treatment to avoid obstruction.

# Thoracic Injuries

Serious intrathoracic injuries are not common in athletes, since impact forces to the well-protected thorax are not sufficient to produce visceral injury. Exceptions are jockeys and race car drivers, who may be subjected to considerable force against the thoracic cage in the event of an accident. In contact sports, however, athletes commonly complain of painful contusions of the lower rib cage. Although the ribs are seldom fractured, these injuries produce considerable morbidity because of pain. When ribs are fractured, athletes often have difficulty breathing and will subsequently refrain from all-out effort because of fear of repeating the injury. Contused areas may involve the cartilaginous portions of the ribs, which do not heal rapidly. Rapid recovery is probably most assured if the athlete continues general conditioning but is withdrawn from actual contact until chest pain begins to subside.

Rib fractures are painful and inhibit respiratory excursion of the involved hemithorax. Chest examination may reveal splinting, which produces a noticeable difference in respiratory excursion between the two sides. The fracture site is tender, so crepitation of the fracture edges should not be attempted in making the diagnosis. Management includes exclusion of injury to underlying organs (hemothorax or pneumothorax). Attempted taping of broken ribs is usually not satisfactory and only inhibits respiratory effort without affording protection or pain relief.

Sports are not usually associated with serious intrathoracic injuries. The most common intrathoracic injury is simple pneumothorax, which is usually associated with a rib fracture and produces an inordinate amount of dyspnea. The pneumothorax is visible radiographically, and treatment is placement of a chest tube. A small pneumothorax may resorb without a chest tube, but faster resolution occurs when air is aspirated via a properly placed tube connected to water-seal drainage. Occasionally, rib fractures are associated with free blood in the pleural cavity either with or without pneumothorax. The hemothorax may be detectable only by chest X-ray even though the rib fracture is obvious clinically. The blood should be removed by tube thoracostomy, for it takes considerable blood to produce an abnormality on the chest film.

Most severe intrathoracic injuries, cardiac contusion, and great vessel injury, are seen in association with automotive trauma and not athletic events.

Foreign-body aspiration occurs occasionally in athletes. They should not have objects in their mouths (chewing gum or tobacco) on the playing field. The techniques for removal of aspirated objects are well standardized, but prevention is certainly the best and least embarrassing method of dealing with this problem.

# Injuries of Abdominal Musculature

Abdominal wall contusions are common and should be treated in the same manner as contusions elsewhere on the body. They are painful and may require prolonged convalescence before maximal activity is again possible.

Hernias should be repaired during the off-season when possible. Most surgeons do not allow significant weightlifting or other physical stress until 6 weeks after hernia repair. At that time, the tensile strength of the wound should be about 90% of normal. Most athletes can resume conditioning training at that point, within limits of discomfort. Activities that cause discomfort should be temporarily stopped until it is certain that no harm is being done to the wound. Gradual increase to normal activity without discomfort should be the rule. Weightlifters, who generate tremendous strain on the abdominal wall, require special care. Gradual resumption of effort seems to be the safest policy.

Acute appendicitis requiring appendectomy is a common affliction of young people. Most surgeons remove the appendix through a transverse lower abdominal incision, which heals readily and is strong in uncomplicated cases. Wound strength is from the overlying abdominal wall musculature, which is merely split and not divided during surgery. These patients may resume some conditioning activities 3 weeks after surgery or whenever the wound becomes painless. Contact sports should not be allowed for approximately 6 weeks after appendectomy.

# Intraabdominal Injuries

Intraabdominal injuries are uncommon in contact sports because the forces generated are insufficient. Although a blow to the abdomen may produce a painful contusion or intramuscular hematoma, injuries to underlying viscera are exceptional.

Athletes suspected of having sustained an intraabdominal injury should be thoroughly examined as soon as possible. This may include laboratory tests to detect bleeding or peritonitis. The organs most commonly injured from blunt trauma are the liver and spleen, because of their considerable size and partial fixation to the abdominal wall. Both organs are soft and vulnerable to laceration by external forces. The injured athlete may show signs of peritoneal irritation, such as rebound tenderness, localized abdominal wall tenderness, or pain in the shoulder, which are suggestive of diaphragmatic irritation. There also may be signs of shock, rapid pulse, and lowering of blood pressure.

Bowel injuries may be associated with a torn mesentery and intraabdominal bleeding. A blowout bowel perforation, leading to generalized peritonitis, can also occur. Increasing abdominal pain, rigidity, and rebound tenderness ensue. Those patients who have signs of intraabdominal bleeding or peritoneal irritation should be transported to an appropriate medical facility and considered for surgery to control bleeding and repair injured organs.

Injury of certain viscera is not associated with much peritoneal reaction. This applies to retroperitoneal organs, kidneys, urinary bladder, pancreas, and duodenum. Patients with genitourinary injuries commonly have hematuria, which should be looked into if it persists for more than a few hours or produces grossly bloody urine. These patients need urinalysis and perhaps even contrast X-rays of the genitourinary system. Contused or minimally lacerated kidneys are usually treated conservatively with bed rest, fluids, and antibiotics, but bladder rupture is more serious. A small retroperitoneal bladder injury can be treated by Foley catheter drainage for 7–10 days, but an intraperitoneal bladder rupture requires surgical closure. Athletes should empty the bladder prior to competition since this may prevent bladder injuries.

# Genital and Lower Urinary Tract Injuries

Women are usually spared genital injuries, although occasionally female athletes sustain a severe mons pubis hematoma. This can be treated conservatively, or if the hematoma is large, aspiration may be required.

Men are more prone to genital injuries, hence the requirement for protective gear. In spite of precautions, contact sports participants are occasionally hit in a way that produces severe testicular injury. Actual testicular fragmentation may occur. This causes immediate and severe pain. On examination, marked swelling is evident, but outright disruption of the testis may not be apparent. With testicular rupture, operative intervention to restore tunica continuity is necessary. After surgery, a support should be worn for comfort and to promote healing. Hormone production by injured testes continues normally, and unilateral injuries do not cause loss of fertility, although bilateral injuries may cause infertility.

The female urethra is short and almost immune from injury. The male urethra is much longer and therefore vulnerable. Injuries to the urethra usually cause severe perineal pain and swelling. Urethrography should be performed to rule out urethral injuries when athletes report severe perineal trauma associated with bleeding from the meatus. Minimal urethral disruptions may be treated with an indwelling catheter. However, complete urethral tears require a suprapubic cystotomy tube with subsequent repair after swelling and hematoma resolve.

Male athletes, like the rest of the male population, are susceptible to hydroceles and varicoceles. These should be repaired in the off-season and proper support should be worn afterwards. Surgical repair does not compromise athletic ability after the operative discomfort and swelling subside.

# Minor Injuries

## Abrasions

Rubbing of equipment against body parts occurs in almost all sports. The resulting injury depends upon the equipment and body part. One of the simplest injuries is skin abrasion, which results from a tight strap. This can be prevented by proper padding. Treatment consists of keeping the involved area clean, using a topical antibiotic, and frequent dressing changes. Although abrasions are uncomfortable, they cause minimal disability.

## Calluses

A more chronic injury, which usually occurs on the feet but may also be seen on the hands, is callus from repeated minor stresses. Keratin build-up occurs at the point of contact. Sharp excision of the callus usually results in pain in the area from which the callus was removed. Thus, it is preferable to treat calluses by shaving with an emery board and softening with a lanolin-base ointment. It is possible, when acute stress is superimposed upon the usual chronic forces over a callus, for a blister to form within or under the callus. Blister therapy takes precedence over long-term treatment of the callus.

## Blisters

Blisters occur when friction is centered over more or less unyielding skin, such as that on the palms and soles. Easily movable skin is more resistant to blistering. Blisters can be induced by prolonged exercise in poorly fitting or new shoes. Shoes, especially, tend to cause blistering because they provide abrasive contact points, warm the skin, and make evaporation of sweat difficult. Slightly moist and warm feet are more susceptible to blistering than cold feet that are either perfectly dry or are very slippery and wet. Blisters on hands and fingers are caused by gripping athletic equipment (tennis rackets) for long periods, allowing friction stresses.

It has been found experimentally that little heat is generated by the force sufficient to produce a blister, so that blistering is not a thermal injury. Typically, the cleft formed by a blister is in the epidermis above the basal cells and usually involves the granular cell layer. Blister fluid forms after the cleft develops, and it depends upon satisfactory capillary pressure. Blister fluid is similar to serum although electrolytes are somewhat lower and calcium content is significantly less. Small amounts of serum proteins are present in the fluid, but fibrin and fibrinogen are usually absent. Immunoglobulins occur in small quantities and abnormal proteins (myeloma protein) are detectable in blister fluid.

Prevention—the best blister management—is not always possible. Intact blisters should be aspirated but not unroofed. If the blister is aspirated within 24 h, the chance that the epidermal layer will again stick to the blister bed is approximately 85%. If the blister is aspirated three times, usually at 2, 6, and 12 h during the first 24 h, the chance that the blister's top will stick to the base is over 90%. Local application of an antibiotic ointment and a protective pad are helpful. Blisters that stick again to the base will do so within 4 days. Withdrawal from athletic events for approximately this time, but with maintenance of general conditioning, is the usual management.

Many blisters are already unroofed by the time they are discovered and are, therefore, more painful. The treatment in this case consists of keeping the area clean, application of antibiotic ointment, and a protective dressing. Blisters usually heal in 4–5 days. Shoe padding protects the healing blister and prevents recurrence.

## Burns

Trivial burns may be inflicted by hot water, electrical appliances, and cigarettes. Skin that is healing from a burn is very susceptible to other minor injury. The newly generated epithelium does not tolerate shearing forces and should be protected from athletic pads and contact with helmet inner linings. An ear newly recovered from a burn should be well padded from the minor trauma of protective headgear. A freshly healed burn does not tolerate sunlight well and should be protected from it by clothing or by an effective sunscreen.

## Warts

Warts can be difficult, especially when they affect the soles of the feet. The temptation to excise plantar warts should be resisted, for a painful wound, worse than the original problem, usually results. Warts may be effectively treated by metatarsal arch bars and the use of mild desiccating agents, such as trichloroacetic acid, applied only to the wart, with removal within an hour. Warts resolve slowly, but with proper foot support and avoidance of radical measures, continued athletic participation is possible.

## Hemorrhoids

Acute hemorrhoids are painful when prolapsed and may cause itching. Athletes should avoid constipation, which aggravates prolapse. Advice about drinking adequate water and use of a stool softener usually alleviates the discomfort. Acutely prolapsed hemorrhoids are best treated with a hypertonic poultice (saturated magnesium sulfate solution), which dramatically reduces the edema. Acute hemorrhoidal thrombosis produces a painful anal nodule that can be incised under local anesthesia for thrombus evacuation.

## Pilonidal Sinus

Pilonidal sinuses may be asymptomatic. However, many eventually become infected, causing a very tender, swollen, inflamed area in the intergluteal fold. An infected pilonidal sinus should be incised and unroofed under local anesthesia. Pus and debris, such as hair, should be removed. A clean wound will heal by secondary intention. With proper cleanliness and padding to the area, prolonged disability does not usually ensue.

## Furuncles

Acute furuncles, localized and very painful, are found in hair-bearing areas. Warm soaks help to localize the infection further. Rapid resolution after incision and drainage under local anesthesia can be expected. Furuncles are almost always caused by staphylococci. When cellulitis or lymphangitis is present, the patient should be given an antistaphylococcal antibiotic for a few days. The drained furuncle heals quickly by secondary intention and usually causes minimal difficulty.

# Trauma to Nipples

Female athletes in particular may develop irritated, tender, bleeding nipples if they participate without supportive garments. This is well known in joggers (joggers' nipples) and can be prevented or treated by use of a proper brassiere or emolient ointment applied before prolonged exertion.

# Chapter 19

# Orthopaedic Aspects of Sports Medicine

by Barry R. Maron

## Commentaries on Athletic Injuries

1. All physical complaints should be considered seriously. The athlete believes he or she has an injury, and the physician should assume a serious disorder is present until proven otherwise. The diagnosis of a psychosomatic condition is made by exclusion.

2. The athletic personality is special. The physician must believe the patient can achieve certain athletic goals, and the physician should do all possible to help in this endeavor.

3. Deterioration in an athletic performance should be investigated to exclude physical or psychologic reasons. A coach who is aware of a player's change in performance should bring this to the physician's attention.

4. An injured joint should be evaluated soon after injury. Most information about the joint and the severity of the injury can then be obtained before swelling, reactive spasm, and guarding occur.

5. Loose joints do not become tighter with time. Developmentally lax ligaments should be protected, and post-traumatic joint laxity should be evaluated. Evaluation of the opposite uninjured extremity usually gives some measure of the looseness and suggests developmental or post-traumatic disorders.

6. An acutely injured extremity should be splinted immediately; failing this, it should be examined and then splinted.

7. The use of X-rays should not be spared, as a missed problem might later lead to legal consequences. An X-ray film, once taken, must be correctly interpreted. If there is any doubt, help should be obtained from a radiologist or orthopaedist.

8. All injured extremities should have immediate and short-term follow-up examination of sensory, motor, and vascular status. Swelling after 4–6 h can cause significant damage to nerves, blood vessels, and musculature.

9. The obvious extremity injury may not be the only one. Careful evaluation is advisable for all the joints above and below the injured area. If a long bone fracture (femur, tibia, fibula, radius, and ulna) is found, an X-ray film of the joint proximal and distal to the fracture should be obtained. A fracture of a forearm could have an associated dislocated radial head. A fractured femur could have an associated fracture or dislocation of the hip.

10. Dislocated joints should be gently reduced as soon as possible. Ideally, an anesthetic should be used for reduction. Muscle relaxation from the anesthetic will decrease the stress of muscle action upon the joint and prevent injury to joint surfaces during reduction.

11. Qualifying sprained joints by degrees (first degree, second degree, third degree) encourages a detailed examination. If there is instability, it is best described by either degrees of opening at the joint surface or by the number of millimeters of joint opening or bone displacement. This allows the physician or subsequent physicians examining the same joint to use common language.

12. Decisions on the open or closed treatment of ligament injury should be made early. Operative treatment, possible for the first 7–10 days, is more ideal within the first 24–36 h.

13. The ideal treatment of the athlete is a return to anatomic and functional normality. Coordination and mechanical advantage that enable participation in athletics may depend on anatomic restoration.

14. Steroids are antianabolic. When applied locally by injection they may impede healing by stopping the first stage, the inflammatory response. If they are injected for tendon inflammation, they should be applied around the tendon and not into the tendon. Steroids should not be injected into acute ligament injuries (sprains). Their use orally for 5–6 days in tapering doses is safer than local injection, and the beneficial effects on healing can be similar. If steriods are used locally, the region into which they are injected should be protected from all but minor stresses for 21 days.

15. Vitamin C does not necessarily prevent the common cold, but it is important in maintaining the structural integrity of collagen in ligaments and tendons. Increased doses of vitamin C used for 14 days after injury can be helpful in healing.

16. Muscle rehabilitation should start immediately after injury. Muscle contractions may be painful, as a result either of direct injury or of joint stresses caused by muscle activity. Both flexor and extensor muscles controlling the joint should be moved by isometric contraction first and then isotonic contractions as the situation improves. Galvanic electrical stimulation of the muscle can help contractions and maintain muscle function. Transcutaneous nerve stimulators, by blocking some pain perception and allowing muscle rehabilitation to proceed, are helpful after injury.

17. A slipped capital femoral epiphysis in adolescents can have dire consequences if the diagnosis is missed. Persistent hip or knee pain should be evaluated by X-ray,

including comparison examination of the opposite extremity. Bilateral slipped epiphyses are not uncommon, however, and it should be kept in mind that both sides may have the same appearance on X-ray films and be pathologic (i.e., bilateral slipped epiphyses).

18. It should always be assumed that a "sprained" knee joint is a complex problem involving more than one ligament, a meniscus, or even a bony structure. The joint may have been dislocated and at examination is already in a reduced state. Stability and peripheral vascular and peripheral nerve function should be examined. A missed knee dislocation with associated arterial damage can cause loss of a limb. Collateral circulation around the knee may initially mask major arterial damage.

19. A bone scan can be helpful in diagnosing a stress fracture when X-ray studies are normal and pain in a bone area exists.

# The Athletic Personality

The complete and successful treatment of an athlete requires that the physician understand the athletic personality. The athlete is anxious to perform physically and is "tuned in" to even minor imperfections in body functions. He or she seeks answers to questions about symptoms that may not have a physiological basis. A sullen and introverted response to an athletic injury can also be expected. Encouragement, in order to keep recovery capabilities within the athlete's reach, is necessary. Reassurance is vital to help the athlete keep faith in returning to the original or an alternative sport. The patient's belief in self and his or her athletic abilities must be shared by the physician with the same enthusiasm to maintain rapport with the patient. The athlete's motivation to get well is great, but a lack of rehabilitation "programs" may delay recovery and there may be excessive stresses of the injured part. Diversions from the injury are necessary, and part of each day should be occupied by physical therapy that is both treatment and diversion. If the injury is not severe but does prevent participation in one sport, substitution of another less stressful activity for a time is suggested. For example, a runner with a foot injury could swim or ride a bicycle until the foot has recovered. Coaches, teammates, teachers, friends, and physician must coordinate their efforts to counteract anticipated depression accompanying serious injury.

# Injury Evaluation

The acute injury gives the examining physician an advantage:

1. The history is recent and the mechanism of injury will be recounted in detail.
2. The earlier a patient is seen after an injury, the easier it is to examine the injured part. There is less edema and less pain and guarding by the patient soon after the injury.

Chronic and recurring symptoms demand detective work to find their cause:

1. Careful history
   a) Onset of symptoms: Was there a specific injury? Were symptoms associated with preparticipation warm-up? What was the duration of play before symptoms began? Can symptoms be predicted or induced by certain activities? What is the duration and frequency of the symptoms? Has there been treatment? What has been the response to treatment (e.g., ice, heat, salicylates, rest)? What other injuries have occurred in the past?
   b) Other medical problems: Has patient ever experienced arthritis, other joint disorders, collagen diseases, metabolic disorders? What has been the family medical history?
2. Detailed examination, including, if possible, evaluation of the patient's performance in sports or during simulated sporting activities.

# Injury Prevention

The best treatment for injuries is prevention. Not all sports are safe for all people. Some will have to be advised to change sports. Others will need counseling regarding their proper place in sports. This counseling should take into consideration the following factors:

1. Injury history
2. Joint mobility
3. Muscle power
4. Ligamentous stability
5. Developmental anomalies
6. Body type (mesomorphic; ectomorphic; endomorphic)
7. Motivation for participation

Generalizations cannot be made, and the patient must be studied. For example, someone with spondylolysis or spondylolisthesis, whether symptomatic or not, would be vulnerable to injury in gymnastics or a collision sport such as football. A distance runner who has been treated for recurrent knee effusions and pain needs help in assessing his or her place in running.

O'Donoghue [1] stresses conditioning and instruction programs. These should include:

1. Proper techniques for the particular sport
2. Protective equipment
3. Calisthenics
4. Endurance training
5. Weight training

Vulnerable parts of the body should be protected with taping and orthotic supports.

# Sprains and Strains

A sprain (ligament injury) and strain (muscle-tendon unit injury) will be part of most injuries. The problem may be acute, with local hemorrhage and swelling from sudden excess stress. The injury may be chronic (recurring) from overuse and associated with pain and limitation of motion with little swelling. Careful examination is necessary to define: 1) functional loss; 2) joint stability; 3) degree of tissue damage. Treatment depends upon grading of the injury and functional loss. Grade I (first-degree) and Grade II (second-degree) injuries are usually associated with little functional deficit and need only protection until spontaneous healing. During healing, the affected muscles should be subjected to isometrics and progressive resistive exercises. This should be carried out until symptoms subside and there is return of confidence and performance.

Grade III injuries (third-degree) are usually associated with significant joint instability or muscle destruction. These injuries may need surgical repair of ligaments or muscles. The decision on operation should be made early before fibrosis and contractures occur.

# Common Acute Spinal Injuries

## Neck Injuries

It is not possible fully to evaluate neck pain on the athletic field. Minor neck symptoms may be associated with major spinal injuries (i.e., spinal fractures or spinal subluxations). Patients with acute neck injuries should be given undivided attention at the scene, even if progress of a sporting event is delayed. The sequence of evaluation and treatment should be as follows.

1. Interview the patient if he or she is conscious. Assess what active function is present in arms and legs. Be certain to note all motor function dependent on intact innervation by the brachial plexus and sciatic nerve.
2. Examine motor function. Look for clonus, plantar responses, and sensory deficits.
3. Support the head with sandbags. Do not try to remove a helmet. Be certain that the airway is patent. It may be necessary to use bolt cutters to remove the face mask from a football helmet without moving the head.
4. Palpate bony prominences for tenderness and instability. Keep the injured patient in the same position until it is established that it is safe to move him or her at all. If establishing an airway by moving the patient into the supine position, be certain that head movement is done slowly. At the same time, speak to the patient and apply gentle traction to the head. Keep track of the conscious patient's ability to move the extremities.
5. Do not ask the patient to turn the head or to flex or extend the neck. Do not passively move the neck. Many times the patient will be turning his or her own head when first seen, removing, at least temporarily, doubt about motion capabilities. There

must be enough assistance available to move the patient to the stretcher. The entire spine should be supported while gentle axial traction is maintained on the neck and lower extremities.

6. Transport the patient to a hospital or office for full X-ray evaluation.

Many patients present neck symptoms when sitting or walking. Their evaluation should be similar, taking full precautions. A collar can be placed around the neck for protection, or the patient can be examined supine. Plain X-ray films may not always be adequate and special studies may be necessary (tomogram, CT scan, or special views). Full support of the injured area must be contained until all serious damage to the cord has been excluded.

*Major neck injuries can progress rapidly, and deterioration in function of the cord can be irreversible.*

When it is safe to do so, flexion, extension and lateral X-rays can be helpful. Always insist on full cervical X-ray pictures, especially to show the C6–7 and C7–T1 levels. Swimmer's views and tomograms are sometimes necessary to see the lower cervical area. The CT scanner can give valuable diagnostic information.

If acute neck symptoms have subsided following treatment and the skeletal evaluation is normal, then early reevaluation is necessary if they recur.

## Stretch Injuries to the Brachial Plexus

The "burner" or "stinger" described by some football players occurs in the neck and shoulder after head or shoulder contact. Shoulder girdle depression, together with neck extension or deviation away from the depressed side, can cause tension and stretching of the brachial plexus. Neurologic function should frequently be evaluated in such patients. They should be advised on strengthening shoulder girdles and neck muscles. These players should also use protective neck rolls during contact or collision sports. Advice should be given as to vulnerability of the brachial plexus to serious injury if continued collisions occur. A small number of players with such complaints will develop selective brachial plexus lesions and functional deficits in the upper extremities.

## Neck Sprains

Various ligaments may be torn by flexion, extension, or rotatory forces. Second- and third-degree injuries are important and potentially deadly. A high level of suspicion by the examiner is necessary to diagnose major sprains. X-ray films are mandatory to assist in making the proper diagnosis.

1. Flexion injuries.
   *Symptoms:* The patient with neck pain will resist active flexion, rigidly holding the neck in extension to the point of fatigue.
   *Signs:* Exquisitely tender posterior interspinous structures may be found by palpation. The patient will not rotate the head to the side.

*Treatment:*   A collar or brace support is applied to prevent flexion of the neck. When symptoms subside, cervical isometrics can begin. Six to 8 weeks are needed for healing a ligament.

Avulsions of the spinous process, subluxations, or dislocations may occur without fracture of the vertebral body or vertebral lamina. The degree of muscle spasm, the limitation of motion, and the history will help in arriving at the correct diagnosis. If dislocation has occurred, all motion of the neck is resisted.

Minor sprains must be protected until fully evaluated and until all symptoms subside. The patient may be symptomatic for 3–8 weeks, depending on the severity of injury. Injured ligaments in the neck are vulnerable to re-injury, especially before complete healing has occurred.

2. Extension injuries

*Symptoms:*   Extension injuries cause varying degrees of anterior pain and tenderness in the neck. Extension of the head is painfully avoided.

3. Rotational injuries

*Symptoms:*   These patients usually present minor pain and limited motion if seen after the injury. As spasm increases over 24 h, the head will be rotated to the injured side and be kept slightly flexed. If subluxation has occurred, motion will be even more limited and spasm will be more acutely prominent. The appearance of the patient is similar to that of a person with a "wry neck," with the head rotated so the chin is upward and toward the opposite side (O'Donoghue [1]). The sternocleidomastoid muscle will be tight on the involved side.

4. Subluxation

*Symptoms:*   Some people are loose-jointed or habitual "neck poppers." They may have subluxation from even minor injury with no acute damage to the ligamentous structures themselves. Reduction of the subluxation reverses most symptoms immediately. The athletic future of these people excludes contact sports. The first subluxation without residual damage should be protected for 6–8 weeks; no sports participation is allowed.

Treatment for neck sprains depends on the severity of the injury. In general, a soft collar, analgesics, ice massage to reduce spasm and pain, and heat applications alternating with the use of ice are indicated. Traction at home or in a hospital is helpful. Muscle relaxants and local injections of anesthetic agents relieve discomfort. Oral cortisone in tapering doses for 2–6 days helps resolve local swelling.

# Common Acute Injuries of the Dorsal and Lumbar Spine

Sprains and strains in the region of the dorsal and lumbar spine may present symptoms and signs similar to those of neck sprains:

1) pain; 2) limited motion away from the injured side; 3) muscle spasm in the region; 4) tilting of the torso toward the injured side.

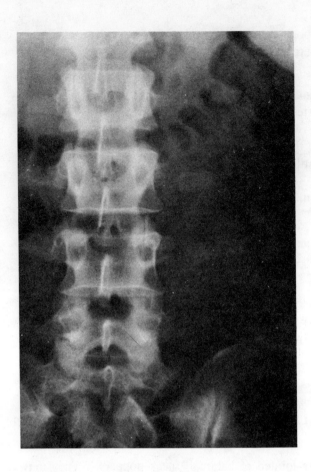

**19–1**  Anteroposterior view of lumbar spine shows displaced fractures of transverse processes of L3–4 and an undisplaced fracture of transverse process of L5.

Treatment begins with rest in bed with the hips and knees flexed over pillows or bolsters. At home, a suitcase with a pillow placed on it can be used as leg support. Ice massage to the area and local anesthetic injections into trigger points, with or without hyaluronidase, may be added. The injection of an anesthetic agent can be repeated if successful. On rare occasions, cortisone may be tried mixed with the anesthetic injection. However, if cortisone is to be used at all, the oral route in tapering doses over 4–6 days is preferable.

Traction and orthotic supports are occasionally helpful. Braces, corsets, and body jacket casts, although unpleasantly warm and heavy, are supportive if used for several days or weeks. Fractures and dislocation of the dorsal and lumbar spine may occur and can be seen on X-ray studies.

Vulnerability to injury may occasionally be predicted from spinal contours. The hyperlordotic person is vulnerable to extension stresses. The kyphotic person is more vulnerable to flexion stresses in the dorsal area and to extension stresses in the lumbar area. It is not unusual to find compensatory increased lumbar lordosis in association with a dorsal kyphosis.

Fractures of the transverse processes (Fig. 19–1) should be treated as sprains, or strains. Failure of union is not uncommon but is usually not a source of discomfort.

Fractures in the region of the pars interarticularis (spondylolysis) may be acute, but they are usually developmental in origin and are brought to attention by an injury. The diagnosis is made by X-ray study (Fig. 19–2). A bone scan is helpful in deciding

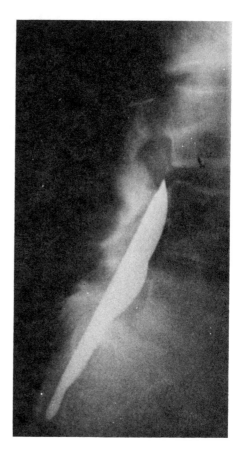

**19–2**   Lateral myelogram of lumbar spine, showing spondylolisthesis defect, Grade I at L5–S1. Pantopaque column is relatively displaced as it passes from L5 to S1 segment.

treatment and prognosis. A hot scan at the spondylolysis area suggests "healing" is possible and can be treated by prolonged body casting (plaster body jacket with or without one thigh included in the cast) or by bracing. If the scan is cold, treatment is as for a sprain. Symptoms may not fully subside, and there is vulnerability to re-injury. Recurring symptoms are a common nuisance. It is often necessary to restrict sports and recommend surgical treatment.

## Disc Lesions

Lumbar disc injuries with degeneration or rupture are important. Symptoms may mimic strains or sprains but are usually associated with radiation of pain to the hip, buttock, or extremity. The signs are similar to those of sprains, but there will usually be sciatic tension signs, sensory deficits, motor weaknesses, and reflex changes. Muscle atrophy may be present.

Disc lesions in the dorsal spine usually present with pain or sometimes lower extremity weakness or clumsiness. In cervical disc lesions, symptoms are similar to those of a sprain or a strain, but they are associated with persistent, usually radicular, pain along one of the brachial plexus dermatomes. Weakness, sensory deficits, and reflex changes in the upper extremity may or may not be present.

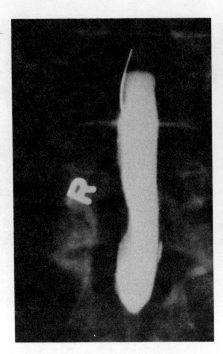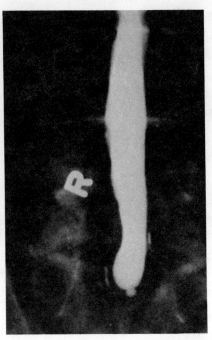

**19–3**   In anteroposterior view of myelogram, large filling defect at level of L5–S1 (*right*) suggests that a herniated nucleus pulposus fragment has entered spinal canal and is deflecting nerve roots.

The diagnosis of a disc lesion is made in part by exclusion after treatment failure for sprains and strains. Once neurologic localizing signs are present, the diagnosis is usually apparent. Tests to confirm the levels of the disc lesions are usually performed, once the decision is made to proceed with surgery. They include electromyography, epidural venography, myelography (Figs. 19–3, 19–4), and CT scan. Persistent or recurring swelling of the articular facet joint or joint of Luschka in the neck may cause radicular symptoms by pressure on nerve roots.

Disc lesions of the dorsal and lumbar region can be treated in similar fashion to sprains and strains. Bed rest in the position of comfort or in hip-flex–knee-flex position decreases nerve root tension and will allow swelling to subside around the roots. After several days, the patient's discomfort is relieved or improved. Anti-inflammatory drugs, with bed rest, are helpful. If oral cortisone is used in tapering doses over 5–7 days, precautions should be taken to minimize irritative effects upon the gastrointestinal tract. Regular meals, antacids between meals, and cimetidine (300 mg) three times daily for the duration of the oral anti-inflammatory therapy are recommended.

*Changes in bladder or bowel habits immediately after the onset of symptoms or even later in the course of disc disease are serious complications.* Pressure from a herniated disc or extruded disc fragment may cause bladder or bowel dysfunction, or both. Early careful evaluation is essential to determine 1) rectal sphincter tone, 2) the bulbocavernosus reflex, and 3) sensation in the region of the genitalia and perineum. This is a medical emergency and demands immediate relief of pressure on nerve roots to preserve bowel and bladder function.

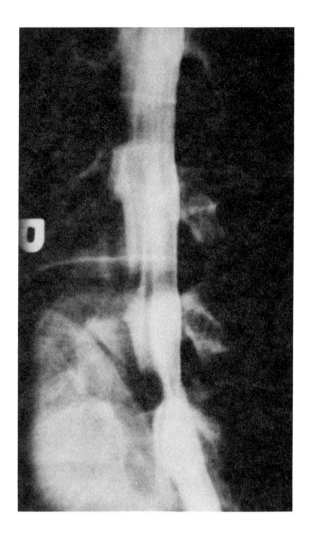

**19–4** Oblique view of myelogram shows larger defect at level of L5–S1 (*right*) that is typical of a large herniated nucleus pulposus in spinal canal, pressing on a nerve root.

## Compression Fractures of the Dorsal and Lumbar Spine

Acute fractures in this area present severe pain. The pain may be accompanied by neurologic deficits in the lower extremity or distal to the lesion (i.e., sensory loss, muscle weakness, reflex changes). Occasionally the pain may be minor and may be erroneously attributed to a sprain or strain.

## Dorsal and Lumbar Injury

The patient is usually in the supine position but is occasionally seated with severe back pain in association with the signs that have been cited. There may also be a loss of bowel sounds. Undivided attention should be given immediately at the scene. If involuntary bowel or bladder evacuation has occurred, there has usually been a major insult to the central nervous system (i.e., concussion, seizure, spinal cord injury). In addition to concentrating on the area of symptoms in the back, a full neurologic evaluation should be carried out, including cranial nerves and peripheral nervous system. The sequence of evaluation and treatment is as follows:

1. Interview the patient. Assess active function in arms and legs by noting movements at first contact.

2. Observe motor function by asking patient to voluntarily move toes, ankles, and knees. If there is no visible motion, palpate muscles to see if there is a flicker of motor response. Look for clonus, plantar responses, and sensory deficits. Gently palpate the spine by slipping a hand underneath the back and moving the fingers gently down the spinous processes. Fracture areas with intact sensation are extremely tender on palpation. Keep the injured patient in the original position until it has been determined that moving the patient will be safe. There should be enough personnel available to support the entire spine while moving the patient.

3. Transport the patient to a hospital or office for full evaluation by X-ray films.

When major neurologic deficits are not present and the patient is ambulatory and functional, flexion and extension lateral X-ray views are helpful in diagnosing residual instability in the spinal column. Sometimes tomographic motion studies are necessary to detect motion at the center of vertebral bodies. This motion is often easier to measure than that noted on plain flexion and extension views or on plain lateral bending films of the spine.

The sprain or strain of the back that remains symptomatic for 10 days or longer and is associated with percussion tenderness should be studied by X-ray to detect the presence of compression fractures. X-ray findings may not give information about the age of the wedging or compression. In this situation, bone scan may be helpful. The scan will usually be "hot" in areas of recent fractures at least 12 h old. The increased uptake of the radioisotopes may persist for 90 days or until there has been complete healing and maturation of tissues.

Always consider Scheuermann's disease (juvenile osteochondrosis) in evaluating an injured spine. This developmental epiphysitis will cause developmental kyphosis. It may be difficult on X-ray studies to separate developmental from post-traumatic wedging of the vertebrae.

# The Shoulder

The shoulder is a ball-and-socket joint. The ligaments surrounding the shoulder are designed to limit movement, but they do not maintain the joint surfaces in apposition. The humerus can be separated from the glenoid passively. The joint is protected by an arch formed by the coracoid process, the acromion, and the coracoacromial ligament (Gray [2]).

# Common Acute Shoulder Injuries

1. Contusion of the shoulder tip

   *Symptoms:* The patient will present difficult abduction pain at the tip of the shoulder (deltoid region) even with slight active motion; passive motion is full with minimal discomfort.

   *Signs:* There is tenderness at the tip of the shoulder, with bruising and tissue swelling; the ability to abduct the shoulder from the neutral position with or without resistance depends upon the degree of injury.

   *X-ray studies:* These are usually normal.

   *Testing:* Infiltration with a local anesthetic agent in the region of tenderness and maximal pain should be tried. If pain is relieved, then the rotator cuff is either intact or in continuity, and abduction of the arm from the neutral position against resistance will be good or excellent. With a moderate or large tear in the rotator cuff or a significant hematoma in the surrounding tissues beyond the area of anesthetic infiltration, abduction will not improve with local anesthesia.

   *Differential Diagnosis:* The possibilities to consider are 1) contusion, or 2) rotator cuff injury.

   *Treatment:* Ice, a sling, rest, gradual physiotherapy exercises, and oral enzymes are recommended. If, after anesthesia, good abduction of the shoulder is possible, then 21 or preferably 28 days should be allowed for the healing of rotator cuff and surrounding tissues. If abduction after anesthetic infiltration remains weak, and this weakness persists for 14–21 days, then a shoulder arthrogram should be obtained to assess the degree of rotator cuff damage. Large and small tears with persistent functional deficit should be surgically repaired.

2. Acromioclavicular (AC) pain

   *History:* The patient reports striking the shoulder tip during a fall.

   *Symptoms:* Pain is present at the AC joint with any motion of the shoulder; there is swelling or deformity of the AC joint region; motion of the shoulders induces snapping at the AC joint area.

   *Signs:* Tenderness is elicited over the AC joint. Clicking or subluxation of the clavicle is induced by palpation on movement of the shoulder and subluxation of the acromion downward with passive application of weight to the involved extremity. There is also apparent subluxation of the lateral tip of the clavicle upward during normal standing, and hypermobility of the clavicle on passive stress of the lateral tip upward.

   *X-ray studies:* Anterio-posterior X-ray films are made of the shoulder while the extremity is weighted or while the patient holds onto an immovable object and tries to lift it (Fig 19–5). There may be hypermobility of the lateral tip of the clavicle (riding cephalad above the acromion). Fracture of the lateral tip of the clavicle may be present. Irregularities or sclerosis of the acromioclavicular joint should be noted.

   *Differential diagnosis:* The following disorders should be considered:
   1. Acute separation of the acromioclavicular joint
   2. Synovitis of the acromioclavicular joint

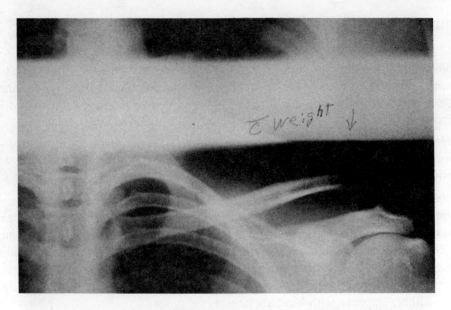

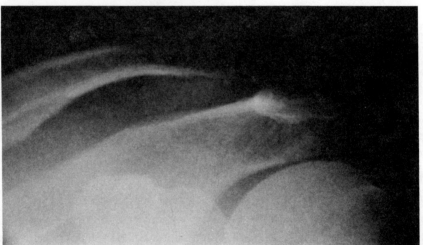

**19–5**   X-rays films of shoulder acromioclavicular separation. Lateral end of clavicle is superior to articular edge of acromion.

3. Acromioclavicular degenerative arthritis aggravated by recent injury
4. Fracture of the lateral clavicle.

In a first-degree acromioclavicular separation, minimal displacement of the clavicular relation to the acromion is found. Third-degree separation shows complete displacement of the clavicle upward from the acromion either with or without applied stress. Also in third-degree separation there is a tear of the acromioclavicular and the coracoclavicular ligaments.

*Treatment:*   Sling rest is helpful. A Kinney-Howard sling splint for severe grade II and grade III separation is recommended along with anti-inflammatory drugs or enzymes orally. Lccal anesthetic injection may help, but no steroid should be injected. Surgery may be needed in third-degree lesions, to insure stability by removal of the

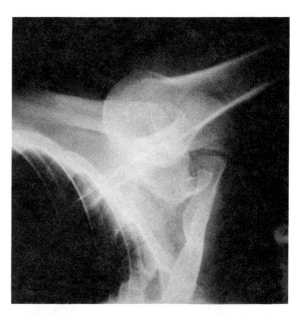

**19–6**  Inferior dislocation of shoulder; luxation erectae type.

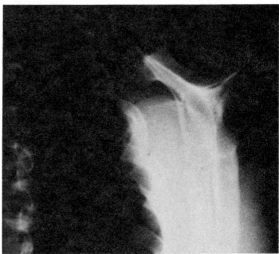

Lateral view of shoulder with anterior inferior dislocation of humeral head. Head of humerus displaced anterior to juncture (*Y*) of scapular spine, coracoid process, and body of the scapula.

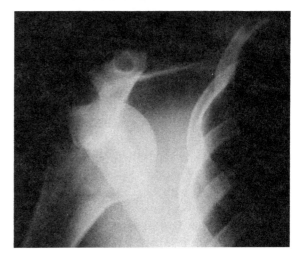

Anterior inferior dislocation of shoulder.

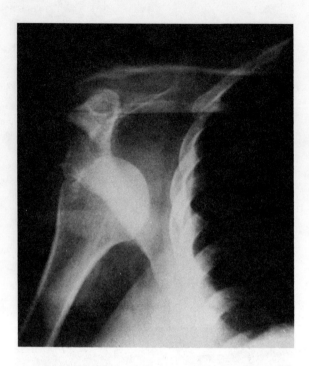

**19–7** Anterior inferior dislocation of shoulder with greater tuberosity fracture.

articular disc and repair of the ligaments. Resection of the lateral tip of the clavicle is sometimes performed together with other stabilizing measures.

3. Anterior dislocation of the shoulder

*Symptoms:*    The arm is usually held by the opposite hand in slight abduction and external rotation. Pain occasionally radiates along branches of the brachial plexus.

*Signs:*    Passive adduction or internal rotation is strongly resisted. The acromion is prominent, and the humeral head can be felt anterior to the acromion and adjacent to the coracoid process. Occasionally the humeral head is located inferior to the glenoid fossa, which can be palpated. The acromion is then more prominent than with a simple anterior dislocation. Posteriorly, the absence of the humeral head is noted by contour and on palpation. The posterior glenoid rim is prominently palpable.

The examiner should check for brachial plexus deficits, and should document impaired nervous function at the time of initial evaluation. The circulatory status will be noted by the appearance of nailbeds and palpation of the radial pulse.

*X-ray Studies:*    Anterior and inferior displacement of the humeral head (Fig. 19–6) will be evident, as well as a fracture, if one has occurred (Fig. 19–7).

*Treatment:*    Attempted reduction should be gentle. If circumstances are not ideal, the patient must be transferred to adequate facilities for reduction of the dislocation. A skilled examiner may attempt on-site reduction after documenting the patient's prereduction neurovascular status, but the possibility should be considered that a fracture might coexist with the dislocation and that the manipulator might later be blamed for it without X-ray documentation before reduction. Reduction under general anesthesia is the most gentle technique, allowing minimal stress to joint surfaces while muscle relaxation is maximal.

*Reduction techniques:*

1. Gentle axial traction alone is used, with countertraction in the form of a sheet around the upper chest held by an assistant pulling in the opposite direction.
2. The patient is prone, with a weight hanging on the arm and the pectoral region raised on a support fashioned from towels or a small bolster. This allows gravity to do the reducing as the muscles relax by fatigue.
3. If the Kocher maneuver is employed, the arm is abducted and externally rotated; adduction and external rotation are then used; internal rotation is the final maneuver. All movements are performed with gentle axial traction at the elbow with one hand, while the wrist is supported on the physician's other hand.
4. When the straight overhead technique is used, the patient is supine. The physician inspires confidence by explaining the plan. Slowly, but steadily and actively, the patient's hand is moved over the shoulder until it touches the sheet just behind the patient's head. The elbow is kept flexed. Gentle pressure is applied to the humeral head, backward and upward with one hand while the other hand guides the arm into flexion overhead. Reduction will be followed by relief of discomfort and easy, active motion of the shoulder joint.

*General anesthesia, intravenous diazepam, or intravenous narcotics are helpful and recommended to insure gentle manipulation.*

Additional injuries found by X-ray studies must be dealt with. Avulsion fractures of the glenoid or fractures of the greater tuberosity or humeral neck may be associated with dislocation of the shoulder. Rarely, the tendon of the long head of the biceps will bowstring across the joint and prevent reentry of the humeral head into the joint area. The post reduction treatment is immobilization by:

1. Sling with a woven elastic wrap around the chest, arm, and forearm, preventing external rotation;
2. Commercial shoulder immobilizer; or
3. Commercial sling and swathe.

The first episodes of anterior shoulder disclocation should be treated by immobilization, in the hope that healing and reestablishment of normal stability will occur. This takes at least 4 weeks. Gradual range-of-motion exercises should then be tried, starting with gravity exercises and progressing to passive and active overhead mobilization. Internal rotation exercises are important to regain shoulder mobility posteriorly. This motion is commonly forgotten. The patient should hold a doorknob with the problem hand and turn away from the treated arm, utilizing body momentum for internal rotation in a posterior direction.

4. Posterior dislocations of the shoulder.

The diagnosis can be missed even after X-ray films have been made, unless the existence of a posterior dislocation has been considered.

*Symptoms:*   The shoulder is painful and there is inability to actively rotate the shoulder externally. Occasionally the pain radiates to the tip of the shoulder, along the distribution of the axillary nerve.

*Signs:*   The arm is held rigidly in internal rotation. Passive motion is strongly resisted. The coracoid process is more prominent than usual and the humeral head can be felt posterior to the acromion. The glenoid fossa can be easily palpated anteriorly. Careful examination is necessary, with attention to circulation and neuromuscular function at the elbow, wrist, and hand.

*X-ray Studies:*  The X-ray films can easily be misinterpreted. If there is doubt, the involved shoulder should be compared with the normal side. A tangential view of the scapula and axial view of the shoulder are helpful. On the tangential view, the humeral head should center at the junction of the scapular spine, glenoid, and acromion projections. Fractures of the glenoid or proximal humerus may accompany this dislocation.

*Treatment:*  Definitive treatment depends upon coexisting fractures. Some fractures need open reduction. Ideally, reduction is attempted under general anesthesia. Gentle axial traction with countertraction by a sheet around the chest and forward pressure to the humeral head with gentle external rotation of the humerus may be successful. Muscle relaxation and analgesia require at least intravenous diazepam or a narcotic. Immediate reduction in the field can be accomplished by a skilled manipulator, but all precautions should be taken (see section on anterior dislocations).

Postreduction management is immobilization for at least 3 weeks, and preferably 4 weeks for the first dislocation. Gravity exercises and increasing range of motion begin after immobilization. The arm can be immobilized in neutral position or in external rotation by means of a modified plaster spica. This type of bandage allows shortening of the posterior capsular distance between the humeral head and the glenoid and may insure more stable healing.

If the dislocation (anterior or posterior is a recurrent one, then immobilization should be only long enough for relief of symptoms. It is improbable that a recurrent dislocation will become more stable with prolonged immobilization after each episode (see section on Common Chronic or Recurring Shoulder Symptoms later in this chapter).

# Fractures of the Humerus

The treatment of fractures of the humerus depends upon location of the fracture, displacement of the segments, and associated nerve or vascular injury. The objective in teenagers and older athletes is to obtain close anatomic reduction and full return of function. Therefore, treatment usually entails one or all of the following at different stages after the injury:

1. Sling and swathe immobilization
2. Hanging cast
3. Coaptation splints
4. Side-arm or over-the-head skeletal traction
5. Open reduction with internal fixation

Open reduction with internal fixation is rarely necessary, but on occasion, nerve exploration, blood vessel repair, or repair of unacceptable shortening or malunion is desirable.

Axial forces applied to the shoulder or direct or rotational forces applied to the proximal humeral region can cause the immature humerus to slip off the proximal humeral

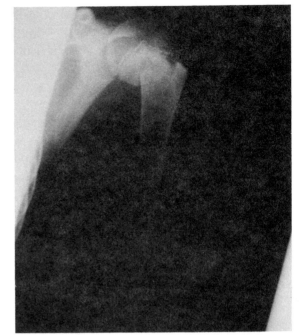

**19–8**  Epiphyseal slip of proximal humeral epiphysis, anteroposterior view. Arm is in external rotation under anesthesia.

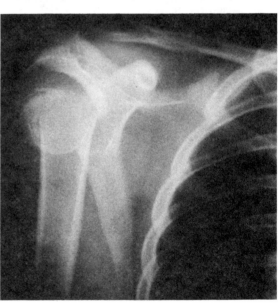

**19–9**  Proximal humeral epiphysis slip with shoulder in internal rotation under general anesthesia.

epiphysis (Figs. 19–8, 19–9). Treatment is reduction without excessive manipulation. The young, immature, proximal humerus will remodel with time if rotational alignment is good. Occasionally anatomic reduction may be obtained under general anesthesia, and the repair is held in place with a percutaneous transfixing pin. A shoulder spica can be applied, with the arm overhead in the "Statue of Liberty" position, with the cast extending to the wrist or palm.

In fractures of the humerus, careful documentation of the status of the neurovascular structures of the extremity is necessary. Blood flow and neural function must be closely observed for 72 h. Injuries to the brachial plexus are not uncommon in association with fractures of the humerus. Injury to the radial nerve may also occur frequently.

# Common Clavicular Injuries

**Sternoclavicular Sprains**  The sternoclavicular joint is a double arthroidial joint. It is formed by the sternal end of the clavicle, the upper and lateral part of the manubrium sternae, and the cartilage of the first rib.

*Symptoms:*  Pain and swelling are present at the medial (sternal end) of the clavicle.

*Signs:*  Tenderness is felt in the area of swelling, and there is fluctuation of the medial end of the clavicle on gentle pressure to the bone of the clavicle. Manipulation of the clavicle outward (anteriorly) will show hypermobility of the medial end.

*X-ray studies:*  Subluxation or dislocation may be evident, but it is very difficult to isolate this joint by routine X-ray films. Tomograms may be necessary if documentation is required. A CT scan will also show this area well.

*Treatment:*  Partial tears (first-degree and second-degree should be treated with ice, rest, and a sling until tenderness subsides. Complete tears (third-degree) involve the sternoclavicular and the costoclavicular ligaments. These are treated by surgical reduction and stabilization.

Many third-degree lesions are missed because of local swelling and minimal deformity. They become manifest later with discomfort and functional limitations.

In posterior dislocations, the medial end of the clavicle is displaced behind the manubrium sternae and locked in that position. Such dislocations will present the same symptoms and, on occasion, swelling of the extremity because of pressure upon major vessels. Posterior dislocation is treated immediately by gentle manipulation of the clavicle forward, preferably under a general anesthesia. Some dislocations will reduce spontaneously and present with a lax sternoclavicular joint and the findings that have been discussed.

**Shaft Fractures of the Clavicle**  Most shaft fractures of the clavicle are treated with a figure-eight splint and a sling support on the injured side. Occasionally, a plaster figure-eight splint is applied to maintain reduction. A plaster splint is no better and no more secure than a soft figure-eight appliance. It is usually not necessary to reduce clavicular fractures surgically except to treat a rare nonunion. Nonunions usually occur in fractures previously reduced surgically. Even comminuted fractures with displaced and rotated butterfly fragments have healed with splinting. If the fragment causes tenting of the skin, the bony protrusion is removed surgically under local anesthesia after healing has occurred.

Acute open reduction and internal fixation may be necessary in cases with a fracture of the clavicle on the dominant side, in athletes involved in throwing or racquet sports. Athletes have special mechanical advantages in the shoulder girdle, which they use with precision. Shortening or slight malrotation of the clavicle can change performance unpredictably.

Some lateral clavicle fractures are treated as a grade III acromioclavicular separation. A Kinney-Howard acromioclavicular splint may be tried. If this splint is successful, X-ray films show acceptable reduction with the splint in place. The splint must be worn day and night for at least 4 weeks. Open repair is occasionally necessary.

For lateral fractures distal to the coracoclavicular ligamentous attachments with intact ligaments, a sling is used for support until swelling and pain subsides. Gradual motion can then be started.

After reductions at the shoulder or clavicle, X-ray studies should be obtained to document the status of the bones after manipulation. If doubt exists about shoulder girdle structures, the films should be sent for consultation to a radiologist or orthopedist. Second opinions of X-ray studies may stimulate thoughts on the ideal treatment of athletes. Poor results can lead to litigation, particularly if consultation was not obtained.

## Common Chronic or Recurring Shoulder Symptoms

Bateman [3] has made some critical evaluations and commentaries about shoulder problems.

1. Subdeltoid or subacromial pain

   *Symptoms:*   The patient suffers aching pain at rest and there is painful and limited range of motion of the shoulder joint.

   *Signs:*   Tenderness is present anterior to the acromion or laterally under the deltoid muscle at the greater tuberosity of the humerus. There is pain with greater than 80° abduction. Pronation or supination against resistance is painless.

   *X-ray studies:*   X-ray films may show calcification in the region of the rotator cuff or capsular structures.

   *Differential diagnosis:*   Among the causes, the following should be considered: 1) tendinitis of the rotator cuff; 2) subacromial bursitis; 3) subdeltoid bursitis.

   *Treatment:*   Initially, a sling, ice, salicylates, and anti-inflammatory drugs are used. Later, local anesthetic injections may be given. Active motion and gravity-assisted passive motion should be encouraged while the anesthetic is effective. Repetitive ice massage helps relieve discomfort and muscle spasm. Oral steroids in tapering doses for 5–7 days are often helpful. Local anesthetic injection can be repeated after 10–14 days, but steroids should not be given again for at least 3 weeks, with no more than three repetitions.

2. Posterior or lateral shoulder pain

   *Sport:*   Football, hockey, or any other sport in which frequent falls and trauma to the deltoid region occur may result in shoulder pains.

   *Signs:*   The victim suffers tenderness of the deltoid muscle; there is function (abduction of 15° against resistance); range of motion is full, but passive.

   *Differential diagnosis:*   Possible causes include hematoma of the deltoid muscle and myositis ossificans.

   *Treatment:*   The hematoma should be aspirated and a local anesthetic agent injected. A sling should be applied and the patient should rest. Ice applications intermittently for 42–72 hours will help. Isometric exercises and pendulum exercises may be used as healing begins.

3. Recurrent pain at the start of throwing or serving in tennis

   *Signs:*   The patient experiences tenderness of the greater tuberosity of the humerus and under the tip of the acromion.

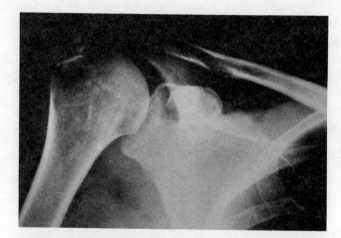

**19–10**   Calcification in rotator cuff of shoulder in calcific tendinitis of rotator cuff.

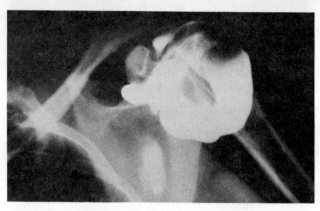

**19–11**   Arthrogram of shoulder, showing tear in rotator cuff with extravasation of contrast material (Conray) out of joint capsule and into subacromial bursa.

*Differential diagnosis:*   The following disorders should be ruled out: 1) rotator cuff tendinitis; 2) subacromial bursitis; 3) subdeltoid bursitis.

*Treatment:*   Throwing frequency should be decreased; salicylates or other anti-inflammatory drugs may be given. Ultrasound treatment and occasionally a diuretic will reduce local swelling.

After the season, local steroid injections around the tendon and into the bursa can be tried while the joint is rested; pendulum and isometric exercises should continue. Local anesthetic injections alone, without the steroid mixture, can be used. Immediately after the local anesthetic injection, 5- to 7-day tapering doses of oral cortisone derivative can be used to reduce inflammation.

X-ray studies may show calcified areas in the region of the rotator cuff (Fig. 19–10). Injections can be made into these areas with the use of fluoroscopy to guide the needle. Large-bore needles are useful for puncturing and aspirating the soft calcium deposits. Recurrent pain should be evaluated by arthrogram to exclude a tear in the rotator cuff (Fig. 19–11). Sometimes surgery is necessary to repair a cuff tear or release the coracoacromial ligament to stop impingement of the humerus against it.

4. Pain at the end of throwing and serving in tennis

*Signs:*   Tenderness is experienced at the posterior glenoid rim.

*Differential diagnosis:* Possible causes are the following: 1) tendon insertion tear (long head of the triceps); 2) tear of the posterior capsule; 3) posterior osteophytes.

*Treatment:* The arm and shoulder should have rest in a sling; anti-inflammatory drugs, ultrasound, and ice massage will help to alleviate pain. A slow return to hard throwing or serving should be made over several weeks. Surgical removal of an osteophyte or loose fragment within the joint may be necessary.

5. Gradual loss of motion of the shoulder with pain during almost all movement

*Signs:* There is loss of some posterior internal rotation and abduction in forward flexion with anterior, lateral, and posterior tenderness at the glenoid rim. Crepitus and stability can be assessed under general anesthesia.

*X-ray studies:* Films may show notching of the humeral head posteriorly; osteophytes of the genoid rim may be present; an osteophyte at the inferior aspect of the humeral head may be present; the humeral head may be distorted.

*Diagnosis:* Post-traumatic osteoarthritis is the likely cause.

*Treatment:* Anti-inflammatory drugs will help, as will active range-of-motion exercises, minimal passive range-of-motion exercises, and heat application. Gentle manipulation of the joint under anesthesia may be necessary, depending on individual circumstances.

6. Anterior shoulder pain

*Signs:* Tenderness is present, and sometimes snapping or crepitation in the bicipital groove. There is some anterior pain with external rotation of the arm while the arm is held abducted 45°, and pain with supination of the forearm against resistance. Bateman [3] noted that anterior shoulder pain is frequently found in underhand pitching, bowling, or overhand throwing activities.

*Differential diagnosis:* The following causes should be considered: 1) bicipital tendinitis; 2) dislocating biceps tendon; 3) subscapularis tendinitis; 4) impingement of the coracoacromial ligament on the biceps tendon; 5) rotator cuff tears; 6) shoulder subluxation.

*X-ray studies:* Films may show a shallow bicipital groove and/or calcification in the rotator cuff tendon.

*Treatment:* Rest in a sling is advisable, as are anti-inflammatory drugs and physical therapy. Occasionally surgery is needed to repair the transverse humeral ligament or to transfer the long head of the biceps tendon or apply tenodesis.

7. Scapular pain, especially at the medial border

*Associated Sports:* The shot-put, discus, javelin may induce scapular pain.

*Signs:* Tenderness is experienced along the medial border of the scapula; there may be crepitation and local muscle spasm

*Diagnosis:* A muscle tear at the medial scapular attachment (rhomboid muscle) or tendinitis of the parascapular region may be the cause.

*Treatment:* Ice massage, sling, rest, local anesthetic injections, ultrasound or other heat may bring relief. Oral steroids with local anesthetic injections can be utilized. Steroid administration should be tapered over 5–7 days.

8. Recurrent forward slipping of the shoulder; recurrent anterior and posterior shoulder dislocation

*Signs:* Occasional tenderness of the biceps tendon may be felt, and there is apprehension on passive 90° abduction and external rotation of the humerus. Forward shift of the humerus is felt by the patient and occasionally by the examiner as the patient contracts his pectoral and latissimus muscle.

*X-ray studies:* Films show loose bodies and/or avulsion fractures of the inferior glenoid rim. They should be compared with prior films taken after past dislocations.

*Diagnosis:* The following situations should be considered: 1) recurrent dislocation of the shoulder (more commonly anterior); 2) subluxation of the shoulder.

*Treatment:* Accurate diagnosis is important. Examination under anesthesia should allow reproduction of the subluxing motion of the humeral head. Prior X-ray documentation of an anterior dislocation does not exclude a new posterior or inferior subluxation. Under anesthesia, the direction of subluxation should be noted. A combination of inferior, anterior, and posterior subluxation may coexist.

Developmental lax ligaments allow recurrent subluxation or dislocations of the shoulder. Hyperextensibility of the elbows or knees and fingers should be looked for. If lax joints are present, the prognosis for results is poor. Orthotic restraints stop maximal abduction or external rotation, which are necessary to subluxate or dislocate the shoulder. Surgical treatment helps most other people by obliterating the lax areas that allow shifting of the humeral head. Surgery can also create mechanical blocks through displacement of the glenoid or of the coracoid process by local osteotomy.

Shoulder dynamics should be kept in mind during examination. The patient should go through the motions that cause symptoms and try to reproduce them in the physician's presence. The tennis racquet, bat, or ball should be used to recreate accurately the symptomatic activity. Overuse syndromes in the shoulder joint are common. Excessive throwing or serving in tennis without proper conditioning and warm-up can cause pain. Fatigue areas develop and muscle tendon units tear without the necessary recovery time. Overuse injuries respond to rest and a transient substitution of one sport for another to allow healing.

Peter Fowler of London, Ontario, Canada (personal communication, 1982) has recently stressed the importance of strengthening the external shoulder rotators when treating shoulder pain syndromes. This muscle group is often forgotten. Dr. Fowler's comments referred to shoulder pain in swimmers.

# Common Acute Injuries to the Elbow Joint

The elbow is a hinged joint. The trochlea of the humerus articulates with the semilunar notch of the ulna. The capitellum of the humerus articulates with the fovea of the head of the radius. There are thickened capsular structures over the ulna, collateral ligament, and radial collateral ligament, which stabilize the joint (Gray [2]).

# Contusion of the Tip of the Olecranon

*Symptoms:*   Pain is experienced on active extension, localized to the olecranon tip.

*Signs:*   Swelling of the olecranon region is present, and fluid in the filled bursa can be felt.

*X-ray studies:*   Films may appear normal, or a small spur may be present at the tip of the olecranon.

*Treatment:*   Ice, a sling, and rest with early active motion help to relieve pain. Bursa aspiration should be done after 36 h and a compression dressing applied. Early compression dressings can be used to prevent recurrent local swelling.

# Fractures of the Elbow

*Symptoms:*   Pain, swelling, and deformity are all experienced. There is occasional loss of normal sensation and function in the hand or loss of the radial pulse early.

*Signs:*   Examine the function of the wrist and hand. Feel radial and ulnar pulses, note blanching at the nailbed, and deformity at the elbow.

*Treatment:*   A splint and ice should be applied immediately and the fracture evaluated by X-ray films.

*Differential diagnosis:*   The following injuries should be ruled out: 1) elbow dislocation, 2) fractures of the distal humerus, proximal radius or proximal ulna.

Radial head fractures deserve special mention. They can be missed by X-ray films. The patient's signs and symptoms should suggest the diagnosis.

# Radial Head Fractures

*Symptoms:*   The patient suffers acute pain and limitation of motion after a fall with an extended elbow and sometimes supinated forearm.

*Signs:*   Tenderness is elicited at the radial head and there is absence of full extension of the elbow. Flexion is possible to approximately 90°. There may be pain with pronation and supination.

*X-ray Studies:*   Films reveal that the fat pad at the anterior aspect of the elbow is displaced proximally and anteriorly by an intra-articular hematoma. A fracture line may not be evident in the head or neck of the radius.

*Treatment:*   A splint is placed for 5–7 days in 90° of flexion, and a sling is applied, allowing gradual range of motion. Some physicians allow immediate motion, using only a sling support. Repeat X-ray films are made in 10–14 days after local absorption of bone has occurred, to see whether a fracture line is evident. If the radial head fracture is displaced, the treatment should be surgical: 1) The fragment can be replaced and fixed in position with pins or small screws, or 2) the radial head can be removed completely, or 3) it can be removed and replaced by a prosthesis.

*Comments:*

1. Intra-articular fractures should be surgically restored to anatomic continuity.
2. Long immobilization of the elbow may be associated with permanent loss of motion. Ideally, motion is started early, while control of fracture segments is still maintained. Sometimes internal fixation is necessary to accomplish this.
3. Epiphyseal injuries not readily apparent on plain X-ray films may occur in the immature elbow. Views of the opposite elbow will facilitate meticulous comparison of the anatomic structures on both sides. Small calcific areas in ectopic sites may indicate an epiphyseal fracture, with avulsion of a portion of bone adjacent to the nonosseous cartilaginous portion of the growth center. X-ray findings should be correlated with clinical swelling, tenderness, and functional deficits.
4. Myositis ossificans or calcification of the elbow joint capsule is not predictable. If surgery is to be carried out, it should be done within the first 24 h or after 21 days to minimize complications.

## The Dislocated Elbow

Dislocation of the elbow is an emergency. Whenever possible, an X-ray film should be obtained prior to treatment to show associated fractures. Without X-ray facilities, treatment can be instituted by skilled manipulation.

*Treatment:*   Ice and a splint are applied immediately. Neurovascular function of the wrist, hand, and antecubital region should be assessed. Additional injuries should also be assessed (especially to the shoulder, wrist, and hand). If the patient is treated at the scene: 1) The radius and ulna are moved gently into alignment by palpation. 2) The elbow is gently extended with one hand at mid forearm or wrist while the other hand is above the elbow. Simultaneously traction is applied at the wrist or hand. If tolerance of pain allows, reduction will occur. Multiple attempts at reduction should not be made. If reduction fails, the patient is transported for X-ray films and reduction under anesthesia. Anesthesia decreases stresses at the articular surface of the elbow joint during reduction maneuvers.

## Elbow Sprains and Strains

First and second degree sprains and strains with little loss of function need only protection, muscle-controlling isometric exercises, gentle range of motion, and progressive resistive exercises until symptoms subside and full function and confidence return.

Third-degree sprains rarely need more than supportive care. Occasionally a complete collateral ligament tear will require surgical repair. Early controlled motion is ideal after operative or nonoperative treatment.

A dislocated elbow is, in fact, a severe third-degree sprain. Evaluation of the collateral ligaments of the elbow joint after the dislocation has been reduced may rarely show ligamentous instability of a degree to warrant surgical correction.

Elbow sprains can be associated with tears of capsular structures. Initially the joint may be painful but with decent range of motion. Gradually pain-free contracture with limitation of motion may develop. In some patients, X-ray studies 3 weeks after injury may show calcification of the capsule. The treatment is gentle, active, controlled motion of the elbow. After tissue matures, gradual stretching can be accomplished through both active and passive motion.

## Chronic, Recurring Elbow Symptoms; Medial and Lateral Joint Pain

These symptoms are called "tennis elbow," epicondylitis, or tendinitis.

*Sport:*  Racquet and throwing sports most commonly cause recurrent symptoms.

*Signs and symptoms:*  Grip is painful, and there is tenderness at the attachment to the epicondylar ridge of the humerus of the common extensor, or common flexor tendon mass. Pain is felt with wrist extension or wrist flexion against resistance at the respective tendon attachment sites at the elbow. There may be weakness of dorsiflexion at the wrist if the lateral region is involved. Lack of full extension of the elbow joint is common.

*X-ray studies:*  The films are usually normal, but there may be calcium deposits along the epicondylar ridge.

*Treatment:*  Rest in a sling or splint, ice massage, and salicylates are recommended. A short course of oral steroids may be tried if symptoms persist; local anesthetic injection may be used later. An elastic clasp band (tennis elbow band) applied at the proximal forearm just distal to the common tendon insertions relieves stress at the attachment sites. As a last resort, operations have been successful. These operations vary from muscle slides (a type of muscle lengthening) to tendon lengthening procedures. Occasionally, entrapment of a branch of the radial nerve has been the source of pain.

## Warning Signs at the Elbow

Lack of full extension is a common elbow sign. When perceived in pre-teenage children, it should be a reminder to observe and evaluate the joint carefully. Myostatic contractures of the elbow flexors can result from overuse of the joint, starting with myositis of the common flexor-pronator group as a result of dynamic overload. The condition then goes on to static contractures.

Valgus deformity of the elbow may be a serious sign in the pre-teenager. Irritation of the medial humeral condyle or, more importantly, of the capitellum can result in osteochondritis dissicans or ischemic necrosis (Panner's disease) with resulting growth disturbances. Such abnormalities have been seen in children overusing the arm in throwing sports. If diagnosed early, the treatment should include: 1) rest; 2) change of sport; 3) alternation of sports; 4) gentle active stretching; 5) physical therapy with heat; 6) salicylates; 7) ice massage after usage.

At times, orthopedic surgery is helpful. Osteotomies or débridements can relieve pain, restore carrying angle, and improve function. Occasionally osteochondral fragments occur within the joint. They can be treated by surgical replacement into their normal anatomic sites or by removing them from the joint.

# Forearm and Wrist Injuries

Contusions, sprains, strains, and fractures are the most common injuries to this part of the body.

## Forearm Fractures

Fractures of the radius and ulna usually present a deformity with exquisite tenderness at the fracture site (Fig. 19–12). Treatment is with splinting and ice application, then transportation for X-ray films and reduction or casting, as necessary.

If marked angulation is present and the circulation or motor function is significantly impaired, immediate reduction of the forearm bones can be performed by a skilled manipulator at the scene.

Before any reduction, the neurovascular status should be documented. After reduction has been performed, sensation, circulation, and motor capabilities of the wrist and hand should be reexamined and documented. A splint or cast should be applied; the extremity should be elevated (wrist higher than elbow and elbow higher than heart level); and ice should be applied for 24–36 h.

Forearm compartment pressure syndromes may result from swelling within muscle compartments that causes ischemia and muscle necrosis. The swelling can be prevented by anticipating a pressure syndrome; splints applied to the wrist and forearm should allow for swelling. A skilled examiner should evaluate the extremity at frequent intervals and note changes in the neurovascular status. Pain should be controlled by ice, aspirin, and splinting. Narcotics should not be used because they mask the pain of incipient muscle ischemia. The fingers should be almost fully extendable, actively or passively, with only minimal discomfort at the fracture site. Sensation to all dermatomes of the hand should be intact.

Two-point discrimination should be tested and compared with the uninjured hand. Any impairment is an indication of possible increasing pressure in the forearm or at the wrist. Capillary filling response of the nailbed should be good when compared with the uninjured extremity. The thumb should oppose the middle finger and index finger with good pinch power. The cast should not hinder thumb motion during this test. The fingers should abduct and adduct with strength sufficient to hold a piece of cardboard between the fingers.

The flexor retinaculum forms the carpal tunnel on the volar aspect of the wrist covering the flexor tendons and the median nerve, and the tunnel can become edematous and press upon the median nerve. The ulnar nerve can become involved in a similar fashion in the ulnar canal of Guyon at the wrist. This is a canal at the distal end of the forearm, through which the ulnar artery and nerve pass to the hand (Spinner [4]). Neurologic deficits in the dermatomes of the median and ulnar nerves will suggest pressure problems. Blockage of conduction of motor or sensory impulses to the hand will be detectable by electrodiagnostic tests. If carpal tunnel or Guyon tunnel syndromes develop and do not respond to elevation of the limb for several hours, further treatment should be considered. Injections of a local anesthetic agent mixed with dexamethasone and hyaluronidase can be used

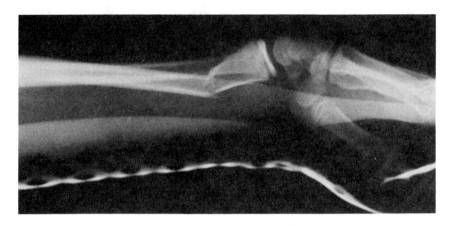

**19–12** X-ray film of wrist, showing dorsally displaced fracture fragment of the distal radius in a 12-year-old boy.

locally with some success. Pressure syndromes are treated by surgical decompression. Injections themselves may temporarily increase the pressure within tight compartments and should not be tried by those with little experience.

Death of muscle is not reversible but is preventable. Most hospitals are equipped with arterial pressure monitoring devices. These can be adapted to measure compartment pressures by comparison with the uninjured limb or by absolute values. Once a syndrome is diagnosed, the treatment is surgical release of the compartment. One should err in releasing a normal compartment rather than in temporizing with a swollen compartment.

Arterial injuries occur at fracture sites. If pulses are not palpable, a Doppler flowmeter should be used. Nailbed filling of capillaries is checked with the arm elevated and arm dependent. Filling and emptying of the veins on the dorsum of the hand are checked by forearm positioning, but swelling of the forearm at the fracture site may prevent such observations.

The adolescent with a forearm fracture needs excellent reduction. Do not hesitate to use open reduction if closed reduction has been less than ideal. It is very difficult for a good athlete to adapt to a poorly functioning forearm that is the result of a malunion of forearm bones.

## Wrist Injuries

The wrist joint is a condyloid articulation. Proximally located are the distal end of the radius and undersurface of the articular disc between the radius and ulna. Distally are the navicula, the lunate, and the triangular bone (triquetrum) (Gray [2]).

Sprains, contusions, and fractures are common injuries of the wrist. The painful swollen wrist should be splinted and then evaluated by X-ray studies. The neurovascular status should be assessed immediately and again at reasonable intervals for the subsequent 24 h. *Carpal bone fractures or carpal fracture with associated intercarpal dislocation can easily be missed.*

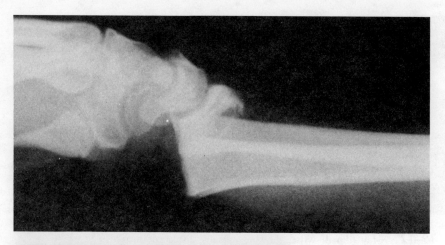

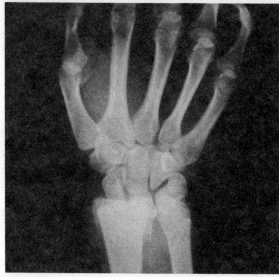

**19–13** Anterioposterior and lateral views of wrist in a 14-year-old roller skater. There is dorsal displacement of the distal radial epiphysis (epiphyseal slip).

Marked swelling and limitation of motion out of proportion to a ''minor injury'' or neurovascular impairment should lead to the suspicion of intercarpal dislocation.

Wrist trauma can cause a carpal tunnel syndrome or swelling within the tunnel of Guyon.

Negative results on X-ray studies, with tenderness at the ''snuffbox'' over the carpal scaphoid bone, suggest a fracture of the scaphoid. The wrist and thumb should be splinted for 14–21 days and then reevaluated clinically and by X-ray films to visualize the scaphoid fracture. This fracture deserves special comment. The healing time in a cast can be greater than 3 months. Some fractures go on to nonunion despite early casting. Some fractures remain undiagnosed and are treated as a sprain for several weeks. Initial treatment for a scaphoid fracture is a long arm-to-thumb spica cast with the forearm in neutral position. Some physicians use only a short arm-to-thumb spica cast. A few incorporate the index and middle fingers into the long cast for more rigid immobilization.

Small chip fractures of the distal end of the scaphoid may be treated as a sprain, with soft immobilization only, until symptoms subside, even though there is the possibility of a fibrous union of that small fragment.

Occasionally an X-ray film will reveal a fracture of the carpal scaphoid bone that already has arthritic changes in and around the radial carpal joint when the diagnosis is finally made. Other missed fractures will have cystic or avascular changes in the carpal scaphoid bone when they are eventually recognized.

The treatment of carpal scaphoid fractures must be individualized. Sometimes early open reduction and internal fixation are recommended. At other times the treatment is staged. Initially a soft wrap is utilized and the patient is allowed to engage in usual activities while internal fixation and bone grafting is planned for a later date. Staging treatment must be done with the informed consent of the patient.

Forced dorsiflexion or forced palmar flexion can cause various degrees of epiphyseal injuries in the immature wrist (Fig. 19–13). If there has not been complete separation or displacement of the growth area, X-ray films may be normal. A swollen wrist with exquisite fracture-type tenderness and significant functional impairment should be considered a fracture and treated as such until proved otherwise. X-ray studies of the uninjured wrist for comparison should be made and compared. The epiphyseal injury will commonly show at least some widening of the epiphyseal line. The only X-ray sign of a slipped epiphysis might be a small, displaced portion of bone at the periphery of the growth line. An inexperienced examiner might conclude that an avulsion fracture has occurred and miss the more serious growth-plate injury.

Treatment for epiphyseal injuries should be immobilization until complete healing. Displacements should be reduced under ideal conditions and as gently as possible, with the aid of appropriate anesthesia. The prognosis for growth will vary, depending on the severity of the epiphyseal trauma. These injuries are graded clinically by the location and extent of the fracture line into the epiphysis and by the degree of compression forces necessary to injure the growth center.

The final measures for sprains and fractures around the wrist include protection during periods of vulnerability and include 1) taping, 2) elastic wrap or leather gauntlet, and 3) commercial splinting.

Avascular necrosis of the carpal lunate bone and early, arthritic changes in the wrist bones will give pain. The best treatment is early recognition and protection from stresses that may cause further injury to the wrist. Later the care, including surgical measures, must be individualized.

# Common Hand Injuries

## Stress to the Carpal-Metacarpal Joint of the Thumb

Initially, thumb injury is treated with a splint, and the patient is transported for X-ray studies. The hand is examined for fractures, subluxation, or dislocation. The degree of stability is assessed, and a local anesthetic injection is given to relieve guarding, if necessary. Treatment must be individualized. If no fracture or subluxation is found, a splint is applied, with the proximal phalanx of the thumb included. Some fractures in this area may need open fixation of fragments and repair of soft tissues.

# Sprain of the Metacarpal-Phalangeal Joint of the Thumb

Gentle stress should be applied to check for joint stability. Local anesthetic injections will facilitate stability evaluation and allow accurate recording of the degree of instability. X-ray films should be obtained while stress is applied to the medial collateral ligament and then the lateral collateral ligament to document the instability. Clinical and X-ray film comparisons can be made with the opposite extremity.

Severe instability due to torn collateral ligaments found after injury should be surgically repaired. Occasionally, avulsion fractures are associated with instability; these can be repaired by internal fixation. Small articular fractures that are not displaced and are associated with minimal or no instability can be treated by casting. Acute injuries without instability should be protected by a splint or cast extending from the distal segment of the thumb to above the wrist, with the hand and wrist in neutral position. Protection should be continued until tenderness subsides, usually after 3 weeks. Later, spica figure-eight taping should be used for at least an additional 3 weeks. Tape protection is offered for all future activities that might injure the thumb again.

# Sprains of the Interphalangeal Joints of the Fingers

Ligament injuries at this level can vary from minor to complete tears of the collateral ligaments, volar capsular plate, or a central slip of the extensor mechanism, with dislocation.

Treatment must be individualized after X-ray studies to examine the degree of stability, and review of the mechanism of injury. Some unstable joints will need open repair of the ligament or fracture fixation. A dislocated interphalangeal joint should be gently reduced and splinted. The position of splinting varies and depends on the mechanism of injury and the areas of instability. Mobilize interphalangeal joint injuries early, usually on the first day after injury if 1) the collateral ligaments are intact; 2) no fracture fragments or only a small volar avulsion fragment is noted with minimal or no displacement; and 3) the central slip of the extensor apparatus allows full, active extension.

If these conditions are found, a ''buddy-taping'' system is recommended: The injured finger is taped to an adjacent finger. A splint is also applied for part of each day, with encouragement to remove it several times a day so that the joint can be moved.

# Avulsion of the Extensor Tendon

Avulsion of the extensor tendon from the distal phalanx (also called mallet finger or baseball finger) can occur with or without avulsion of a small fragment of bone from the extensor surface of the distal phalanx. Avulsion occurs at the tendon insertion. Most such injuries can be treated by a small volar splint across the distal interphalangeal joint, with the joint in hyperextension. Open reduction and internal fixation are indicated when a large fragment is avulsed or an early postsplinting X-ray film shows persistence of the bony fragment in a dorsally displaced position.

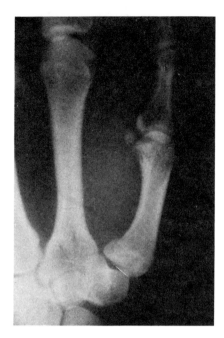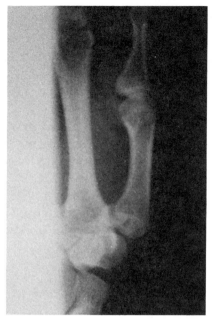

**19–14**   X-ray film of first metacarpal bone, showing minimally displaced intra-articular fracture of base of first metacarpal bone.

In some cases, percutaneous pinning across the extended distal interphalangeal joint can be carried out. If there is excellent extensor function at the distal interphalangeal joint, and good 15°–25° active flexion despite the presence of a large displaced fragment, splinting alone is sometimes the best treatment.

*Despite treatment, there may still be persistent tenderness or fullness at the insertion of the tendon on the dorsum of the distal phalanx.*

There may also be persistent extensor lag (mallet deformity). Operative treatment may lead to limitation of flexion at the distal interphalangeal joint, even though the extensor lag has been reduced or corrected. Careful evaluation of the patient's functional needs for the hand is necessary. If the distal interphalangeal joint becomes stiff and flexion is lost, serious impairment may occur.

## Fractures of the Metacarpal Bones and Phalanges

These fractures are considered individually after X-ray studies and clinical evaluation (Fig. 19–14). Special attention should be given to epiphyseal injuries in children. After the initial evaluation and treatment, patients should be seen for follow-up two or three times per week until healing occurs, to insure that proper rotation and alignment are maintained. Children heal rapidly, and malpositions must be corrected while fracture motion still exists.

## Nerve and Vascular Injuries

Direct trauma to the palm or wrist that is simultaneous with hyperextension can injure the palmar arterial arch, ulnar artery, and median or ulnar nerves. These injuries should be kept in mind when a swollen wrist or hand is undergoing examination. If blood vessels have been injured, there will usually be point tenderness over the involved arteries. Commonly, vascular injury occurs in the region of the hamate bone at the ulnar border of the hand, in the vicinity of the tunnel of Guyon.

The circulation to the nails or fingers can be checked by Allen's test. This is performed by having the patient elevate the hand and clench the fist, to exsanguinate the hand. While the fist is clenched, the examiner's fingers are applied to occlude the radial and ulnar arteries. The patient's hand is then opened and pressure is released one vessel at a time. If the hand blushes as blood enters it, then that vessel is patent.

# Rib-cage Injuries

Rib fractures usually present with painful respirations. The chest should be inspected to note the presence of decreased inspiratory excursion. Palpation will define areas of exquisite fracture-type tenderness and subcutaneous emphysema. Auscultation may reveal impaired ventilation and also the presence of subcutaneous emphysema. Percussion may be dull, as a result of bleeding into the peripleural space. Supportive care depends upon respiratory impairment until chest and rib X-ray films can be obtained. Sternochondral and costochondral injuries should be suspected when pain and tenderness are present in these areas.

Treatment consists of ice, local anesthetic injection, and elastic binder for temporary pain relief. The physician should ascertain that the patient's respirations are not significantly impaired by the binder. Evaluation of the chest must be complete, for any force violent enough to fracture or dislocate ribs can cause intrathoracic injury.

Some sternochondral or costochondral injuries need open repair. Others present chronically with the sensation of snapping, pain, and instability. Chronic injuries often need surgical treatment.

A painful chest area, with or without clinical signs of tenderness or instability, needs exact localization of pain distribution. Selective intercostal nerve blocks may help in localizing the level of discomfort.

Rib fractures may be present with initially negative X-ray films. Reliance on symptoms and clinical findings is thus important. The conclusion that a fractured rib is present often can be based on symptoms only. Follow-up X-ray studies at 3–4 weeks will usually show fracture callus.

Radicular pain from an injured dorsal spine can radiate along the distribution of an intercostal nerve. The spine must be completely evaluated when symptoms or signs of rib injuries are being treated.

# Injuries to the Sternum

The sternum may suffer contusions, sprains, dislocations, and fractures. The physician should palpate and localize tender areas over the sternum. X-ray studies are less important in this region. It is difficult to see sternoclavicular or even costosternal relationships on plain X-ray films. Tomograms or CT scans will help identify injuries.

Dislocations of the manubrium sterni can occur. Usually reduction is spontaneous, and the patient presents with pain, tenderness, and shallow respirations. Dislocations that do not spontaneously reduce usually involve the body of the sternum. They are depressed and associated with anterior prominence of the distal edge of the manubrium. These dislocations should be reduced under general anesthesia. Open reduction is sometimes necessary.

Fractures or subluxations involving the sternum can be associated with intrathoracic injuries resulting from the same force, and cause progressive impairment of function. Close evaluation in the hospital for 24–48 h is recommended after a proven dislocation of the sternum.

# Common Injuries to the Pelvis and Hip

## Contusions and Strains

Contusions and strains are the dominant injuries of the pelvis. The most important contusion is called a "hip pointer." A hematoma forms at the point of contact along the iliac crest. The best prevention is the use of appropriate protective padding. Once a hip pointer occurs, treatment consists of ice applications, compression, and local injection of a long-acting anesthetic agent and hyaluronidase. Ultrasound is also helpful. The deep structures are not usually involved.

Strains vary in degree, depending on the extent of tearing of a tendon insertion away from the iliac bone. The common aponeuroses of the external oblique muscles can be torn completely from the iliac crest. Occasionally distraction or compression stresses to the immature pelvis will cause an epiphyseal injury. This will show on an X-ray film as widening of the growth apophysis of the iliac bone. This injury is similar to an avulsion fracture in which a separation occurred at the cartilaginous growth area instead of bones being torn from the parent bone (O'Donoghue [1]).

Major tears of the aponeuroses present with guarding and difficulty in straightening the torso. There is localized tenderness. Treatment is determined by the degree of tear. Most will respond to supportive treatment and no strenuous activities until symptoms subside. Abdominal binders or tight adhesive taping is helpful. Occasionally, surgical repair will be necessary to restore anatomic continuity of tissues. If the normal aponeurotic planes are reestablished surgically, there is less morbidity.

A large segment of scar tissue in the torn aponeuroses or immature fascial tissue in the region of the tearing is often painful when stressed. Surgical repair prevents pathologic scar tissue formation. For most contusions and deep hematomas in the vicinity of the pelvis, ice is applied for 15–30 min separated by 30-min intervals. This procedure is continued for the first 24 h after injury. Ice can then be used periodically for a week to relieve symptoms and encourage deep drainage of the resolving hematoma.

## Pelvic Fractures and Sprains

Fractures of the pelvis are not uncommon in sports. They result usually from compression of the iliac wing, either by a lateral force or by an anterior force. The ischium and pubic bones are also vulnerable to hard, direct pressure. More frequent, but still uncommon, are avulsion fractures of the anterosuperior iliac spine or ischial tuberosity. Unusual, violent muscle contractions of the sartorius and tensor fasciae latae in jumping or running sports can avulse the anterior iliac apophysis (O'Donoghue [1]).

Forced hip flexion with the knee extended can apply stress to the common origin of the hamstrings at the ischial tuberosity. This injury can be seen in hurdlers and other track and field athletes. Straddle injuries can lead to avulsion of the common adductor tendon from the pubic bone, with or without a small bone segment. Forced extension and internal rotation of the hip can cause injuries to the iliopsoas muscle, leading to an avulsion of the lesser trochanter. X-ray studies are necessary for diagnosis.

*Clinical Findings:*   Exquisite tenderness is present at the fracture site. There is pain with contraction of the involved muscle and relief on relaxation. Holding the extremity passively in the position achieved by maximal contraction of an involved muscle relieves tension on that muscle. For example, the sartorius muscle is at rest with hip flexion, knee flexion, and external rotation of the hip joint. The adductor muscles are at rest when the thighs are together in adduction. The hamstring muscles are at rest when the knee is flexed and the hips are slightly extended while the patient is lying sideways.

*Treatment:*   The treatment for avulsion injuries around the pelvis is usually ice, rest, and occasionally casting of the involved extremity in the position of least stress on the involved muscle. Widely separated fractures can be treated by surgical reattachment and internal fixation. Late surgical treatment is possible if the patient remains symptomatic, but it is less satisfactory because of muscle shortening and intrinsic scar formation. These make reattachment of the avulsed area difficult.

Fractures of the sacrum can escape diagnosis and heal while treated as a contusion. X-ray films of the sacrum should be obtained, especially if disability is excessive for a "contusion." The athlete and coach can then better plan the future, once the true nature of this injury is recognized. Full healing of the sacrum is important before allowing stress to the region.

Sprains in the pelvic area are common, especially at the sacroiliac region. *(A disc lesion can present presacral or sacroiliac pain also.)* Acute sprains in this region are associated with tenderness. Lumbosacral disc herniations may cause pain or pressure or a burning discomfort, but otherwise palpation is negative. The sacroiliac joint can be stressed in a side-lying (decubitus) position. Rocking of the sacroiliac joint occurs if the hip on the side against the table is held hyperflexed while the opposite hip is passively extended. Pain in this position is not always diagnostic of sacroiliac irritation. This test should be part of the general examination that includes hip-roll stressing, straight-leg

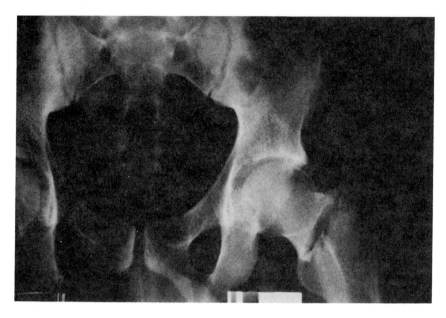

**19–15**  X-ray film of hip, showing minimally displaced fracture at
base of femoral neck in a 25-year-old patient injured while skiing.

raising, and compression and separation of the iliac wings. All these maneuvers apply
stress to the sacroiliac joints. A neurologic evaluation of the lower extremities is also
necessary in order to determine, especially, sciatic tension signs, reflex changes, sensory
deficits, and motor weaknesses. Discrepancy in leg length should be noted by accurate
measurement from the umbilicus to the medial malleolus or from the anterosuperior iliac
spine to the medial malleolus.

Stress injuries to the perineum can cause severe sprains of the pubic symphysis. Unless
actual separation of the bones has occurred these respond to simple, supportive measures,
which include rest, ice, and avoidance of thigh abduction. Injuries to the urethra or bowel
can occur from the same injuries to the perineum. Voiding should be tested and rectal
examination carried out. Urinalysis and cystogram may be necessary to assess the injury
completely. Consultation with a urologist or gynecologist may be necessary.

## Fractures and Dislocations Around the Hip Joint

Proximal fractures of the femoral neck, intertrochanteric or subtrochanteric region present
severe pain and inability to bear weight (Fig. 19–15). If displacements have occurred,
these will be (in the supine position) external rotation deformity of the involved extremity
and resistance to internal rotation or flexing of the leg. Initial treatment is splinting of the
extremity, utilizing the opposite extremity or a broomstick. Definitive treatment is
traction or surgical fixation.

Acute anterior dislocations of the hip present with fixed deformity in flexion and
external rotation. Attempts at passive internal rotation are met with resistance and cause
marked discomfort. Posterior dislocation of the hip presents with fixed flexion, adduction,

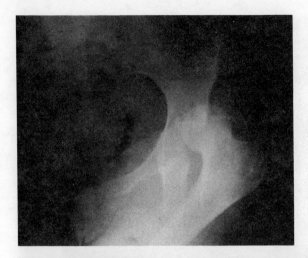

**19–16a**  Posterior dislocation of hip, with a fracture of posterior wall of acetabulum.

Reduced fracture of hip, with posterior fragment of acetabulum still displaced.

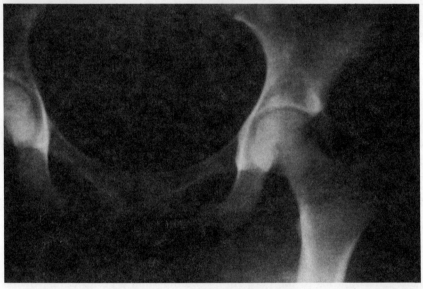

and internal rotation (Fig. 19–16). Attempts to move the hip are met with pain and resistance.

In the adolescent, the "sprained hip" may represent a slipped capital femoral epiphysis (Fig. 19–17). Occasionally this presents pain in the knee (especially the medial aspect of the knee). Objective examination reveals a normal knee but limited hip motion, especially internal rotation and flexion. This is a not uncommon abnormality in overweight adolescents.

In general, X-ray studies are important in hip injuries. Tomograms or CT scans may be necessary to show an otherwise invisible fracture or osteochondritis dessicans within the hip joint. If a slipped capital femoral epiphysis is found on one side, the other side should be examined also. The asymptomatic side should be observed at intervals thereafter to detect an early slip.

Treatment for slipped capital femoral epiphysis is usually internal fixation. Treatment for hip dislocations is closed reduction under general anesthesia.

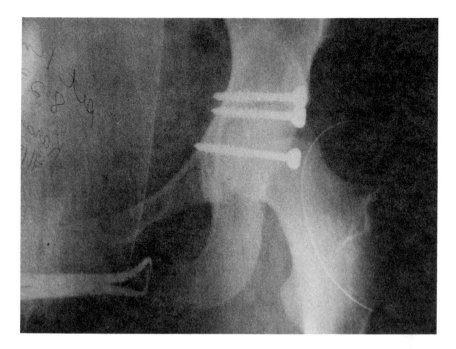

**19–16b**   Postoperative film showing screw fixation of posterior wall of acetabulum and reduced hip joint.

# Common Acute Injuries to the Thigh

## Contusion

A contusion of the thigh presents swelling and often discoloration in the region of the bruise. Palpation defines the area of muscle or subcutaneous hematoma. Treatment varies, but no definitive measure will prevent organization and calcification rather than absorption of the hematoma.

Treatment may include the following steps:

1. Rest, by splinting or crutches and ice applications. (The rest period should extend for the duration of symptoms and while painful isometric contractions persist. Oral enzymes are utilized to facilitate hematoma breakdown and absorption. Later, physical therapy and heat are helpful.)
2. Aspiration of the hematoma, injection of a local anesthetic agent, and hyaluronidase solution to aid hematoma absorption.
3. Regional nerve blocks once or twice daily for 2 or 3 days to relieve spasm and allow pain-free hip and knee motion and isometric muscle contractions. (The blocks are used in conjunction with ice applications and supportive analgesics.)

Contusions, treated early, will do well. If treatment is started after 72 h, the patient may have a greater tendency to scar formation or calcification in the region of the hematoma.

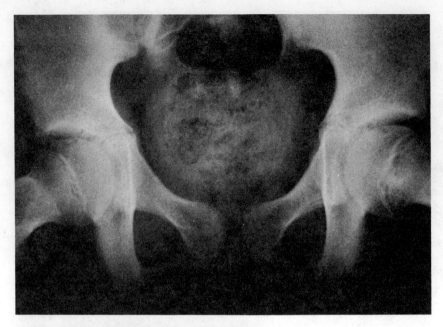

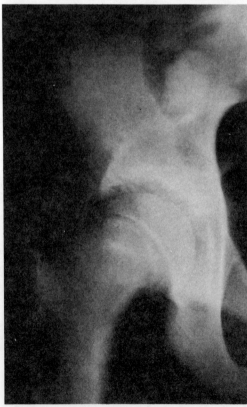

**19–17**  Frog lateral and anteroposterior views of hip in 11-year-old female with Grade I slippage of capital femoral epiphysis.

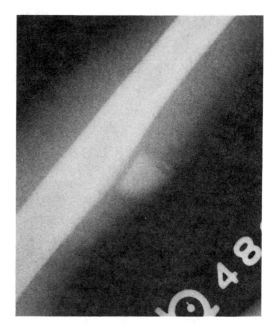

**19–18**   Myositis ossificans of arm at site of muscle contusion.

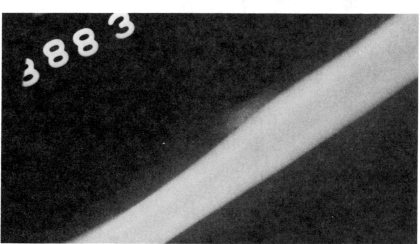

# Muscle Tears

Hamstrings, quadriceps, or adductor muscles can tear partially or completely. Initial treatment is ice and compression wrap. For complete tears, early repair of the muscles should be done before muscle shortening and fibrosis occurs. Sometimes local or general anesthesia is necessary to assess fully the degree of muscle damage.

Partial tears should be protected for 4–6 weeks to allow complete healing before returning to athletics.

Rarely, isolated fascial tears can occur without muscle damage. The tear allows bulging (herniation) of the muscles through the rent in the fascia. Small bulges can be painful. If symptoms persist, surgery is indicated to enlarge the rent in the fascia, dissipate the forces of herniation, and render the area asymptomatic.

## Femoral Shaft Fractures

Fractures of the femoral shaft are initially treated by splinting and ice application. Definitive treatment requires hospitalization.

# Myositis Ossificans

This unpredictable calcification of injured muscle requires varied treatment (Fig. 19–18). The ectopic bone must fully mature before it is removed. Maturation takes 9–12 months and can be monitored by bone scan. The calcified area should not be more active than the other bone. Once maturation has occurred, the bone can be removed surgically with less likelihood of recurrence. Diphosphonates or irradiation may be used to decrease recurrence of myositis ossificans. These measures are considered experimental and need fully informed consent.

# Knee Injuries

The knee joint is a hinge joint or ginglymus joint, but because of its rotational capacity, it is more complex. The articular surfaces of the femur and tibia are connected by ligaments (Gray [2]):

1. Medial and lateral capsular ligaments
2. Ligament of the patella
3. Oblique popliteal ligament
4. Arcuate popliteal ligament
5. Tibial collateral ligament
6. Fibular collateral ligament
7. Anterior cruciate ligament
8. Posterior cruciate ligament
9. Medial and lateral menisci
10. Transverse ligament
11. Coronary ligaments

## Sprains at the Knee

*Medial injuries:* These involve the medial capsular ligament. The mid one-third of the ligament (medial collateral ligament) has a deep and a superficial layer. First-degree tears will cause pain and limited motion (''stiff knee''). On examination, there is tenderness along most of the course of the ligament from the adductor tubercle to just below the joint line. A tear of the medial meniscus can coexist with injury to the medial collateral ligament.

A second-degree tear can comprise a complete tear of the deep layer and a partial tear of the superficial portion or a partial tear of both segments. Instability may be minimal when valgus stress is applied to the knee while the knee is flexed 15°–20°.

Third-degree tears are complete tears, involving both superficial and deep layers of the medial collateral ligament. These sprains allow opening of the mid joint line with valgus stress when the knee is in flexion of 15°–20°. The normal laxity of the joint can be noted by testing the uninjured knee. X-ray documentation is important. Films should be obtained to show the degree of joint line opening with valgus stress. In third-degree tears, swelling of tissues surrounding the joint may be minimal. The disruption of the capsular structures allows diffusion of inflammatory exudates into the surrounding tissues. There will not usually be a joint effusion.

The ability to open the medial joint line with valgus stress while the knee is fully extended (0° of flexion) implies posterior cruciate insufficiency or a tear.

It is rare to have a "simple" ligament injury to the knee. Usually, there are injuries to at least two other major knee structures. Careful and systematic examination should be performed to assess fully the extent of injury.

*Lateral injuries:*    These injuries involve the lateral capsular ligament. Varus knee stress can tear the capsule or avulse a bone fragment from the tibia or femur. These fragments can be seen on plain films of the knee or varus stress films. Signs will include tenderness of the lateral joint line with some lateral opening of the joint when there is varus stress with the knee flexed 15°–30°. Avulsion of the lateral-collateral ligament and biceps femoris muscle attachment from the fibular head can occur from the same type of force. Swelling may be minimal, as a result of the severity of tearing and diffusion of blood into soft tissues. Documentation of the varus laxity should be made by varus stress X-ray studies. Peroneal nerve injuries can occur in association with lateral ligament disruption.

The more severe the ligament injury, the less pain is felt with stress examination of the ligament. Minor tears are more painful and are associated with more guarding to prevent the stress of the examination. If an acute peroneal palsy is present, the implications must be discussed with the patient. Most peroneal palsies recover with time, but some do not. Stretch injuries or tears of the nerve should be diagnosed early and repaired or decompressed by utilizing microscopic techniques. Electromyographic studies early and late after injury are important to evaluate function fully.

*Cruciate ligament injuries:*    Forced hyperextension, forced internal rotation of the thigh upon a planted foot with a flexed knee, or sudden hyperflexion with posterior directed stress can cause tears of either or both cruciate ligaments. These are severe injuries, associated with immediate pain and instability. The patient usually cannot walk unassisted. The degree of instability will be determined by the severity of ligament involvement. It should be noted that there is rarely a simple injury to the ligaments of the knee. Always assume that cruciate ligament injury is complex, involving other knee structures as well. An on-the-spot examination will give most information before swelling, pain, spasm, and guarding make assessment difficult.

# The Knee Examination

*Inspection:*   Attitude of the knee should be determined. Is it flail? Is it held flexed, or is it lying fully extended with valgus or varus attitude? What is the color of the foot or leg? Is there joint swelling with obliteration of normal contours? Is the patella floating (ballottable)? Is the kneecap in its normal anatomic position?

*Palpation:*   Is the pedal pulse present? Is sensation normal? Are active toe and ankle motion normal with good strength? The heel should be gently lifted to note hyperextension at the knee. The joint-line should be palpated to note tender areas above and below or just at the joint-line. Is there tenderness at the fibular head? With the knee straight, valgus or varus stress is applied and joint opening noted. The degree of opening (in millimeters) is estimated and recorded. An anterior drawer sign is elicited with the knee fully extended by gently applying anterior force below the knee (pulling leg forward) and counter force posteriorly above the knee. The patient is requested to flex the knee slowly while a hand supports the popliteal region. With the knee flexed 15°–20°, valgus and varus stresses are applied to check stability and note joint openings medially or laterally. The posterior drawer sign should be checked with the knee flexed. Gentle force is applied posteriorly (pushing leg backward) just distal to the joint to determine whether the tibia moves posteriorly in relation to the femur.

Similarly, the anterior drawer sign is rechecked with the patient supine and the involved extremity on the side of the examiner. With the patient's knee held between full extension and 15° flexion and slight external rotation at the hip, the femur is stabilized with one hand while firm pressure is applied to the posterior aspect of the proximal tibia in an attempt to translate it anteriorly (Torg [5]).

The anterior drawer sign is again checked with the knee flexed almost to 90° and the leg held first internally and then externally rotated at the knee. If the anterior drawer sign is abolished by forced internal rotation, this implies that the posterior cruciate ligament is intact. If anterior drawer is present with external rotation the implication is that the anterior cruciate ligament is torn.

If a tibia is posteriorly displaced due to a posterior cruciate ligament laxity or tear, the anterior drawer maneuver will bring the tibia to its normal position. This can be misinterpreted as a positive anterior drawer sign.

The popliteal, posterior tibial, and dorsalis pedis pulses should be palpated. The hands are moved slowly across the hamstrings medially and laterally to check for swelling, tenderness, and spasm. The condyles are gently palpated in the supracondylar region of the femur to note crepitation, bony irregularities, and exquisite fracture tenderness.

A developmentally "tight joint" may have a cruciate ligament injury with no clinical instability.

After the initial examination has been completed, the extremity is splinted until definitive treatment, X-ray studies, or further examination under anesthesia can be performed. If the injury is not examined within 6 h, guarding and spasm will prevent adequate assessment. Spinal or general anesthesia may be necessary to define the injury fully. A subtle posterior cruciate injury can be missed. Clues to the presence of a posterior cruciate lesion are as follows.

1. Straight posterior laxity (posterior drawer sign).
2. Valgus opening of the medial jointline with the knee fully extended. (Examination will further define whether there is an acute straight instability or rotational instability at the knee.)
3. Failure to stop an anterior drawer sign with forced internal rotation of the tibia.

## The Acutely Swollen Knee

Joint effusion appearing immediately after an injury is due to blood accumulation within the joint (hemarthrosis). Hemarthrosis is a significant injury. The patient will be unable fully to extend and lock the knee. There will be a limp and, very likely, assistance in walking will be needed. Because the joint has contained the blood within, the likelihood of an acute third-degree tear of the capsular ligament is less. Third-degree tears will allow diffusion of blood into soft tissues outside the joint. Possible causes of an acute hemarthrosis are as follows:

1. Meniscus tear (medial or lateral)
2. Anterior cruciate tear
3. Dislocation or subluxation of the patella
4. Synovial pinching or tearing
5. Osteochondral fracture

*Treatment:*   After examination has established the diagnosis, the joint is aspirated under aseptic conditions, and frequent reevaluation is necessary. X-ray studies should be obtained as soon as pain tolerance allows. When possible, X-ray studies should include anteroposterior views; 45° flexion lateral view; tunnel view; skyline view of the patella; and weightbearing anteroposterior view. Oblique views may help reveal avulsion fractures from the articular margins. Arthrography and arthroscopy should be considered in the first 24 h after injury for precise diagnosis. If there are clear indications of instability, surgery becomes necessary and arthrography can be avoided. Arthroscopy may precede the surgical procedure if there is no evidence of capsular tearing (which could cause extensive soft-tissue swelling from fluid extravasation). At surgery a thorough joint examination should also be done.

The surgical objective is to reestablish anatomic continuity of torn structures and restore stability to the knee.

## Patellar Dislocation or Subluxation

Some knees are more vulnerable to lateral displacement of the patella because of developmental variations, such as 1) genu valgum, 2) patella alta, 3) vastus medialis insufficiency, 4) increased quadriceps angle (Q-angle), 5) externally pointing patellae.

## The Acute Patellar Dislocation or Subluxation

Many patellar dislocations or subluxations will spontaneously reduce, and the patient will have a swollen, painful knee. On palpation, there is a hemarthrosis and tenderness at the medial capsule. Efforts to move the patella laterally, while gently, passively extending the knee will be met with resistance and anxiety. Because of the hemarthrosis, the knee cannot flex past 60°–80°, nor can it be extended beyond 15° flex position.

The history is often that the patella shifted or snapped with an associated sudden pain, causing a fall. A careful history may reveal similar, but less severe previous episodes.

A patient with recurrent dislocations may present only with a swollen knee, without tenderness along the medial capsule or vastus medialis. In such patients, soft tissues have already been stretched from prior episodes and were not significantly injured during the last, acute injury.

Patellar dislocations can cause a chondral or osteochondral fracture of the articular surface of the patella or of the lateral femoral condyle. X-ray films should be obtained at the initial evaluation and after reduction.

A patella presenting in a dislocated lateral position must be reduced. It is best to use general anesthesia or, alternatively, to fill the joint, under sterile conditions, with local anesthetic solution in addition to a regional block of the femoral nerve. The anesthetic allows minimal forces to the articular surface of the patellofemoral joint during reduction. After spontaneous or therapeutic reduction the joint hematoma should be aspirated, ice should be applied, and the knee splinted. Isometric exercises should begin immediately. Some acute capsular tears are best treated by surgical repair to decrease the chance of recurrence.

If an osteochondral fracture is seen on X-ray films, surgery should be performed to assess the damage, replace or remove the fragments, and repair torn soft tissues.

Systematic examination for associated ligamentous injuries should always be performed, as outlined. Attention should not be focused only at the obvious kneecap injury while an associated ligamentous tear with potential instability is missed.

## Bursitis of the Knee

All the bursae around the knee can become acutely swollen or inflamed. The bursae are as follows:

1. Suprapatellar
2. Prepatellar
3. Superficial infrapatellar
4. Deep infrapatellar
5. Anserine
6. Semimembranous
7. Bursa at the head of the fibula
8. Bursa between the fibula collateral ligament and the popliteus tendon
9. Bursa between the lateral gastrocnemius head and the lateral femoral condyle
10. Bursa just anterior to the popliteus muscle

*Treatment:*

1. Warm compresses
2. Aspiration, culture, and gram stain of the aspirate
3. If no infection is found, local steroid injection
4. Short immobilization if necessary

Bursitis can occur from direct contusion or overuse due to rubbing of the bursa during athletic activity.

It is necessary to distinguish between a deep infrapatellar bursitis and an irritation of the patellar fat pad. Hyperflexion of the knee will increase pressure within the bursa but not in the fat pad. Passive or active knee extension will stress the fat pad but will not usually increase pressure in the bursa. The relatively superficial position of the bursa makes it easier to compress it on palpation and cause pain. It is more difficult to compress the fat pad palpably (O'Donoghue [1]).

# Injuries to the Menisci

The medial meniscus is injured more commonly than the lateral meniscus. The coronary ligament connects the meniscus medially to the tibia and to the medial one-third of the capsular ligament. Laterally there is no capsular attachment of the meniscus; only the coronary ligament attaches to the tibia. Because of more adherence to collateral structures medially, the medial meniscus is more vulnerable to injury. Peripheral tears of the menisci in or near the coronary ligament potentially heal with time if stress to the area is decreased. A tear within the substance of the meniscus will be prevented from healing by local stresses and a poor blood supply in this region. Tears may be longitudinal, oblique, and transverse. Meniscus lesions that cause recurring pain or recurrent locking of the joint are detrimental to the joint. Such functional impairment may cause destruction of areas of articular cartilage and can predispose the knee to ligamentous injury by increasing its vulnerability to trauma.

Menisci are useful weight-bearing cushions and stabilizing elements in the knees. The function of the knee joint is more effective with the menisci intact. When the meniscus is injured, causing joint effusion, unreduced locking, recurrent locking, or pain at the joint line with activity, orthopaedic evaluation and treatment may be necessary.

The acutely injured meniscus may present as one of the following:

1. A locked knee (unable to extend fully and unable to flex fully)
2. A swollen knee (hemarthrosis)
3. Joint-line tenderness in the vicinity of the meniscus tear

The patient's history will often show previous "catching" episodes, knee sprain or knee effusions (water on the knee). The knee should be systematically examined, as for sprain. Blood should be aspirated and the knee reexamined. A locked knee can be reduced by skilled manipulation with or without a general anesthetic. Weight-bearing should not be allowed until the joint is movable again. The locked knee is not protected during weight-bearing. Weight-bearing causes impingement of the tibial cartilage surface against the femoral cartilage surface rather than the usual gliding of the cartilaginous surface. The

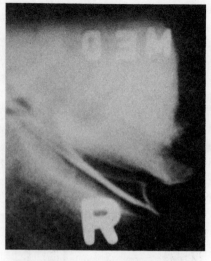

**19–19** Arthrography of medial compartment of knee shows anterior (a), posterior (b), and midvertical (c) tearing of medial meniscus, in which contrast material flowed between body of meniscus and its peripheral attachment. The tear is complete, of bucket-handle type, and is unstable, with a tendency for central portion to be displaced into joint, causing locking or knee buckling.

a

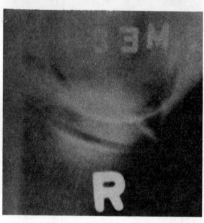

b

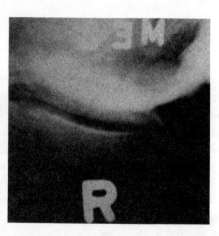

c

true stability of the knee (especially the status of the anterior cruciate ligament) cannot be determined while the knee is "locked."

## Diagnosis of Acute Meniscus Problems

It is best to assemble as much information as possible about an injured knee within the first 24 h. This will allow a definitive decision about knee stability and whether ligament repair will be necessary. The following situations should be checked:

1. If the knee is not locked, or if it can be unlocked without anesthesia, the joint is examined as it is for sprains, discussed earlier in this chapter, and signs of meniscus hypermobility are noted. If there is no instability, but signs of meniscus tear are found, an arthrogram (Fig. 19–19) and arthroscopy will further define the problem.
2. If the arthrogram shows no lesions of the meniscus, then treatment is supportive (splint, isometric exercises, progressive resistance exercises, gradual range-of-

motion activities, and follow-up in 1 week).

3. If the arthrogram shows a tear in the meniscus, with the substance of the meniscus and the cruciate system apparently intact, then treatment is individualized. There is no urgency to remove a torn meniscus, so long as the knee is not locked. Supportive care is necessary, however, with a splint, crutches, isometric exercises, and gradual range-of-motion exercises. Weight bearing may be permitted in some cases, and the patient is followed up in 1 week. Arthroscopy will be helpful.

4. If the arthrogram shows absence of the cruciate ligament, examination under anesthesia, arthroscopy, and surgery may be necessary.

5. If there is repetitive pain and locking, in association with positive results on an arthrogram, arthroscopy and surgery are performed.

6. If anesthesia is necessary to unlock the knee, arthroscopy is performed; definitive surgery often follows.

7. Many physicians are using diagnostic and operative arthroscopy to definitively treat meniscus pathology early.

## The Chronic Meniscus Lesion

Patients suffering chronic problems of the meniscus present a history of the knee "giving way," "catching," or locking, in association with recurrent effusions (water on the knee). Quadriceps atrophy will often be noted by comparison with the opposite side at a fixed-distance point above the knee joint. Squatting may be difficult. The cutting maneuver or pivoting maneuver may cause pain or snapping. Joint-line tenderness in the area of a meniscus tear is usually found. This must be differentiated from tenderness along the entire medial collateral ligament, which is seen with a sprain of the ligament. A sprain of the medial collateral ligament may coexist with a meniscus lesion.

The McMurray maneuver, the Apley grind test, or the Apley distraction test can reproduce symptoms by causing the meniscus to move at the tear.

The McMurray test is used to diagnose a lesion of the posterior or mid third segment of the meniscus. The patient is supine, and the knee is flexed maximally toward the buttock. One hand steadies the knee, and the other hand holds the heel. To test the lateral meniscus, the leg is turned with internal rotation, and slight varus stress is applied. To test the medial meniscus, the leg is externally rotated while slight valgus stress is applied. While the knee is forcibly rotated, the leg is extended slowly. A painful click will be felt and sometimes heard as the meniscus moves in and out of its normal position or the femoral condyle moves over an irregularity in the meniscus.

The Apley grinding test is performed while the patient is lying prone. The knee is flexed 90° and rotated while a compression force is applied. This causes pain if a meniscus is torn.

The Apley distraction test is performed while the patient is prone. The examiner holds the patient's thigh on the table with his own knee, then applies rotation and distraction to the patient's knee. Pain indicates that a ligament rather than the meniscus has been injured (Helfet [6]).

Treatment of a symptomatic, isolated meniscus lesion should include consideration of the following points:

1. The athletic objectives of the patient
2. The stability of the knee before meniscus surgery (rotatory instability of the knee may be increased by removal of the meniscus)
3. Frequency of pain, catching, or swelling
4. Partial meniscus excision with intact peripheral rim
5. The status of the articular cartilage (as noted on X-ray studies and by arthroscopy) to determine whether the meniscus is reparable
6. The possibility of treating torn segments by operative arthroscopy
7. Loose bodies within the knee joint

The presence of loose fragments on X-ray films and their anatomic relationships may allow correlation with clinical instability. Avulsion fracture fragments usually, but not always, necessitate surgical repair of an involved ligament. Common avulsion fracture sites are the following:

1. Tibial spine (anterior cruciate ligament)
2. Posteromedial aspect of the femur (posterior cruciate ligament)
3. Tibial tubercle (patellar tendon insertion)
4. Lateral rim of tibial plateau (lateral capsular ligament)
5. Inferior tip of patella (patellar ligament insertion)
6. Upper pole of patella (quadriceps insertion point)

# Patellofemoral Arthralgia

In patellofemoral arthralgia (also called chondromalacia of the patellofemoral articulation), pain on the articular surface of the kneecap is difficult to cure. It is probably the most common knee complaint in practice and occurs more often in females. Symptoms are caused by areas of surface irregularities of the patella alone or of the patella and the femoral groove.

*Symptoms:*

1. Pain at anterior aspect of knee with walking or running
2. Anterior pain on descending stairs, squatting, or ascending stairs
3. Recurrent effusion, depending upon activity
4. Crepitation (the feeling of grating), as knee is actively flexed and extended
5. Rarely, symptoms at rest

*Signs:*

1. Crepitation as patella is passively moved within femoral groove while pressure is simultaneously applied
2. Easy lateral subluxation of patella with lateral stress
3. Pain and recurrence of symptoms with passive movement of and simultaneous pressure to patella within the femoral groove
4. Pain with contraction of quadriceps as patella is held in groove (patella inhibition test)
5. Quadriceps angle (Q-angle) greater than 10°, often 15°–20°

6. Tenderness on palpation of lateral patellofemoral ligament. (This can be elicited in supine position. It is more easily done while patient is prone. The patella is gently moved out of femoral groove while pressure is applied to lateral soft-tissue attachments of kneecap.)
7. Genu valgum deformity
8. External tibial torsion with external rotation of tibial tubercle
9. Femoral anteversion combined with external tibial torsion (malalignment syndrome)

The articular pathology should be graded by both clinical assessment and by arthroscopic evaluation. Grade I is softening of the articular surface. Grade II is fissuring of the articular surface. Grade III is fragmentation of the articular surface. Grade IV is eburnation or hard, bony exposure with loss of articular cartilage.

*X-ray signs:*

1. Patella alta
2. Shallow femoral groove
3. Shallow patellar articular angle
4. Tilting of patella on skyline view

*Treatment:*

1. Development of strong quadriceps and hamstring muscles by isometric exercises and progressive resistive exercises
2. Avoidance of stair climbing and squatting whenever possible
3. Small doses of aspirin on a regular basis
4. Pull-on elastic knee support or restraining brace for patella
5. Orthotic inserts to alter stress at knee by balancing foot
6. Surgery as a last resort, utilizing realignment measures; shaving and drilling; elevation of tibial tubercle; resurfacing; or patellectomy

## Osteochondritis Dissecans of the Knee Joint

This osteochondral defect (bone and cartilage fragment) is usually localized to the lateral articular edge of the medial femoral condyle. The fragment is usually not displaced or is only minimally elevated from the surrounding articular cartilage. Rarely, it has been noted in other areas of the articular surface of the knee joint. The etiology of osteochondritis dissecans is not known, but vascular compromise and trauma have been suggested. It presents as a painful knee. Symptoms are associated with running, kicking (especially side kicks and cross-over kicks, common in soccer). Objective findings may be minimal: 1) joint effusion; 2) pain on placing the heel of the symptomatic leg on the opposite knee in a cross-knee fashion and passively forcing external rotation at the hip.

The diagnosis is made by X-ray studies (Fig. 19–20) (especially the tunnel view of the knee). The joint surface can be inspected by arthroscopy.

*Treatment:* The patient's age, symptoms, and the degree of elevation and separation of the fragment from articular cartilage determine the type of treatment. The preteenager can be treated with casting, splint, and isometric exercises, with reasonable chances of

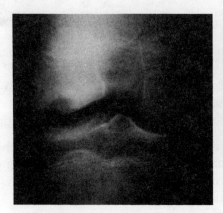 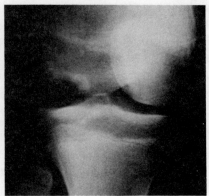

**19–20** Anteroposterior and oblique views of knee, showing large osteochondritis dissecans defects in articular surface of lateral femoral condyle.

healing. Older patients will need individual considerations. Symptomatic lesions in older patients are usually removed surgically. Some fragments may be held with internal fixation pins or suture material.

## Osgood-Schlatter Disease

The symptoms of Osgood-Schlatter disease occur in the immature knee and can be due to inflammation of the deep infrapatellar tendon bursa or to irritation or fragmentation of the anterior proximal tibial epiphysis (epiphysitis).

The patient presents activity-induced discomfort and tenderness, localized to the tibial tubercle. The symptoms usually subside after epiphyseal closure and tissue maturation in the region of the tibial tubercle. On rare occasions, symptoms persist into adulthood and are associated with the persistence of bone or cartilage fragments in the region of the tibial tubercle.

*Treatment:*

1. Decreasing activities to tolerance
2. Ice applications to tibial tubercle before and after activities
3. Strengthening quadriceps and hamstring muscles
4. Use of knee-immobilizing splint periodically to rest knee while isometric exercises are continued for quadriceps and hamstrings
5. On rare occasions, an injection of local anesthetic agent with steroids into region of patellar tendon insertion
6. Surgical removal of fragments of epiphysis (to be done only after bone has matured.) (This procedure can cause premature anterior tibial epiphyseal closure with a resulting recurvatum deformity of the knee.)

## Recurrent Knee-Joint Effusion

The cause of the effusion must be sought systematically by the following means.

1. A check for mechanical reasons (chondromalacia, meniscus lesions, knee instability, and loose bodies)
2. Aspiration of fluid for analysis (cell count, mucin clot test, crystals, uric acid level, complement and enzyme studies)
3. Blood tests (sedimentation rate, rheumatoid factor, antinuclear antibodies, uric acid levels, HLA-B27)
4. Culture of aspirate (routine aerobic and anaerobic organisms, acid fast organisms, fungus, and brucella)

*Treatment:*    Therapy should be directed at etiology. If no diagnosis is made, symptomatic treatment and maintenance of function should be instituted:

1. Immobilization with splint or cast
2. Isometric and progressive resistive exercises
3. Oral anti-inflammatory drugs (aspirin, acetominophen, and newer anti-inflammatory medications)
4. Rare steroid injection if tuberculosis and other infections have been excluded
5. Outpatient saline washout with 1000–2000 cc saline run through joint by irrigation tubes
6. Diagnostic arthrography and arthroscopy to search for mechanical causes or to obtain synovial biopsy

## Minor Knee Symptoms

Lateral joint-line pain associated with distance running can be caused by bursitis, popliteal tendinitis, iliotibial band irritation, meniscus tears, or meniscus cysts. These can be treated by rest, ice massage, gradual increase in running tolerance by decreasing distances, and increasing sprinting. Rarely, local injections of an anesthetic agent, with or without a steroid preparation, can be tried. A podiatric evaluation with foot balancing sometimes solves the problem.

## Complete Dislocation of the Knee

Tibial-femoral dislocation is, fortunately, an uncommon injury in athletes. Before examination there has usually been spontaneous reduction of the dislocation. On occasion, the patient has already been splinted and is ambulatory on crutches at the time of the examination. The knee should be systematically evaluated, and sensory function and circulation distal to the knee should be carefully examined. If, after the examination, the clinical assessment is that of anterior and posterior cruciate ligamentous tears, then it may be assumed that dislocation of the knee has occurred. It is imperative to assess and follow

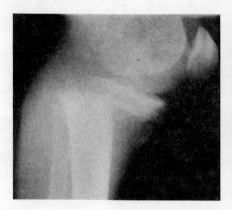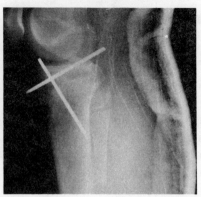

**19–21** Epiphyseal slip of proximal tibial epiphysis. Distal segment displaced posteriorly, causing arterial injury. Arterial repair was necessary in this case.

Post reduction film, showing pin fixation of epiphysis to maintain stability while arterial repair and healing occurred.

carefully for 24–36 h the blood supply to the involved extremity. It is not uncommon for trauma to the popliteal vessel to allow good blood flow initially and then for obstruction of flow to occur after several hours. The collateral circulation around the knee may often carry enough blood to the foot and ankle, which remain pink with good capillary supply to the nailbed and palpable dorsalis pedis and posterior tibial pulses. It is important to quantitate the pulses by comparison with the opposite extremity and by correlation with the patient's blood pressure.

Doppler flow studies or arteriograms are worthwhile during the first 24 h to document patency of the popliteal vessel and an uninjured trifurcation (peroneal artery, posterior tibial artery, and anterior tibial artery).

Treatment of the dislocated knee is surgical, to establish anatomic continuity of torn structures. If vascular compromise is discovered, vessels should be repaired by a vascular surgeon and the knee stabilized by temporary internal or external fixation until the repaired vessels have healed.

In the immature knee, the same force that would cause a dislocation can lead to a major displacement (slippage) of the proximal tibial epiphysis. If the shaft of the tibia is displaced posteriorly, the popliteal artery can be injured (Fig. 19–21). With this injury, the knee ligaments are usually not torn.

# Common Leg Injuries

## Compartment Syndromes

Overuse can cause swelling within leg compartments. The anterior and lateral compartments are frequently involved. This disorder is common in runners. It can also occur with leg contusion or fractures of leg bones. The patient usually presents pain after running. The pain will respond to ice and rest. Sometimes the swelling within the compartment does not subside before causing signs of neurovascular compression: weakness of dorsiflexion or in extension of the large toe, or decrease in peroneal muscle function and hypalgesia in the first web space or over the entire dorsum of the foot. Rarely, the posterior or deep intermediate compartments can be involved, causing weakness of plantar flexion, flexion of the large toe and lateral toes, and hypalgesia along the distribution of the posterior tibial and plantar nerves on the sole of the foot.

If the condition is seen while in the acute stage, the diagnosis can be made by pressure studies from within the compartment and by comparing results with the opposite side (see section on Forearm Fractures earlier in this chapter).

*Treatment:*   If a compartment syndrome has been documented by pressure studies and if compression of neurovascular structures compromises function, then surgical release of the fascial covering may be necessary. The deep intermediate compartment is decompressed by removing a portion of the fibula.

## Shin Splints

A pain syndrome of multiple causes, usually localized to the anterolateral aspect of the leg or posteromedial aspect of the calf and associated with overuse of the extremity is known as "shin splints." Sometimes relatively little activity may induce the symptoms. The syndrome is most common in long-distance runners.

Several theories have been proposed to explain shin splints:

1. Stress fractures of the tibia or fibula
2. Partial tear of the muscle fascia of the gastrocnemius or posterior tibial muscle
3. Compartment syndrome
4. Stretch irritation of branches of the peroneal nerve because of muscle swelling or repetitive muscle contraction
5. Periostitis of the fascial attachment to the tibia

*X-ray studies:*   Occasionally stress fractures of the tibia or fibula are seen in the region of symptoms. "Looser zones" may be noted. If so, follow-up X-ray studies should be made at 6-week intervals until these defects either resolve or show signs of callous formation, indicating a stress fracture had been present. A bone scan may be helpful.

*Treatment:*   Treatment varies with the etiology. If no one cause can be found, the treatment includes one or more of the following steps:

1. Gentle stretching of both anterior and posterior musculature (especially the calf, heel cord, and hamstring)
2. Ice massage or ice packs before and after activities
3. Gentle, progressive resistive exercises to build muscle tone (especially the dorsiflexors of the foot)
4. Gradual build-up of endurance in running or jumping sports
5. Regular use of salicylates taken just before or during sports. (Some athletes improve with this regimen.)

6. Repetitive ultrasound application
7. Taping and elastic wrap of the calf, with padding over involved muscles
8. Holistic approaches, including acupuncture and vitamin and calcium supplements. (There are no data to support this therapy.)
9. Long rest or change of sports. (This procedure may be helpful and protective of the muscle compartments.)
10. Release of anterior and lateral compartments in runners with persistent symptoms. (There is no documentation of the efficacy of this treatment.)

## Muscle Tears

The most common tear occurs usually medially or centrally in the gastrocnemius fascia. The plantaris muscle tendon unit can also tear, but this is more often suspected than it actually occurs. The treatment is supportive (ice, elevation, crutches, gradual weight bearing, elastic stocking). Occult venous thrombosis can occur after injury. Increased swelling or pain should be studied by venography or phlebography.

# Common Ankle Injuries

The ankle joint is a hinge. The joint is composed of the lower end of the tibia, the tibial malleolus, the fibular malleolus, and the dome of the talus. These bones are connected by the 1) deltoid ligament, 2) calcaneofibular ligament, 3) anterior and posterior talofibular ligaments, and 4) articular capsule (Gray [2]).

## Sprain

Acute soft-tissue injuries of the ankle are usually the result of inversion stress to the anterolateral capsule and to the lateral collateral ligament. With the inversion stress, there is internal rotation and plantar flexion of the foot in relation to the leg. This causes tearing of the anterolateral capsule and swelling and partial tearing at the origin of the muscle mass of the short extensor muscles of the toes. There is also tearing of the fibulocalcaneal ligament (lateral collateral ligament of the ankle). The injury to the collateral ligament can be of first to third degree.

The patient presents a swollen, painful ankle; the tenderness and swelling are mostly on the anterolateral and direct lateral aspects. Occasionally there is swelling of the medial joint line in the vicinity of the deltoid ligament. A hematoma will rapidly dissect along tissue planes of the foot, causing ecchymotic discoloration in many areas.

The history is important. The patient may describe many prior, similar sprains, each one with symptoms and signs.

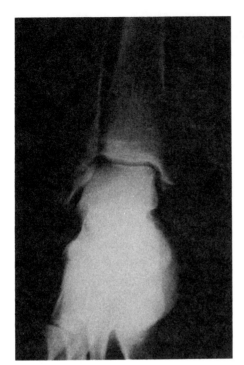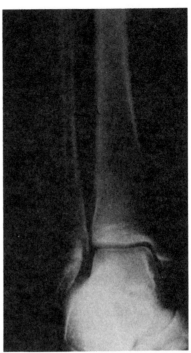

**19–22**   Anteroposterior view of ankle showing minimally displaced fracture of distal fibula at level of tibial-talar joint line.

*Clinical Examination:*   First-degree injury shows no signs of instability on anterior or posterior draw stress (draw sign) or with inversion stress. The instability of second- and third-degree injuries will depend on the amount of tissue tearing.

*X-ray studies:*   The X-ray films may reveal an avulsion fracture of the tip of the lateral malleolus (Fig. 19–22) with associated fractures of the medial malleolus or distal fibula. There may be calcifications in soft tissue that suggest old and recurrent ligamentous trauma. Inversion stress films should be obtained to record the amount of talar tilt. A comparison should be made with the opposite ankle, though it is not uncommon for both ankles to have been involved in recurring sprains so that stress X-ray studies show bilateral laxity.

*Treatment:*   The type of care is determined by stability. A stable and minimally swollen ankle with no signs of recent fracture or dislocation requires 1) elevation, 2) ice, 3) soft ankle wrap (sheet wadding or cotton covered with an Ace bandage or covered with an Unna paste boot), 4) use of crutches to avoid bearing weight.

After 5–7 days a heavy pull-on elastic stocking, elevation of the foot most of the time, some weight bearing with the use of a cane or crutches as necessary, will help to encourage ankle motion. Swimming is good ankle exercise. The patient should regularly do isometric and progressive resistive exercises for calf and anterior leg muscles.

If swelling is marked and the ankle is clinically stable, the balloon distention effect can mask instability temporarily. Severely swollen ankles should be casted or splinted, with the foot in neutral position. Elevation of the leg should be encouraged, and the leg reevaluated in 7–10 days.

Treatment of the unstable ankle is individualized. Many recreational and professional athletes have unstable ankles because of recurrent lateral and anterolateral tissue tears that have not been surgically treated. Decent function with an unstable ankle is possible, provided supportive taping or above-ankle shoes are utilized. Lateral or anterolateral injuries that cause ankle instability can be treated as follows:

1.  The first episode associated with anterolateral or straight varus (inversion) instability without fractures requires the use of a cast for 3–6 weeks, or the torn ligaments should be surgically repaired.
2.  Acute lateral or anterolateral injury, with a past history of recurrent similar injuries and associated instability, should be treated with ankle taping; pull-on elastic ankle support; and crutches or a cast for 7–10 days. Surgical treatment might necessitate reconstructive measures to create anterior and lateral stabilizing elements.
3.  The first episode of lateral or anterolateral injury associated with instability can be treated with a pull-on elastic support or with taping alone, provided the swelling is not severe and the patient is cooperative and will utilize crutches. Starting early ankle motion while participating in progressive resistive and isometric exercises for calf and anterior compartment structures is essential. This treatment requires the patient's informed consent and knowledge of alternative therapies.

The application of a short walking cast to the leg is a good standby for treatment. However, the cast can cause increased morbidity, including stiffness of the ankle and phlebitis as a result of the immobilization.

Late reconstructive measures for chronic and recurring anterolateral and lateral ankle instability are successful. A choice in treatment programs short of surgery is therefore possible at an early time. Closed treatment, however, cannot predict that healing of the torn capsule and ligamentous structures will be good. Periarticular disarray of torn ligaments may never allow end-to-end joining of ligamentous structures, and fibrous bridging strong enough to give the ankle stability may not be possible. The athlete and the family, in the case of minors, should help in deciding treatment choice.

Medial ligament injuries (deltoid ligament) are less common. Third-degree tears of this ligament are associated with complete instability on eversion or valgus stress to the ankle. X-ray studies and palpation will document the condition. The draw sign may not be present with anterior and posterior stress in the neutral position of the foot. Treatment for third-degree deltoid ligament lesion is surgical repair. Most likely this ligament will be displaced between the medial malleolus and the talus, preventing adequate healing despite immobilization. Third- and second-degree tears are treated as lateral injuries.

## Tears of the Achilles Tendon

Injuries to the Achilles tendon deserve special comment. This muscle tendon unit stabilizes the lower extremity. Partial or complete tear of the Achilles tendon can be diagnosed by careful systematic evaluation. The patient will complain of weakness on plantar flexion of the foot or inability to stand upon the toes of the involved foot only.

On examination there will be swelling, tenderness, and sometimes a palpable defect where the tendon is torn. When the patient is in the prone or kneeling position, complete discontinuity of the Achilles tendon can be shown when the calf muscle is squeezed. In response to this maneuver, the foot should slightly plantar flex, or at least the Achilles tendon at the point of attachment to the calcaneous should become prominent. Failure of this response implies a complete tear of the Achilles tendon.

To assess the degree of tear, infiltration with local anesthetic solution into the area of tenderness and hematoma relieves pain and allows active plantar flexion of the foot against resistance if minimal first- or second-degree tearing of the tendon has occurred. The power of plantar flexion can be compared with the opposite extremity.

*Treatment:* Treatment for complete ruptures of the Achilles tendon in an athlete is surgical repair. Nonoperative treatment can be utilized, but the patient must understand that morbidity is prolonged and function of the gastrocnemius-soleus tendon complex may in the end be inadequate for athletic demands. Nonoperative treatment for complete tears of the Achilles tendon is a long leg cast with the knee flexed 15°–20°, and the foot plantar-flexed at the ankle. The cast should be worn for at least 6 and preferably for 8–10 weeks. Alternative treatments for partial tears include crutches, no weight bearing, but isometric exercises for the calf. Restrictive taping can be used for partial tears.

## Peroneal Tendon Subluxation or Dislocation

When this injury is acute, it may be confused with an ankle sprain. Forced dorsiflexion and eversion of the foot during sports can tear the retinaculum surrounding the peroneal tendons, and the long peroneal or short peroneal tendon can then move out of its normal groove behind the lateral malleolus. If the foot is brought into plantar flexion and inversion, the tendons will usually reduce.

*X-ray studies:* The X-ray films may show an avulsion fracture in the region of the distal fibular, but usually only soft-tissue swelling is present, without bony abnormality in this region.

*Diagnosis and treatment:* If the diagnosis is suspected, local anesthetic infiltration with sterile technique will allow painless reproduction of the injury and permit the tendon to slip free of its normal groove passively during dorsiflexion and eversion of the foot. The treatment is operative repair of the retinaculum or deepening of the peroneal groove, depending upon the findings at surgery.

Nonoperative treatment is supportive. A felt pad to fit over the peroneal tendons is placed under taping, or a plaster cast is applied over the felt to maintain the position of the tendons for at least 21, but preferably 28, days. During this time the foot should not be brought into eversion without a cast, and the patient should not bear weight.

*The recurring problem:* Treatment for chronic subluxation or dislocation of the peroneal tendons is usually surgical reconstruction of the retinaculum or deepening of the peroneal groove behind the lateral malleolus. Supportive taping with a felt pressure pad over the tendons has been successful on occasions. If the movement at the ankle is strong, however, external supporting will not suffice.

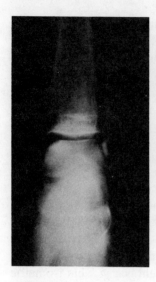
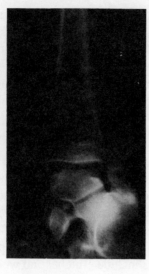

**19–23** Anteroposterior (a) and oblique (b) views of ankle, showing osteochondritis dissecans of superior and medial aspect of talus.

## Osteochondral Fractures

The most common location for osteochondral fragment lesions at the ankle are the superomedial or superolateral aspects of the talus. The possibility that these lesions exist within the ankle joint should be kept in mind when an ankle injury in the acute or chronic phase is being evaluated. Sometimes the first X-ray films will not show the fragments because the fragments have not displaced from the bony bed and no bone resorption has occurred at the fracture line. Follow-up X-ray films at 14–21 days will usually show the defect.

X-ray studies of the ankle should include anteroposterior and lateral and oblique views. True mortise views can be taken with the foot in maximal plantar and maximal dorsiflexion to show different areas of the talar dome. Suspicious areas in the talus on plain films can be evaluated more closely by tomograms or CT scan.

Osteochondral fracture should be suspected if morbidity after a "sprain" is excessive (Fig. 19–23).

*Treatment:* The osteochondral fracture fragment can be removed by surgery, or if circumstances permit, the segment may be replaced. Often there will be no bony involvement, only a surface cartilage lesion.

## Fractures Around the Ankle

Treatment of fractures in the vicinity of the ankle demands individualization (Fig. 19–24). Because of the weight-bearing and built-in rotational components of the joint, anatomic restoration of structures is important. Failure to obtain this can seriously affect weight-bearing relationships between the tibia and talus, causing serious mechanical consequences and early degenerative arthritis.

Even slight displacement of fractured segments of the lateral malleolus can affect the support and rotation of the talus.

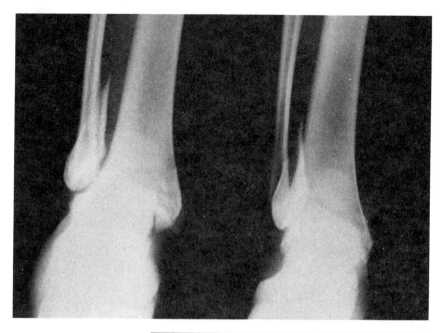

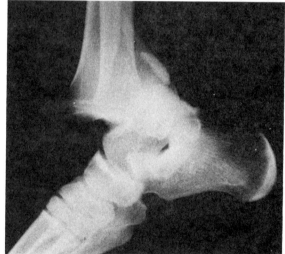

**19–24** Anteroposterior view of fracture dislocation of right ankle. There is a fracture through distal fibula, above syndesmosis and fracture of posterior tibial plafond, with posterior dislocation of talus.

Lateral view of trimalleolar ankle fracture with dislocation of talus seen above.

# Common Foot Injuries

Many foot problems of athletes are direct results of developmental variations of the lower extremity. The stresses upon the foot most often result from static alignment and dynamic relationships among the hip, knee, and ankle. For example, femoral anteversion, genu valgum, genu varum, and tibial torsion all will have direct effects on foot function.

Developmental changes within the foot are very often a consequence of proximal forces. The low-arched foot (flat foot) or the high-arched foot (cavus foot) will often predispose athletes to symptoms during activity.

# Sprains of the Foot

Any foot ligament can be torn by repetitive stresses or forced torsion of the foot. Ligamentous injuries will vary in location and can be classified into first-, second-, or third-degree sprains, as elsewhere in the body. A third-degree sprain is a complete dislocation between bones connected by the affected ligaments. In the mid and hind foot, the subtalar and midtarsal joints can be involved in third-degree sprains. The only symptom or sign may be a swollen foot. Violent high-torque injuries can cause tarsal-metatarsal dislocations. X-ray studies are important in evaluating a swollen foot to assess bone and joint relationships.

*Treatment of acute injuries:*   Ice, elevation, and supportive wrap are all helpful. The wrap may be sheet wadding or cotton roll covered by muslin or roller gauze and finally covered by a woven elastic (Ace) wrap, with minimal pressure within the elastic wrapping.

The markedly swollen foot demands an accurate check of the neurologic status of all branches of the plantar and peroneal nerves and of the posterior tibial dorsalis pedis pulses and capillary filling of nail beds. It is not uncommon for a swollen foot to lead to a compartment syndrome of the foot. This can destroy the plantar musculature by circulatory compromise. The potential for compartment syndrome is greater if a third-degree sprain has occurred. The treatment of compartment syndrome is surgical release.

Sprains involving the plantar ligament deserve special comment. With weight bearing, stress is automatically applied to the span of the plantar ligament. Treatment for plantar ligament sprains is initially ice, elevation, and avoidance of weight bearing by using crutches. Local anesthetic injections and hyaluronidase sometimes disperse the hematoma and promote early healing. Ultrasound applied daily for 10–14 days is sometimes helpful in dispersing inflammatory fluids. When symptoms subside, protective taping should be applied to decrease distraction stress on the plantar surface of the foot. After the injury has recovered, an arch support is good protection. Sometimes, supportive taping must be applied indefinitely to prevent recurrence.

Sprains of the foot with weight bearing at the transverse metatarsal arch can cause recurring symptoms after an acute injury. Initial treatment is by rest and avoidance of weight bearing until symptoms subside. During the rest period, isometric and isotonic exercises of the foot can be carried out: curling the toes and picking up small objects with the toes to maintain good muscle function. Supportive taping should be utilized in a circumferential fashion at the level of the metatarsal heads. This may prevent recurrences. Orthotic inserts in the shoe to support the longitudinal and the transverse arches are also helpful.

Acute lateral ligament injuries are treated by ice and taping. During healing, lateral heel and sole wedges decrease tension on the lateral ligaments by lessening inversion stress.

# Neuromas of the Feet

Irritation of nerves can occur at any point in the foot. Shoes can rub superficial sensory nerves, causing symptoms. Loss of static intermetatarsal ligamentous and muscular support can cause stress upon digital nerves or proximal branches of the plantar nerve as they pass between the metatarsal heads. Irritation occurs frequently at the junction of the medial and lateral plantar nerves, in the regions of the third and fourth metatarsal heads. This irritation is referred to as a Morton's neuralgia.

*Symptoms:*    Intermittent (shocklike) recurring pain or tingling along the lateral aspect of the distal foot, especially the adjacent sides of the third and fourth toes. If sudden pressure is applied to the transverse intermetatarsal arch, pain can radiate to the web space between the third and fourth toes.

*Signs:*    Compressing the foot around the transverse arch will reproduce the pain. Pressure by the thumb applied to the space between the third and fourth metatarsal heads will often reproduce symptoms also. Hypalgesia may be found between the third and fourth toes and in some cases hyperpathia in the same region.

*X-ray studies:*    The X-ray films are often normal. Special studies in weight bearing will usually show the absence of the transverse arch.

*Treatment:*    Balancing of the foot is important. Longitudinal and intermetatarsal arch support proximal to the metatarsal heads is often helpful. Occasionally local injection of an anesthetic will give relief for a long period of time. A metatarsal bar on the shoe can distribute the force of the weight away from the metatarsal heads. Cortisone injections can be tried with some reservation. They may cause subcutaneous tissue atrophy and increase symptoms. Surgical treatment is a last resort and is often curative. However, caution must be used. Scar tissue is produced by surgery, and early weight bearing may cause prolonged morbidity from repetitive irritation of scar tissue.

## Bursitis and Blister Problems

Overuse of the foot, with irritation from the shoe, will frequently cause blisters and irritation of various bursae. Commonly affected bursae are those between the skin and the calcaneous and at the Achilles tendon insertion (O'Donoghue [1]).

Bony prominences on the plantar aspect of the foot (especially the metatarsal heads) can lead to painful callosities in the unbalanced foot. This is especially true if the transverse arch is inadequate, leading to excessive stresses. Treatment is foot-balancing techniques and counter-pressure pads to decrease stress. Injections of steroids and local anesthetics into the bursae can be tried. However, they can cause atrophy of subcutaneous tissues. Ice massage should be utilized for acute pain, and ultrasound helps disperse inflammatory fluids. Blisters may be aspirated and coated with tincture of benzoin. The blister area may then be surrounded by a ''doughnut'' of thin felt to avoid pressure.

## Fractures of the Foot

*Comments:*

1. Most nonarticular fractures of the phalanges of the toes can be treated by taping to an adjacent, uninjured toe (Fig. 19–25). Supportive cotton or felt should be placed

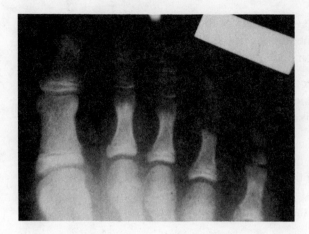

**19–25** X-ray film of toes in a child, showing nondisplaced transverse fracture of middle segment of fifth, and congenital fusion of distal, interphalangeal joints.

between the toes. Toe fractures needing reduction can be manipulated with or without anesthetic before taping. Documentation of the fracture by X-ray studies before and after manipulation is important.

2. Undisplaced fractures of metatarsal bones can be treated with supportive care. If the patient is more comfortable without a cast, using crutches alone, this is acceptable. Motion of the toes and bathing or swimming during convalescence is beneficial. Follow-up X-ray films at 7–10 days and then again in 3 weeks to check alignment of the fracture segment is important. If the patient is unreliable or, for convenience, needs a cast support, then a short-leg walking cast will usually suffice (Fig. 19–26).

3. Fracture at the base of the fifth metatarsal bone (dancer's fracture or Jones's fracture) is best treated with casting until healing occurs. The development of nonunion of this fracture is increased if cast support is not utilized.

4. Stress fracture can occur in any of the metatarsal bones but usually involves the second, third, and fourth metatarsals at the metatarsal neck region. Fractures may occur with repetitive trauma, such as running, or occasionally in an athlete who overuses the foot. If the initial X-ray films are negative but fracture tenderness exists in the symptomatic area, the foot should be treated as for a metatarsal fracture and followed by reexamination with X-ray studies and further clinical evaluation in 14–21 days. At that time fracture callus should be present or the absorption of bone at the fracture line will make the diagnosis.

5. Fracture dislocation of the midfoot may not be readily apparent on routine films, and only by comparison with the other foot can the dislocation be noted (Fig. 19–27).

6. Anatomic reduction is preferable. Malunion of the metatarsal bones can change the stresses at the metatarsal heads, causing painful callosities or midfoot discomfort.

7. When necessary, surgical pin fixation of acute foot fractures should be used. Intra-articular fractures can result in painful spurring, deformity, and degenerative arthritis.

8. Painful joints as a result of malunion or arthritic changes may need reconstructive measures, such as joint fusion or excisional arthroplasty.

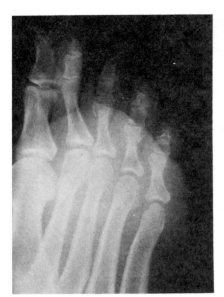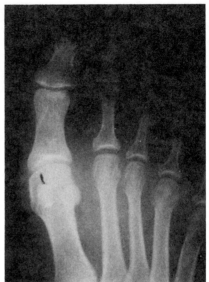

**19–26** X-ray films of foot, showing comminuted but minimally displaced fractures of distal ends of proximal phalanges of third and fourth toes.

## Developmental Variations Affecting Function

If symptoms are in the foot, examination from the waist down, at least, is necessary to evaluate the "whole" athlete. If the symptoms are in the hip, examination should be from the neck down. If examination is restricted to the area of pain only, the cause of the problem may be missed.

The body will adapt to structural variations. There may be a limit, however, to how long effective function with adaptations will continue. The examiner should note the following points:

1. Are the joints lax or tight? Can the elbow hyperextend? Can the knee hyperextend (back knee)? Can the thumb be brought back against the forearm?
2. Is there structural or functional scoliosis? Does the patient stand in a slouched fashion or erect? Is there hyperlordosis (sway back) with prominent buttocks?
3. Are there tight hamstrings? Can the patient easily touch the toes with knees extended?
4. Is there hip flexion contracture? Is the tightness due to a tight iliopsoas or to a tight rectus femoris? Are there structural abnormalities on X-ray films of the hips?
5. Is the walk toed-in (pigeon-toed) or toed-out (duck walk)? Do the kneecaps point forward or inward during gait?
6. Is there increased stability by internal rotation of the hip? Can the patient sit comfortably in the "squat sprawl" position (knees on the floor, hips internally rotated and buttocks resting on the heels)?
7. Are there genu valgum (knock-knee) or tibia vara (bowleg) deformities?
8. Is there internal tibial torsion or external tibial torsion?
9. Is there excessive heel valgus or foot pronation? Are there bunion deformities?

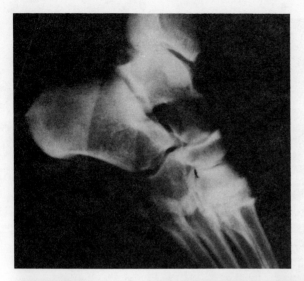

**19–27**    Lateral view of midfoot dislocation. Tarsal-metatarsal joints are dislocated, and first metatarsal bone is displaced
dorsally.

Midfoot dislocation of tarsal-metatarsal
joints shows widening of joint space between first metatarsal and first cuneiform
bones.

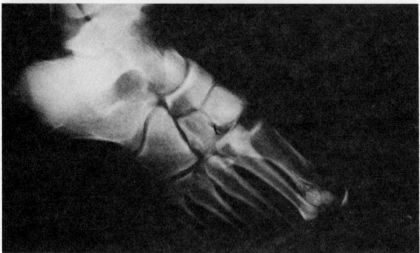

All the foregoing questions should be answered in deciding the causes of symptoms. Pain
is often caused by compensatory stresses in response to malalignment.

Tight muscles should be stretched gently and regularly. Posture exercises should be
encouraged to decrease lumbar lordosis stresses. A lower extremity malalignment syndrome should be treated from proximal to distal. Most fixed deformities in the lower
extremities can be corrected or improved only by muscle reeducation and orthotic
appliances in the shoes. Occasionally, surgical measures can be used to realign an
extremity, but the basic defects must first be defined.

In younger patients, developmental problems have a better prognosis. The "kinetic
chain" from proximal to distal can be altered in the growing child by stretching, muscle
education, and orthotic devices. Once deformities are fixed and adaptations have occurred, the problems are more difficult to solve.

The exact cause of osteochondritis is yet to be found. Freiberg's disease of the second
metatarsal head in teenagers and Sever's disease of the calcaneal apophysis in pre-
teenagers could be related to compensatory stresses in these regions. Osgood-Schlatter

disease likewise could be secondary to developmental forces on the patellar ligamentous insertion. The treatment of all these bony changes is supportive. Splinting, taping, orthotic pads, or crutches are utilized until symptoms subside. Occasionally surgery is utilized in the older patient.

# Returning to Sports After Injury

The decision on whether an athlete should return to a particular sport is the responsibility of his physician. It may rest upon consultation between an orthopedist, neurosurgeon, family physician, team physician, and team coach. Some injuries lead to vulnerability for re-injury in that sport. The athlete must then consider a change. "Athletic performance" should be the primary consideration. The athlete must have confidence in his or her ability in the chosen sport. Physicians and coaches must feel that the patient's physical capability will allow safe continued participation. Objective testing should be obtained before return with isokinetic measuring methods of extremity musculature. This method compares the injured extremity with the opposite extremity or with its pre-injury capabilities. Before contact sports are undertaken a coach should spend time with the individual athletes to assess performance and effectiveness in the field. When necessary, protective equipment such as braces, pads, or taping should be designed for the athlete to protect vulnerable areas.

# References

1. O'Donoghue, D.H. 1970. Treatment of Injuries to Athletes, 2nd Ed. W.B. Saunders Co., Philadelphia, pp 11–33, 405, 442, 446, 493, 671.
2. Gray, H. 1959. Anatomy of the Human Body. C.M. Goss, ed (27th Ed.). Lea & Febiger, Philadelphia, pp 356, 360, 366, 380, 390.
3. Bateman, J.E. 1969. Shoulder injuries in the throwing sports. In: Symposium on Sports Medicine. C.V. Mosby Co., Saint Louis, pp 87-96.
4. Spinner, M. 1972. Injuries to the Major Branches of Peripheral Nerves of the Forearm. W.B. Saunders Co., Philadelphia, p 114.
5. Torg, J.S., Conrad, W., Kalan, V. 1976. Clinical diagnosis of anterior cruciate ligament instability in the athlete. Am J Sports Med 4(2): 84-91.
6. Helfet, A.J. 1963. Management of Internal Derangements of the Knee. J.B. Lippincott Co., Philadelphia, p 80.

# Chapter 20

# Muscle Testing for Sports

## by Vivian H. Heyward

# Introduction

The importance of muscular fitness for successful performance in sports has led to widespread use of weight training and physical conditioning programs to supplement the skills training of athletes. Understanding how to assess various components of muscular fitness can be useful to the coach, athletic trainer, and sports physician in the following ways: 1) to evaluate the athlete's potential for a particular sport or position within that sport, 2) to plan a supplementary program of weight training and physical conditioning to improve muscular fitness and performance, 3) to pinpoint muscular imbalances that lead to an increased risk of injury, and 4) to determine loss of muscle function due to injury.

In this chapter, tests and performance norms that can be used to assess various components of muscular fitness for athletes are presented. Factors that influence muscular fitness, as well as problems associated with muscle testing, are discussed.

# Definition of Terms

Three important components of muscular fitness are: strength, endurance, and power. *Strength* is the ability of a muscle group to exert maximum contractile force against resistance; whereas, *muscular endurance* is the ability of that muscle group to exert submaximum force for extended periods of time. *Power,* or the rate of doing work, is a function of strength and speed (power = force × velocity). Often in athletics, the term "explosive strength," is used to describe muscular power. The extent to which each of these components is needed for successful performance is highly specific to the sport. For example, high jumping requires leg strength and power, whereas, a high level of muscular endurance is needed for long-distance running.

In addition to determining the physical demands of the sport, a number of important factors must be considered when selecting tests to assess the athlete's strength, muscular endurance, or power. First, the muscle groups and the type of muscle contraction used in the performance must be identified. The type of muscle contraction may be *static* or *dynamic* depending on the resistance encountered. When the resistance is immovable, the muscle contracts statically (or *isometrically*). In other words, the change in muscle length is minimal (*iso* = same; *metric* = length), and there is no visible movement at the joint. When there is visible joint movement, however, the muscle is contracting dynamically.

The specific type of dynamic contraction (*concentric* or *eccentric*) is dependent on the magnitude of the muscle force and the resistance. When the force exceeds the resistance, the muscle will shorten as it moves the bony lever (concentric contraction). When the resistance exceeds the muscle force, the bony lever will rotate in the opposite direction as the muscle lengthens and exerts tension (eccentric contraction). Eccentric contraction produces a braking force that decelerates rapidly moving body segments and resists gravitational acceleration during the movement. In the past, the term, *isotonic* (*iso* = same; *tonic* = tension) *contraction* was used to describe both concentric and eccentric muscle contraction. In actuality, however, there are large fluctuations in muscle force throughout the range of motion, even though the external resistance or weight being raised or lowered stays the same. This fluctuation in muscle force is due to the change in muscle length and angle of pull as the bony lever is moved (Kreigbaum and Barthels [1]). As a result, the term *dynamic* is more widely accepted to describe the concentric and eccentric contractions of a muscle group.

*Isokinetic contraction* is a special type of dynamic muscle contraction in which the speed of contraction is controlled mechanically so that the limb rotates at a predetermined velocity (e.g., 60°/sec). Isokinetic contraction involves maximum contraction of the muscle group at a constant speed throughout the entire range of motion. Electromechanical or hydraulic mechanisms vary the resistance so that it matches fluctuations in muscle force due to the changing muscle length and angle of pull. Thus, with the aid of isokinetic exercise devices, the muscle group encounters variable maximum resistances throughout its complete range of motion.

# Assessment of Muscular Fitness

Strength, muscular endurance, and power are measured using dynamometers, cable tensiometers, force platforms, isokinetic devices, and constant resistance or variable resistance exercise machines. The selection of the test instrumentation depends on the type of test (strength, endurance, or power), the muscle group being evaluated, and the type of muscle contraction (static, dynamic, or isokinetic). In addition, certain practical factors such as transportability of equipment, time allotted for testing, ease of test administration, and availability and expense of equipment should be taken into consideration. Sources for muscle testing equipment are included at the end of this chapter.

# Assessing Static Muscle Function

Although most sports are dynamic in nature, it may be desirable, for certain sports or events, to evaluate strength and muscular endurance during static contractions of muscle groups. In gymnastics, for example, successful performance of an iron-cross maneuver on the stationary rings is highly dependent on the static strength and endurance of the shoulder abductors/adductors and elbow flexors/extensors. Likewise, strength and endurance of the grip-squeezing muscles are important in sports such as tennis, squash, and racquetball. When the body or sports implement must be maintained in a stationary position either momentarily or for extended periods of time, a certain degree of static strength and endurance is a prerequisite for successful performance. Static strength and endurance can be measured using dynamometers, cable tensiometers, and electromechanical devices.

**Dynamometers, Test Protocols, and Norms**   A handgrip dynamometer and back/leg dynamometer can be used to measure static strength and endurance of the grip-squeezing muscles and leg and back muscles. The handgrip dynamometer measures forces between 0 kg and 100 kg in 1-kg increments, whereas, the back and leg dynamometer measures forces ranging between 0 lb and 2500 lb in 10-lb increments. Both dynamometers are spring devices that move the indicator needle on the dial an amount corresponding to the force applied to the instrument.

Prior to measuring grip strength or endurance, the handgrip size of the dynamometer is adjusted to a position that is comfortable for the individual. Alternatively, a caliper can be used to determine an optimum grip size (Montoye and Faulkner [2]). To measure static grip strength the individual stands erect with the arms at the sides. With the forearm in a neutral position and the dial facing away from the body, the individual squeezes the handle as hard as possible without moving the arm. Three trials, with a 1-min rest between trials, are administered for each hand. Static grip strength is measured as the maximum force registered on the dial.

To assess the static endurance of the grip-squeezing muscles, the subject is instructed to squeeze the handle as hard as possible for a 60-sec period. The force is recorded every 10 sec. The greater the endurance, the less the rate of decline in force. The relative endurance score is the final force divided by the initial force multiplied by 100. An alternative static endurance test requires the individual to maintain a submaximum force level that is a designated percentage of his or her maximum voluntary contractile strength (e.g., 60% MVC). The relative endurance score is the amount of time that this tension level is sustained. The subject must watch the dial of the dynamometer to monitor the appropriate force level during the test.

To assess static leg strength, the subject stands on the platform of the back and leg dynamometer. The knees are flexed to an angle of 130° to 140°, keeping the trunk erect. The crossbar is held using a pronated grip and the chain is adjusted so that the handbar lies across the thighs. As the knees are slowly and vigorously extended, the indicator needle on the dial moves a corresponding amount. The maximum indicator needle remains at the peak force achieved. This score is then converted to kilograms. Usually two to three trials are administered with a 1-min rest between trials.

**Table 20–1**   Static Strength Norms*

| Classification | Left Grip (kg) | Right Grip (kg) | Back Strength (kg) | Leg Strength (kg) | Total Strength | Strength/BW (kg) |
|---|---|---|---|---|---|---|
| **Men** | | | | | | |
| Excellent | >68 | >70 | >209 | >241 | >587 | >7.50 |
| Good | 56–67 | 62–69 | 177–208 | 214–240 | 508–586 | 7.10–7.49 |
| Average | 43–55 | 48–61 | 126–176 | 160–213 | 375–507 | 5.21–7.09 |
| Poor | 39–42 | 41-47 | 91–125 | 137–159 | 307–374 | 4.81–5.20 |
| Very Poor | <39 | <41 | <91 | <137 | <307 | <4.81 |
| **Women** | | | | | | |
| Excellent | >37 | >41 | >111 | >136 | >324 | >5.50 |
| Good | 34–36 | 38–40 | 98–110 | 114–135 | 282–323 | 4.80–5.49 |
| Average | 22–33 | 25–37 | 52–97 | 66–113 | 164–281 | 2.90–4.79 |
| Poor | 18–21 | 22-24 | 39–51 | 49–65 | 117–163 | 2.10–2.89 |
| Very Poor | <18 | <22 | <39 | <49 | <117 | <2.10 |

*From Heyward, V. 1983. Designs for Fitness. Burgess Publishing Co., Minneapolis. In press. Reprinted with permission of the publisher.

The back and leg dynamometer also is used to assess static back strength. Standing on the platform with the knees fully extended and the trunk erect, the individual grasps the handbar using a pronated grip for the right hand and a supinated grip for the left hand. The handbar is positioned across the thighs and is pulled upward using the trunk extensor muscles. The shoulders are rolled backward during the pull. The maximum score, as indicated on the dial, is converted to kilograms. Two trials are administered with a 1-min rest between trials.

Norms for these dynamometric tests for men and women are presented in Table 20–1. The right grip, left grip, leg strength, and back strength scores are totaled to determine the overall static strength score. Before adding the scores, however, the leg and back strength scores must be converted from pounds to kilograms. The total strength score is divided by the body weight (in kilograms) to determine the relative strength.

**Cable Tensiometry**   The static strength of approximately 38 different muscle groups throughout the body can be measured using cable tensiometry, which consists of a tensiometer, steel cables, strength table, wall hooks, straps, and a goniometer. The cable is attached to the wall or table hooks, and the other end is attached to the body segment being tested, using a strap. The cable is always positioned at right angles to the bony lever. After the tensiometer is positioned on the tightened cable, the individual is instructed to pull as hard as possible. The force exerted on the cable depresses the riser of the tensiometer and the indicator needle registers the maximum force produced. Forces ranging between 0 lb and 400 lb can be measured using large tensiometers. For a more precise and accurate assessment of forces ranging between 0 lb and 100 lb, a smaller tensiometer is used.

The standardized testing procedures, as described by Clarke and Clarke [3], should be followed carefully. Since static strength is specific to the joint angle and muscle group being tested, cable tensiometer test batteries usually include three to four different sites to provide an adequate estimation of overall static strength. A goniometer is used to measure the specified joint angle for each test item. Test batteries for males (9 yr–college age) include the following three items: shoulder extension, knee extension, and ankle plantar flexion strength. For senior high school and college women, the test battery includes shoulder flexion, hip flexion, and ankle plantar flexion strength. Norms for these test batteries are provided elsewhere (Clarke [4]; Clarke and Monroe [5]).

**Electromechanical Devices**    If a high degree of precision is needed, electromechanical systems can be used to assess static strength and endurance of muscle groups. Linear voltage differential transformers and strain gauges can be used to transform the applied mechanical force to an electrical voltage. This change in voltage is recorded and parameters such as peak force, rate of force production, and time to peak force can be extracted from the recorded output. The system can be designed to test the static strength and endurance of many muscle groups. Due to the expense, these electromechanical devices are not very practical. The degree of sophistication afforded by these instruments, however, is well-suited for research purposes.

## Assessing Dynamic Muscle Function

Dynamic strength, muscular endurance, and power can be assessed using constant resistance or variable resistance exercise modes. With the constant resistance mode, the resistance that the muscle encounters does not vary with the changing mechanical and physiological advantage of the musculoskeletal system. The maximum weight that can be moved through the full range of motion is no greater than the weight that can be lifted at the weakest point in the range. Equipment such as free weights, dumbbells, and some stations of the Universal Gym Machine provide a constant resistance.

To overcome this shortcoming, exercise machines have been designed that vary the resistance during the movement. These variable resistance exercise machines have a moving connection between the point of force application and the resistance. As the weight is lifted, the mechanical advantage of the machine decreases and more force must be applied to continue the movement. These machines attempt to compensate for the changing mechanical advantage of the muscle during the movement. They do not compensate, however, for the decreased physiological advantage that occurs as the muscle shortens during the movement.

Nautilus makes a complete line of variable resistance machines that can be used to test dynamic muscle function. These include abdominal, rotary torso, hip/back, hip abductor/adductor, leg curl, leg press, leg extension, pullover, double chest, neck, shoulder, compound arm curl, and multiexercise machines. Some models of the Universal Gym Machine also provide variable resistance at the bench press, leg press, and shoulder press stations.

**Dynamic Strength Test Protocols and Norms**    Typically, dynamic strength is measured by determining the maximum weight that can be lifted for one complete repetition of a movement. This is known as the "1-RM value" and is obtained through trial and error. After a successful attempt at a given weight, the subject should rest 2 to 3 min before trying to lift a heavier weight. Usually, the weight is increased by 5 to 10 lb for each trial. Pollack et al. [6] recommend using the Universal Gym Machine to determine the 1-RM strength of four muscle groups: bench press, standing press, arm curl, and leg press. Performance norms for men and women are based on body weight (Table 20–2).

**Table 20–2** Optimal Strength Values (in Pounds) for Various Body Weights, Based on the 1-RM Test*†

| Body Weight (lb) | Bench Press Male | Bench Press Female | Standing Press Male | Standing Press Female | Curl Male | Curl Female | Leg Press Male | Leg Press Female |
|---|---|---|---|---|---|---|---|---|
| 80 | 80 | 56 | 53 | 37 | 40 | 28 | 160 | 112 |
| 100 | 100 | 70 | 67 | 47 | 50 | 35 | 200 | 140 |
| 120 | 120 | 84 | 80 | 56 | 60 | 42 | 240 | 168 |
| 140 | 140 | 98 | 93 | 65 | 70 | 49 | 280 | 196 |
| 160 | 160 | 112 | 107 | 75 | 80 | 56 | 320 | 224 |
| 180 | 180 | 126 | 120 | 84 | 90 | 63 | 360 | 252 |
| 200 | 200 | 140 | 133 | 93 | 100 | 70 | 400 | 280 |
| 220 | 220 | 154 | 147 | 103 | 110 | 77 | 440 | 308 |
| 240 | 240 | 168 | 160 | 112 | 120 | 84 | 480 | 336 |

*From Pollack, M.L. et al. 1978. Health and Fitness Through Physical Activity. John Wiley & Sons, New York. Reprinted with permission of the publisher.
†Data collected on Universal Gym apparatus. Information collected on other apparatus could modify results.

**Table 20–3** Strength/Body Weight Ratios for Selected Dynamic Strength Tests*

| Bench Press | Arm Curl | Lateral Pull-down | Leg Press | Leg Extension | Leg Curl | Points |
|---|---|---|---|---|---|---|
| **Men** | | | | | | |
| 1.50 | .70 | 1.20 | 3.00 | .80 | .70 | 10 |
| 1.40 | .65 | 1.15 | 2.80 | .75 | .65 | 9 |
| 1.30 | .60 | 1.10 | 2.60 | .70 | .60 | 8 |
| 1.20 | .55 | 1.05 | 2.40 | .65 | .55 | 7 |
| 1.10 | .50 | 1.00 | 2.20 | .60 | .50 | 6 |
| 1.00 | .45 | .95 | 2.00 | .55 | .45 | 5 |
| .90 | .40 | .90 | 1.80 | .50 | .40 | 4 |
| .80 | .35 | .85 | 1.60 | .45 | .35 | 3 |
| .70 | .30 | .80 | 1.40 | .40 | .30 | 2 |
| .60 | .25 | .75 | 1.20 | .35 | .25 | 1 |
| **Women** | | | | | | |
| .90 | .50 | .85 | 2.70 | .70 | .60 | 10 |
| .85 | .45 | .80 | 2.50 | .65 | .55 | 9 |
| .80 | .42 | .75 | 2.30 | .60 | .52 | 8 |
| .70 | .38 | .73 | 2.10 | .55 | .50 | 7 |
| .65 | .35 | .70 | 2.00 | .52 | .45 | 6 |
| .60 | .32 | .65 | 1.80 | .50 | .40 | 5 |
| .55 | .28 | .63 | 1.60 | .45 | .35 | 4 |
| .50 | .25 | .60 | 1.40 | .40 | .30 | 3 |
| .45 | .21 | .55 | 1.20 | .35 | .25 | 2 |
| .35 | .18 | .50 | 1.00 | .30 | .20 | 1 |

| Total Points | Strength Fitness Category |
|---|---|
| 48–60 | Excellent |
| 37–47 | Good |
| 25–36 | Average |
| 13–24 | Fair |
| 0–12 | Poor |

*From Heyward, V. 1983. Designs for Fitness. Burgess Publishing Co., Minneapolis. In press. Reprinted with permission of the publisher.

Another test battery has been devised that evaluates the 1-RM value as a percentage of the individual's body weight (Table 20–3). The six test items are: bench press, arm curl, lateral pull-down, leg press, leg extension, and leg curl. For each exercise, the 1-RM value is divided by the body weight to determine the strength/body weight ratio, and the corresponding point value is noted. The overall strength is assessed by totaling the points accumulated for each exercise.

**Dynamic Muscular Endurance Test Protocols and Norms**    The individual's muscular endurance is highly dependent on strength. Therefore, most muscular endurance tests are designed so that the athlete performs as many repetitions as possible using a weight that is a designated percentage of the 1-RM strength value for that exercise. Another method uses a weight that corresponds to a percentage of the athlete's body weight. This method is less desirable, however, since a larger body weight does not always reflect a larger muscle mass.

To date, there are no good performance norms for evaluating dynamic muscular endurance. Pollack et al. [6] recommend using a weight that is 70% of the 1-RM for each exercise. They suggest that the average person should be able to complete 12 to 15 repetitions at that intensity. The competitive athlete, however, should be able to complete 20 to 25 repetitions.

**Dynamic Muscular Power Tests and Norms**    At present, there are few practical tests that yield valid and objective measures of dynamic power. In the past, performance tests such as the sitting shot put, medicine ball throw, vertical jump, standing long jump, and sprints were used to assess upper and lower body power. These tests, however, are not recommended to assess muscular power, since their validity has not been established (Considine [7]).

In addition, it is not easy to measure muscular power using conventional constant resistance exercise equipment. Because power is a function of force and velocity, both the magnitude of the weight and the speed of the movement must be measured. Accurate measurement of the speed of movement, however, is difficult, time-consuming, and expensive. Typically, high speed cinematography is used to record the performance and to determine both the distance that the weight is moved and the movement speed through frame-by-frame analysis of the film. There is a new, experimental device, however, that attaches to a standard weight stack (Wilmore [8]). The device, a microprocessor, measures the elapsed time and the distance that the weight travels, thereby computing the power (force $\times$ distance/time). When this device becomes readily available, it should facilitate accurate and rapid assessments of dynamic muscular power.

Force platforms can be used to assess leg power during jumping events. The force applied to the platform and the time of force application can be recorded to the nearest .01 sec. The power is calculated using the following equation (Considine [7]): $P = \frac{1}{8}F \times gT^2 \div T_2$; where F = body weight of subject, g = gravitational acceleration, T = total elapsed airborne time, and $T_2$ = length of time force is applied.

Margaria et al. [9] devised a practical test to measure leg power. This test, as modified by Kalamen [10], involves running upstairs, three steps at a time, as quickly as possible. A switchmat is placed on the third and ninth steps, and is used to trigger a timer that records the elapsed time to the nearest .01 sec. Power is computed using the following equation: $P = W \times D \div T$; where P = power (kg-m/sec), W = body weight of athlete

**Table 20–4**    Norms for Margaria-Kalamen Leg Power Test*

| Classification | 15–20 | 20–30 | 30–40 | 40–50 | Over 50 |
|---|---|---|---|---|---|
| | **Men** | | | | |
| | **Age Group (years)** | | | | |
| Poor | Under 113† | Under 106 | Under 85 | Under 65 | Under 50 |
| Fair | 113–149 | 106–139 | 85–111 | 65–84 | 50–65 |
| Average | 150–187 | 140–175 | 112–140 | 85–105 | 66–82 |
| Good | 188–224 | 176–210 | 141–168 | 106–125 | 83–98 |
| Excellent | Over 224 | Over 210 | Over 168 | Over 125 | Over 98 |
| | **Women** | | | | |
| | **Age Group (years)** | | | | |
| Classification | 15–20 | 20–30 | 30–40 | 40–50 | Over 50 |
| Poor | Under 92 | Under 85 | Under 65 | Under 50 | Under 38 |
| Fair | 92–120 | 85–111 | 66–84 | 50–65 | 38–48 |
| Average | 121–151 | 112–140 | 85–105 | 66–82 | 49–61 |
| Good | 152–182 | 141–168 | 106–125 | 83–98 | 62–75 |
| Excellent | Over 182 | Over 168 | Over 125 | Over 98 | Over 75 |

†Units of measurement are kg-m/sec.
*Based on data from Margaria et al. [9] and Kalamen [10].

(kg), D = vertical distance (m) for six steps (between third and ninth steps), and T = elapsed time (sec). Performance norms have been established based on age, sex, and fitness level of the individual (Table 20–4).

## Assessing Isokinetic Muscle Function

Isokinetic dynamometers provide an accurate and reliable assessment of the athlete's strength, endurance, and power. One major advantage of using isokinetic equipment is that the dynamometer keeps the speed of limb movement at a constant preselected velocity. An increase in muscular force results in increased resistance rather than increased acceleration of the limb. Thus, fluctuations in muscle force are matched by an equal counterforce or resistance. This capability is known as "accommodating resistance" and is produced electromechanically by controlling the velocity of movement during the contraction. Since it has been documented that the muscle group is capable of generating less force at faster speeds of contraction (Coyle et al. [11]; Gregor et al. [12]; Lesmes et al. [13]; Scudder [14]; Thorstensson et al. [15]), speed settings for isokinetic strength, muscular endurance, and power tests have been recommended (Table 20–5). Another advantage of isokinetic dynamometers is that muscular function, at speeds of movement that closely simulate those used during the actual sports performance, can be evaluated using the speed control feature of these devices.

**Isokinetic Equipment**    The Cybex II (Fig. 20–1) is an isokinetic dynamometer that measures muscular torque production of the shoulder, elbow, forearm, wrist, hip, knee, and ankle joints at speeds varying between 0° and 300°/sec. The resulting torque output, along with range of motion data, are recorded on a dual channel recorder.

Other isokinetic devices made by Cybex include the bench press, leg press, and Orthotron. The Orthotron is similar to the Cybex II but lacks the recording capability.

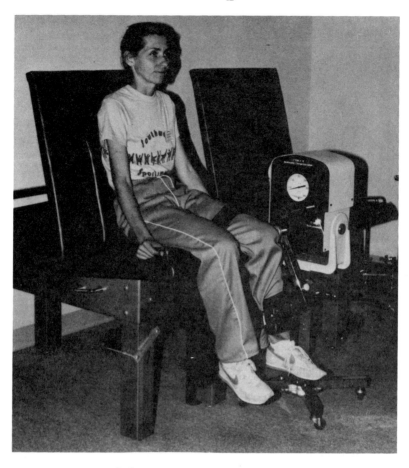

**20–1**    Cybex II Isokinetic Dynamometer.

However, it can still be used effectively for testing and evaluating muscle function. For purposes of exercise training and rehabilitation, the Orthotron is better suited than the Cybex II, since it is more durable and less expensive.

Mini-Gym makes a complete line of variable speed, isokinetic equipment that can be used for training and rehabilitation. These machines include wall pulleys, bench press, and leg press, as well as specialized devices designed to simulate movement patterns used during running, jumping, throwing, swimming, and gymnastics. Compared to Cybex dynamometers, Mini-Gym equipment is considerably less expensive; however, the speed control is not as accurate or precise.

**Isokinetic Strength Test Protocols**    Standardized test protocols and guidelines have been recommended by the Cybex manufacturer for assessing muscle function. Isokinetic strength is measured as the peak torque (ft-lb, kg-m, or N-m) at speeds of either 30° or 60°/sec depending on the joint action and muscle group being tested (Table 20–5). Prior to testing, two submaximum practice trials are administered to familiarize the athlete with the equipment and testing procedure. This is followed immediately by three maximum contractions in both directions (e.g. pronation/supination or flexion/extension). When the Orthotron is used to measure isokinetic strength, the speed is set at either 2½ (30°/sec) or 3 (60°/sec).

**Table 20–5**   Recommended Speed Settings
for Isokinetic Muscle Testing (in Degrees/Second)*

| Joint Actions | Strength | Endurance and Power | |
|---|---|---|---|
| | | Nonathletes and Female Athletes | Male Athletes |
| Shoulder | | | |
| Extension/Flexion | 60° | 180° | 240° or 300° |
| Abduction/Adduction | 60° | 180° | 240° or 300° |
| Int./Ext. Rotation | 60° | 180° | 240° or 300° |
| Elbow | | | |
| Extension/Flexion | 60° | 180° | 240° |
| Forearm | | | |
| Pronation/Supination | 30° | 120° | 180° |
| Wrist | | | |
| Extension/Flexion | 30° | 120° | 180° |
| Hip | | | |
| Abduction/Adduction | 30° | 120° | 180° |
| Extension/Flexion | 30° | 120° | 180° |
| Int./Ext. Rotation | 30° | 120° | 180° |
| Knee | | | |
| Extension/Flexion | 60° | 180° | 240° |
| Tibial Rotation | 30° | 120° | 180° |
| Ankle | | | |
| Plantar/Dorsiflexion | 30° | 120° | 180° |
| Inversion/Eversion | 30° | 120° | 180° |

*From Cybex. 1980. Isolated Joint Testing and Exercise. Cybex. A division of Lumex, Inc., RonKonKoma, N.Y.

**Isokinetic Endurance Test Protocols**   To assess the isokinetic endurance of the muscle group, repetitive maximum effort trials are used. Endurance is measured as the number of successive repetitions performed before the torque reading decreases to 50% of the initial maximum torque value. The athlete with greater muscular endurance will be able to maintain torque levels above this level for a longer time, thereby completing a greater number of repetitions. Appropriate speed settings range between 120° and 180°/sec for nonathletes and female athletes and between 180° and 300°/sec for male athletes (Table 20–5).

**Isokinetic Power Test Protocols**   Power is a function of force and velocity and is measured by the maximum torque produced through the range of motion at a fast contractile velocity. The speed of movement varies between 120° and 300°/sec depending on the joint action and athletic classification of the individual. After two submaximum practice trials, the athlete is instructed to perform three maximum effort contractions in both directions (e.g. adduction/abduction). Power is measured as the peak torque (ft-lb or N-m) achieved in each direction of joint rotation. Alternatively, power can be measured using a digital work integrator that is attached in series to the Cybex II instrumentation system. This device integrates the area beneath the torque-time curve; thus, an accurate assessment of the total work accomplished during the movement is provided. In addition, power can be measured as the product of force and velocity using the following equation: $P = T \times V/57.29$; where $P =$ power (ft-lb), $T =$ torque; $V =$ speed of movement (°/sec), and 57.29 is a constant.

**Isokinetic Norms**   Performance norms have not been established to evaluate isokinetic strength, endurance, and power of athletes. Meaningful comparisons of means and standard deviations reported in the literature for maximum torque, endurance, and power output are not readily made, since standardized testing procedures concerning the velocity of the movement, limb position, and muscle group tested, were not always followed. In general, the following observations are warranted based on data reported in the literature:

1. The overall isokinetic strength, as measured by the maximum torque produced during isokinetic bench press and leg press exercises, is significantly greater for men than for women, even when differences in body size are controlled statistically. This is predominantly due a difference in upper body strength rather than lower body strength (Hoffman et al. [16]).

2. The isokinetic bench press and leg press strength of men is significantly greater than that of women athletes (basketball and volleyball), even when differences in body size are statistically controlled (Morrow and Hosler [17]).

3. Isokinetic strength decreases as the speed of movement (0° to 300°/sec) increases for normal, healthy men (Lesmes et al. [13]; Scudder [14]), habitually active men (Thorstensson et al. [15]), competitive male athletes (Coyle et al. [11]; Thorstensson et al. [18]), and competitive female athletes (Gregor et al. [12]).

4. Isokinetic power, measured as the product of maximum torque and angular velocity, increases as the speed of joint rotation increases for normal, healthy men and women (Perrine and Edgerton [19], and male and female athletes (Coyle et al. [11]; Gregor et al. [12]).

5. The rate of decline in torque production during an isokinetic endurance test is directly related to the initial isokinetic strength (Clarkson et al. [20]; Patton et al. [21]). In other words, high-strength individuals tend to have less isokinetic endurance (a faster rate of fatigue and greater loss of strength) than low-strength individuals.

# Muscle Fiber Types and Performance

In humans, two distinct fiber types have been identified based on contractile characteristics and histochemical myofibrillar ATPase activity of skeletal muscle. Fast-twitch (FT) fibers have a faster contraction time, higher force production capability, greater anaerobic capacity, and a more rapid rate of fatigue than slow-twitch (ST) fibers. Thus, FT fibers are highly recruited in and better suited for strength and power performances. ST fibers, on the other hand, have a greater aerobic capacity, slower contraction time, and a slower rate of fatigue, making them well-suited for endurance activities (Gregor et al. [12]; Thorstensson et al. [18]); Prince et al. [22]; Clarkson et al. [23]; Costill et al. [24, 25]; Dons et al. [26]; Gollnick et al. [27]; Komi et al. [28]).

When muscle fibers are classified on the basis of both myofibrillar ATPase and SDH activities, three fiber types are identified: 1) fast-twitch-glycolytic (FG), 2) fast-twitch-oxidative-glycolytic (FOG), and 3) slow-twitch-oxidative (SO) (Prince et al. [22]). The FOG fiber is an intermediate fiber type. It has an oxidative capacity that is greater than that of the FG fiber but less than that of the SO fiber. However, the contractile characteristics of the FOG are similar to that of the FG fiber.

In many research laboratories, muscle biopsies are taken routinely as a part of the athlete's physiological profile. Data indicate that there is a tendency for strength and power athletes, such as weightlifters, sprinters, and jumpers, to have a predominance of FT fibers. Endurance athletes such as long-distance runners and cross-country skiers tend to have a greater percentage of ST fibers. There is, however variability in fiber type between athletes within a given sport or event (Prince et al. [22]; Edstrom and Ekblom [29]), as well as intraindividual variation in the muscle groups of each athlete (Clarkson et al. [23]).

These observations have stimulated research into muscle fiber type and sports performance in an attempt to predict an athlete's potential for a given sport. These efforts have focused on 1) the degree to which fiber type distribution is genetically determined, 2) the influence of aerobic training and weight training on fiber type distribution, relative fiber size (FT/ST ratio), and muscle metabolism of fiber types, 3) the importance of fiber type and size to the strength, muscular endurance, and power capabilities of the athlete, and 4) the prediction of fiber type composition from physical performance measures.

## Influence of Heredity and Training on Fiber Type

Results of research indicate that fiber type distribution is genetically determined. For males and females, respectively, heredity accounts for 99.5% and 92.5% of the variability in fiber type (Komi et al. [30]). It also has been confirmed that the percent fiber distribution does not change as a result of endurance, anaerobic, or weight training (Costill et al. [25]; Dons et al. [26]; Gollnick et al. [31]). Although FT to ST fiber interconversions cannot occur, data suggest that interconversions within FT fibers are possible due to weight training (FOG to FG conversion) and aerobic endurance training (FG to FOG conversion) (Prince et al. [22]).

With regard to fiber size, there is evidence that supports the selective hypertrophy of FT fibers due to weight training (Prince et al. [22]; Costill et al. [25]; Thorstensson et al. [32]). In addition, comparisons of relative size of FT and ST fibers of power and endurance athletes show that power athletes tend to have a greater relative size of the FT fibers. The FT fibers of endurance athletes are smaller, while the ST fiber size of endurance athletes is similar to that of power athletes (Gregor et al. [12]; Clarkson et al. [23]; Edstrom and Ekblom [29]. This same trend has been observed for both male and female athletes, although the size of the ST fibers relative to FT fibers tends to be greater for females than for males (Gregor et al. [12]).

## Relationship of Fiber Type to Muscular Performance

The importance of fiber type to muscular performance has been studied extensively. The following summary is based on a review of research dealing with the relationship of fiber type to strength, muscular endurance, and power.

It has been noted that the percentage of FT fiber distribution is not significantly related to the static (isometric) strength of the knee extensors (Gregor et al. [12]; Thorstensson et al. [15]; Clarkson et al. [20, 33]; Dons et al. [26]). Komi et al. [28], however, observed a statistically significant but low correlation (r = .38) between percentage of FT fibers and relative, static leg strength. Clarkson et al. [23] concluded that the relationship of fiber type and static strength depends on the muscle group studied and the type of athlete. They reported that the correlation between percentage of ST fibers in the vastus lateralis and static knee extensor strength was significant for power athletes (r = .80) but not significant for endurance athletes (r = .63). In contrast, the percentage of ST fibers in the gastrocnemius was noted to be negatively related to the static strength of the ankle plantar flexors for power athletes (r = − .94).

Percent fiber distribution is not related to dynamic strength (1-RM) of the knee extensors (Dons et al. [26]). However, Dons et al. reported after 7 weeks of strength training, the correlation between the increase in strength per unit of cross section of the muscle and the percentage of FT fibers was r = .80.

A number of investigators have reported significant correlations between percentage of fiber type and isokinetic strength, especially for high speeds of movement (Coyle et al. [11]; Thorstensson et al. [15, 18]; Nilsson et al. [34]). These correlations range between .44 and .81. Gregor et al. [12] compared the isokinetic strength of the knee extensors at three different speeds of movement. National caliber, female track and field athletes were divided into two groups, those having greater than or less than 50% ST fiber distribution in the vastus lateralis. Gregor et al. [12] noted that the maximum torque of the > 50% ST group was significantly less than that of the < 50% ST group at all speeds of movement (96°, 192°, and 288°/sec). In addition, the relative fiber size (FT/ST area) was significantly related to torque production at all three speeds. Thorstensson et al. [15] also observed that the maximum speed of isokinetic contraction was significantly related to percentage of FT distribution (r = .50) and to relative area of FT fibers (r = .50).

When field tests such as the Margaria Leg Power Test and the Sargent Jump Test are used to assess power, dynamic leg power is not related to percentage of fiber type (Komi et al. [28]; Komi and Karlsson [35]; Campbell et al. [36]). On the other hand, Nilsson et al. [34] noted that percentage of FT fibers was significantly related to isokinetic power assessed as the work per unit of time. Likewise, Coyle et al. [11] reported that the isokinetic power, measured as relative peak torque, was significantly greater for the FT group (> 50% FT) than for the ST group (< 50% FT) at velocities of 115°, 200°, 287°, and 400°/sec.

There has been little work done on the influence of fiber type on static and dynamic muscular endurance. In one study, Dons et al. [26] observed that percentage of fiber distribution was not related to performance on a variety of tests used to assess static and dynamic muscular endurance of the knee extensors. Clarkson et al. [37] reported that a higher percentage of ST fibers was associated with a slower rate of fatigue during static exercise of the plantar flexors of endurance and power athletes. The authors were unable, however, to demonstrate a similar relationship for the knee extensors. In isokinetic exercise, a higher percentage of FT fibers appears to be linked to a faster rate of fatigue and less isokinetic endurance (Thorstensson and Karlsson [38]).

Significant correlations between percentage of FT fibers and relative decline in peak torque (r = .75), work (r = .64), and power (r = .73) have been reported for knee extensors (Nilsson et al. [34]). In contrast, Clarkson et al. [20] were unable to support

**Table 20–6**    Sources for Muscle Testing Equipment

| Product | Manufacturer's Address |
| --- | --- |
| Cable Tensiometer<br>(static) | Pacific Scientific Co. Inc.<br>Anaheim, CA 92803 |
| CAM II<br>(variable resistance) | Keiser<br>1603 E St.<br>Fresno, CA 93706 |
| Cybex II, Orthotron<br>(isokinetic) | Cybex<br>2100 Smithtown Ave.<br>Ronkonkoma, NY 11779 |
| Free Weights<br>(constant resistance) | York Barbell Co.<br>Box 1707<br>York, PA 17405 |
| Handgrip Dynamometer<br>(static) | C. H. Stoelting Co.<br>424 North Homan Ave.<br>Chicago, IL 60624 |
| Hydra-gym<br>(variable resistance) | Hydra-gym Athletics Inc.<br>2121 Industrial Rd.<br>Belton, TX 76513 |
| Leg/Back Dynamometer<br>(static) | Nissen Corp.<br>Cedar Rapids, IA 52406 |
| Mini-Gym<br>(isokinetic) | Mini Gym Inc.<br>P.O. Box 266<br>Independence, MO 64051 |
| Nautilus<br>(variable resistance) | Sports/Medical Industries<br>P.O. Box 1783<br>DeLand, FL 32720 |
| Total Gym<br>(variable resistance) | Total Medical Systems<br>7161 Engineer Rd.<br>San Diego, CA 92111 |
| Universal Gym Machine<br>(constant and variable<br>resistance) | Kidde<br>Box 1270<br>Cedar Rapids, IA 52406 |
| Versa-Gym<br>(constant resistance) | Versatile Fitness Equipment. Inc.<br>798 Holbrook Ave.<br>Simi Valley, CA 93065 |

those observations. The authors suggested that the lack of relationship between fiber type and isokinetic endurance was most likely due to the limited sample size used in their study ($N = 8$).

## Prediction of Muscle Fiber Type

The ability to predict muscle fiber composition from performance measures would eliminate the need for muscle biopsies; and, the trauma and expense of the procedure could be avoided. To date, however, researchers have been unsuccessful in predicting fiber type from performance measures such as bicycle ergometer power tests, Sargent Jump Test, and $\dot{V}O_{2max}$ tests (Campbell et al. [36]).

# Problems Associated with Muscle Testing

A number of factors can influence the measurement of strength, muscular endurance, and power. Each of these factors, listed below, should be controlled to insure valid, reliable, and objective assessments of muscle function whenever possible.

1. No single test can be used to assess overall strength, muscular endurance, or power. These factors are highly specific to the muscle group, type of muscular contraction (static, dynamic, or isokinetic), the limb position, joint angle tested during static tests, and the speed of movement during isokinetic tests. To evaluate a specific muscle function, it is recommended that a test be selected that matches the requirements of the performance. For example, in high jumping, the coach or trainer should assess the dynamic strength and power of the hip, knee, and ankle extensor muscle groups of the take-off leg, using patterns and speeds of movement that closely simulate those used during the high-jumping performance.
2. To assess total body strength, a minimum of three measures should be taken, due to the highly specific nature of strength. The test battery should include measures of abdominal, upper body, and lower body strength.
3. Strength and power measurements are influenced by body size and body composition. These scores, therefore, should be expressed in relative, as well as absolute terms. The performance should be evaluated relative to lean body weight or total body weight, especially if between-group comparisons (e.g. male versus female athletes or football versus basketball players) are to be made.
4. Absolute measures of muscular endurance are dependent on the strength of the individual. Therefore, it is recommended that tests that are proportional to maximum strength or to lean body weight of the athlete be used to assess muscular endurance.
5. When administering strength, muscular endurance, and power tests, standardized procedures should be followed. Factors such as body position of the athlete, joint angle, speed of movement, number of practice and performance trials, and the way in which the function is measured (best trial versus average of trials) should be noted.

6. Strength, muscular endurance, and power tests require maximum effort on the part of the athlete. Therefore, factors that influence maximum performance need to be controlled. These include time of day of testing, sex of the experimenter and subject, temperature, humidity, altitude, sleep, drug usage, and motivation of the subject. To control motivation, each subject should be treated in a similar manner by the experimenter. This means that the instructions, verbal encouragement given during the test, and knowledge of results given either during or after the test should be standardized.

7. Assessing the athlete's potential for a given sport or event is hampered by a lack of performance norms. Strength, muscular endurance, and power norms need to be established for male and female athletes in all sports.

# References

1. Kreigbaum, E., Barthels, K.M. 1981. Biomechanics: A Qualitative Approach for Studying Human Movement. Burgess Publishing Co., Minneapolis.

2. Montoye, H.J., Faulkner, J.A. 1964. Determination of the optimum setting of an adjustable grip dynamometer. Res Q 35:29–36.

3. Clarke, H.H., Clarke, D.H. 1963. Developmental and Adapted Physical Education. Prentice-Hall, Englewood Cliffs, N.J.

4. Clarke, D.H. 1975. Exercise Physiology. Prentice-Hall, Englewood Cliffs, N.J.

5. Clarke, H.H., Monroe, R.A. 1970. Test Manual: Oregon Cable Tension Strength Test Batteries for Boys and Girls from Fourth Grade Through College. University of Oregon, Eugene.

6. Pollack, M.L., Wilmore, J.H., Fox, S.M.III. 1978. Health and Fitness Through Physical Activity. John Wiley & Sons, New York.

7. Considine, W.J. 1971. A validity analysis of selected leg power tests, utilizing a force platform. In: Copper, J.M., (ed): Biomechanics. The Athletic Press, Chicago, pp 243–249.

8. Wilmore, J.H. 1982. Training for Sport and Activity: The Physiological Basis of the Conditioning Process. Allyn and Bacon, Boston.

9. Margaria, R., Aghemo, I., Rovelli, E. 1966. Measurement of muscular power (anaerobic) in man. J Appl Physiol 21:1662–1664.

10. Kalamen, J. 1968. Measurement of maximal muscular power in man. Unpublished doctoral dissertation, Ohio State University, Columbus.

11. Coyle, E.F., Costill, D.L., Lesmes, G.R. 1979. Leg extension power and muscle fiber composition. Med Sci Sports 11:12–15.

12. Gregor, R.J., Edgerton, V.R., Perrine, J.J., Campion, D.S., DeBus, C. 1979. Torque-velocity relationships and muscle fiber composition in elite female athletes. J Appl Physiol 47:388–392.

13. Lesmes, G.R., Costill, D.L., Coyle, E.F., Fink, W.J. 1978. Muscle strength and power changes during maximal isokinetic training. Med Sci Sports 10:266–269.

14. Scudder, G.N. 1980. Torque curves produced at the knee during isometric and isokinetic exercise. Arch Phys Med Rehabil 61:68–73.

15. Thorstensson, A., Grimby, G., Karlsson, J. 1976. Force-velocity relations and fiber composition in human knee extensor muscles. J Appl Physiol 40:12–16.

16. Hoffman, T., Stauffer, R.W., Jackson, A.S. 1979. Sex differences in strength. Am J Sports Med 7:265–267.

17. Morrow, J.R., Hosler, W.W. 1981. Strength comparisons in untrained men and trained women athletes. Med Sci Sports Exerc 13:194–198.

18. Thorstensson, A., Larsson, L., Tesch, P., Karlsson, J. 1977. Muscle strength and fiber composition in athletes and sedentary men. Med Sci Sports 9:26–30.

19. Perrine, J.J., Edgerton, V.R. 1978. Muscle force-velocity and power-velocity relationships under isokinetic loading. Med Sci Sports 10:159–166.

20. Clarkson, P.M., Johnson, J., Dextradeur, D., Leszczynski, W., Wai, J., Melchionda, A. 1982. The relationships among isokinetic endurance, initial strength level, and fiber type. Res Q Exerc Sport 53:15–19.

21. Patton, R.W., Hinson, M.M., Arnold, B.R., Lessard, B. 1978. Fatigue curves of isokinetic contractions. Arch Phys Med Rehabil 59:507–509.

22. Prince, F.P., Hikida, R.S., Hagerman, F.C. 1976. Human muscle fiber types in power lifters, distance runners and untrained subjects. Pflügers Arch 363:19–26.

23. Clarkson, P.M., Kroll, W., McBride, T.C. 1980. Maximal isometric strength and fiber type composition in power and endurance athletes. Eur J Appl Physiol 44:35–42.

24. Costill, D.L., Daniels, J., Evans, W., Fink, W., Krahenbuhl, G., Saltin, B. 1976. Skeletal muscle enzymes and fiber composition in male and female track athletes. J Appl Physiol 40:149–154.

25. Costill, D.L., Coyle, E.F., Fink, W.F., Lesmes, G.R., Witzmann, F.A. 1979. Adaptations in skeletal muscle following strength training. J Appl Physiol 46:96–99.

26. Dons, B., Bollerup, K., Bonde-Petersen, F., Hancke, S. 1979. The effect of weightlifting exercise related to muscle fiber composition and muscle cross-sectional area in humans. Eur J Appl Physiol 40:95–106.

27. Gollnick, P.D., Armstrong, R.B., Saubert, C.W., Piehl, K. Saltin, B. 1972. Enzyme activity and fiber composition in skeletal muscle of untrained and trained men. J Appl Physiol 33:312–319.

28. Komi, P.V., Rusko, H., Vos, J., Vihko, V. 1977. Anaerobic performance capacity in athletes. Acta Physiol Scand 100:107–114.

29. Edstrom, L., Ekblom, B. 1972. Differences in sizes of red and white muscle fibres in vastus lateralis of musculus quadriceps femoris of normal individuals and athletes. Relation to physical performance. Scand J Clin Lab Invest 30:175–181.

30. Komi, P., Vitasalo, J., Havu, M., Thorstensson, A., Sjödin, B., Karlsson, J. 1977. Skeletal muscle fibers and muscle enzyme activities in monozygous and dizygous twins of both sexes. Acta Physiol Scand 100:385–392.

31. Gollnick, P., Armstrong, R., Saltin, B. Saubert, C., Sembrowich, W., Shepard, R. 1973. Effect of training on enzyme activity and fiber composition of human skeletal muscle. J Appl Physiol 34:107–111.

32. Thorstensson, A., Hulten, B., vonDobeln, W., Karlsson, J. 1976. Effect of strength training on enzyme activities and fibre characteristics in human skeletal muscle. Acta Physiol Scand 96:392–398.

33. Clarkson, P.M., Kroll, W., Melchionda, A.M. 1981. Age, isometric strength, rate of tension development and fiber type composition. J Gerontol 36:648–653.

34. Nilsson, J., Tesch, P., Thorstensson, A. 1977. Fatigue and EMG of repeated fast voluntary contractions in man. Acta Physiol Scand 101:194–198.

35. Komi, P.V., Karlsson, J. 1978. Skeletal muscle fibre types, enzyme activities and physical performance in young males and females. Acta Physiol Scand 103:210–218.

36. Campbell, C.J., Bonen, A., Kirby, R.L., Belcastro, A.N. 1979. Muscle fiber composition and performance capacities of women. Med Sci Sports 11:260–265.

37. Clarkson, P.M., Kroll, W., McBride, T.C. 1980. Plantar flexion fatigue and muscle fiber type in power and endurance athletes. Med Sci Sports Exerc 12:262–267.

38. Thorstensson, A., Karlsson, J. 1976. Fatiguability and fibre composition of human skeletal muscle. Acta Physiol Scand 98:318–322.

Chapter 21

# Massage and Sports

by Carol A. Kresge

## Introduction

"Massage is a vital part of systematic training. It is a *must* in basic conditioning." Thus begins a 1979 article in *Track and Field News*; an accompanying article, by Bob Beeten, head of the United States Olympic Committee Sports Medicine program and a massage advocate, is entitled "But Not in U.S." (Nordqvist [1]). These articles aptly describe the state of massage in athletics here and abroad: Massage is extensively prescribed and researched in European countries, including those of the Communist bloc, while in the U.S., it was replaced for a long period by technologic aids and has only recently begun to reappear.

This chapter examines the role massage can play in the athlete's life. Basically, it can be an adjunct to training in three ways:

1. By enabling the athlete to recover from injury more rapidly and completely, with less likelihood of chronic problems
2. By maintaining muscles in their best state of relaxation, flexibility, and nutrition and
3. By reducing muscle soreness, enabling athletes to recover more quickly, and to train at a higher level, thus pushing back that fine line between maximum training and over-training.

An overview of the research of massage physiology as therapy is provided in this chapter, as well as the athletic implications of such research. The reader should note that "massage" throughout refers to the technique of Swedish massage (including effleurage, pétrissage, friction, and tapotement) as well as sustained pressure on trigger points, compression in the form of muscle pumping, and cross-fiber massage on specific points on injuries or entire muscle groups.

367

**Table 21–1**   Effects and Implications of Massage

| Organ or Tissue | Effects of Massage | Implications/Applications |
|---|---|---|
| Vascular system | Manually increases blood flow | Increases cellular nutrition |
| | Reflex vasodilation | Decreases edema |
| | Increases diameter and permeability of capillaries | Increases toxin removal |
| | | Decreases muscle soreness |
| | Increases RBC | Decreases pain |
| | Decreases blood pressure | Decreases muscle fatigue |
| | Increases systolic stroke volume | Increases work capability |
| | | Increases metabolism |
| | Decreases pulse | |
| Lymph | Manually empties | Decreases edema |
| | | Decreases tendency toward fibrosis |
| Muscular system | Relaxes | Increases flexibility |
| | Manually separates fibers | Decreases spasm |
| | Can stimulate contraction | Decreases undesired adhesions |
| | | Decreases pain |
| | | Increases body awareness |
| Skeletal system | Increases retention of nitrogen, sulphur, and phosphorous | Aids fracture healing |

## Physiology of Massage Therapy

The therapeutic value of massage lies in its numerous and combined physiologic effects. These effects and their implications, as they apply to the systems important to athletic activity, are outlined in Table 21-1.

## Circulatory Effects of Massage

Massage has been reported more effective than shortwave diathermy or ultrasound in removing $^{133}$Xe from muscles (Hansen and Kristensen [2]), but other investigators in similar experiments found no net increase in blood flow, and the increased disappearance rate of $^{133}$Xe from muscles was attributed to the mechanical emptying and refilling of vascular beds (Hovind and Nielsen [3]). Still other investigators (Wolfson [4]) reported a great initial increase in blood flow with massage, and then a decrease while the treatment was still in progress. The total volume was no greater, but more complete emptying occurred associated with greater influx of fresh blood, suggesting more frequent shorter duration massages are more beneficial.

Wakim et al. [5] found inconsistent increases in blood flow, but a definite decrease in edema in all subjects, indicating that perhaps the lymph plays a greater role in the physiologic effects of massage.

Bell [6] found that blood volume and flow doubled and did not begin to drop until 40 min. after completion of massage. This reported discrepancy between no lasting effect on circulation and a sustained increase is due to two different circulatory effects. The first is mechanical, or manual, pushing of venous blood. The second is reflex, and results from release of acetylcholine and histamines that cause sustained vasodilation (Scull [7]; Meagher and Boughton [8]).

Increased blood flow and systolic stroke volume, and decreased blood pressure and heart rate plus increased blood flow in the nontreated homologous limb have been reported in response to deep massage in athletes (Severini and Venerando [9]), suggesting possibilities for increasing blood flow through limbs in casts.

Wakim [10] cites other massage effects on circulation, including a study by Krogh that showed increased diameter and permeability of capillaries from mechanical stimulation. Experiments using "windows" in rabbit ears showed that massage increased the speed of circulating elements as well as the rate of exchange of substances between cells and circulating blood, thus improving metabolism (Wood [11]).

Massage raises red blood cell count temporarily (Scull [7]) by mobilizing stagnant blood cells in the splanchnic circulation rather than by increased production (Schneider and Havens [12]). This temporary increase in oxygen-carrying capacity supports increased metabolism.

## Lymph Flow

Massage is more effective than passive motion or electrical muscle stimulation in increasing the lymph flow (Ladd et al. [13]).

## Massage, Muscle Relaxation, and Performance

Massage has been shown to consistently relax muscles and increase flexibility (Nordschow and Bierman [14]), an effect achieved through generalized massage in which no special attention was given to specific tension areas palpable in 4 out of 5 normal subjects. Massage in a clinical setting tailored to an individual's tension areas should have an even more profound effect. The effect of muscle relaxation on performance is especially noteworthy when considering athletics:

> . . . the muscles of the back are kept at a tension beyond that required to hold the body in any plane, as judged by the fact that the reduction of this tension does not interfere with the function of the body, and indeed permits the performance of these functions with greater ease (Nordschow and Bierman [14]).

## Muscle Recovery and Efficiency

Massage of muscles tired from running or bicycle riding has been found to reduce recovery time, as shown by a faster decline in pulse rate and quicker recovery of muscle

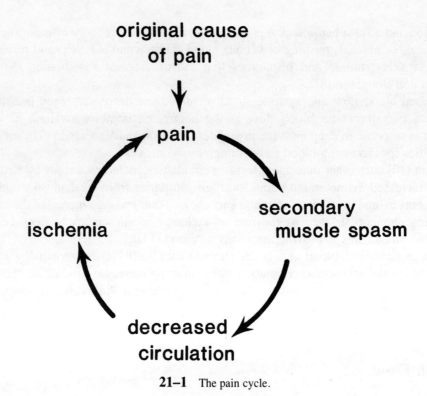

**21–1**    The pain cycle.

efficiency (Muller et al. [15]). Massage instead of usual rest periods enabled the subjects to almost triple their work capacity. At some point, inadequate "fuel" was thought to limit work. Quicker muscle recovery and greater work capacity were also achieved experimentally through massage by two other investigators (Wood [11]; Licht [16]).

## Skeletal System

Cuthbertson [17] showed that local massage in those with fractures of long bones increased significantly the retention of nitrogen, sulfur, and phosphorus necessary for tissue repair.

## Clinical vs. Experimental Results

It has been frequently noted that clinical results of massage are often more dramatic than experiments with massage would indicate. Massage, however, tends to have a cumulative effect that is not shown in short-term experiments. It is a science and an art combining a variety of strokes in infinite ways to best suit individual situations, while scientific experiments must employ standardized, repeatable procedures.

# Massage and the Injured Athlete

Massage can play an important role in the treatment of pain, edema, and decreased range of motion secondary to myofascial injury.

## Pain

Massage may be an effective treatment for pain that tends to create more pain regardless of its cause (Fig. 21-1). A painful stimulus results in reflex muscle contraction and localized muscle splinting or guarding, which restricts movement and local circulation. The subsequent ischemia creates more pain. Muscle splinting is intensified and the cycle repeats itself (Jacobs [18]).

Experimental production of localized pain results in a more generalized secondary pain as splinting and the pain cycle begin, and the secondary, more generalized pain may *outlast* or *exceed* the original discomfort (Jacobs [18]). Thus, it becomes important to treat the original cause and also the secondary muscle contraction. Massage effectively breaks the pain cycle by relaxing muscles (Nordschow and Bierman [14]), increasing circulation (Scull [7]; Wakim [10]), and removing metabolic wastes (Wakim [10]; Muller et al. [15]).

Anxiety and stress aggravate the secondary pain of muscle contraction (Jacobs [18]), and massage intervenes by promoting relaxation (Nordschow and Bierman [14]) and sense of well-being (Nordschow and Bierman [14]; Jacobs [18]).

## Edema

The localized swelling of soft-tissue injuries creates pain, pressure, stiffness, and impaired motion, and increases the tendency toward fibrosis (Scull [7]). It slows healing by reducing the metabolic circulation from the capillary across the interstitial space into the cell and back. As the distance from the cell to the capillaries is increased by excess extravascular fluid, diffusion time is increased by the square of the distance. Thus, with swelling doubling the distance, diffusion time is increased by four (Ladd et al. [13]). Massage is an effective means of reducing edema and thus speeding metabolic circulation.

## Compensation

Muscle splinting secondary to pain not only causes localized spasm, but may change the carriage of the body as a whole, resulting in distant compensatory problems. This is often the cause for chronic injuries in athletes who resume activity too soon with altered posture and create new areas of biomechanical stress. Massage can find and clear these areas before new injury occurs.

Limping, casting, and splinting likewise create compensatory muscle spasm in distant body parts. Foot casts create a functional long leg/short leg and may cause knee, hip, and lower back problems. These areas should be massaged while the cast is in place and afterward as gait and stance are changing.

## Healing

The effects of massage on injured muscles was studied by producing crushing injury to animal muscle followed by massage to one group and no treatment to another group (Wood [11]). Microscopic examination of the untreated muscle showed dissociation of the muscle fibers, hyperplasia, sometimes a swelling of the connective tissue, areas of increase in connective tissue nuclei, interstitial hemorrhages, and hyperplasia of adventitial layers of blood vessels. The sarcolemma was usually intact, but, in one section, increased interstitial nuclei gave the appearance of myositis. In the massaged limbs, muscle fibers appeared normal. Fibrous thickening of vessel walls was not seen, muscle bulk was greater, and there were no hemorrhages. Thus, massage seems to promote healing of injured tissued.

## Range of Motion

Early restoration of normal range of motion to an injured area is not only a therapeutic aim, but it is also excellent therapy. Motion decreases adhesion formation (Jacobs [18]), increases blood flow and nutrition to the area, and reduces healing time. Massage helps to increase range of motion by breaking the pain cycle and reducing edema. When active or passive motion is inappropriate, cross-fiber massage (Meagher and Boughton [8]; Cyriax [19, 20, 21]) can create the necessary movement.

## Cross Fiber Massage

Longitudinal scars that parallel muscle fibers interfere less with normal contraction and strength and are less subject to re-injury and chronic pain than are transverse scars which may cause adherence of adjacent fibers or of muscle fibers to bony structures (Cyriax [19]).

Adhesions between individual fibers limit contraction. Gross scarring across an entire muscle is often asymptomatic once healed, since equal tension is present on all parts of the muscle as it contracts. However, random adhesions within a muscle can cause chronic pain because of the variations of tension during contraction in areas where normal tissue joins scar tissue.

To create strong scar tissue longitudinally and limit transverse adhesions, movement mimicking the muscle's normal use is most appropriate. This motion can be active

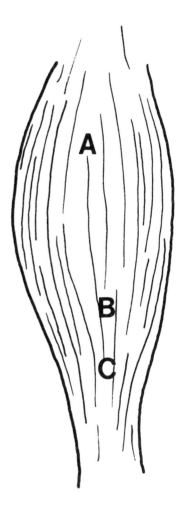

**21–2** The closer a muscle lesion is to an immobile structure, the less effective is movement or local anesthesia, and the more effective is cross fiber massage. A, B, and C refer to lesions nearing the joint. The lesion in C would best be treated by cross fiber massage. (Adapted from Cyriax [19]).

(nonweightbearing, weightbearing, or resisted), passive, or manual (as in deep cross-fiber massage).

During observation of scar tissue formation under the microscope, it was noted that the arrangement of fibrils was dependent upon mechanical factors, especially movement (Cyriax [19]). Thus, appropriate movement within the muscle as it is healing inhibits unwanted adhesion formation and creates a strong scar where it is needed.

Cross-fiber massage becomes a more important treatment modality the closer a muscle injury is to an immobile structure, since active movement is less effective in fiber spreading in this situation (see Fig. 21-2).

Muscle tears heal best with cross-fiber friction massage followed by active movement, initially in a relaxed, nonweight-bearing isometric contraction (Cyriax [20]).

When ligaments at joints under voluntary control are injured, i.e., ankle sprains, chronic reinjury occurs as adhesions form between the ligament and bone. This limits the proper motion of the ligament over the bone and during later strenuous use predisposes the ligament to chronic injury. Appropriate rehabilitation includes cross-fiber massage, manually moving the ligament over the bone followed by passive motion under local anesthesia (Cyriax [20]).

Tendons with sheaths are subjected to tenosynovitis, a roughening between the surface of the tendon and its sheath, caused by longitudinal friction. Appropriate treatment is cross-fiber transverse friction with the tendon held taut. In this instance, passive and active movement should be avoided, since motion creates the longitudinal friction that caused the tenosynovitis (Cyriax [20]).

Tendonitis in a sheathless tendon can also be treated with cross-fiber friction massage, although the mechanism of benefit in this situation is not as clearly understood (Cyriax [20]).

J. Cyriax, the orthopedic surgeon pioneering cross fiber massage, maintains that there are a number of lesions in which cross-fiber friction massage is the *only* effective means of treatment. These lesions include injury of the following (Cyriax [20, 21]):

1. subclavius belly
2. supraspinatus, musculotendinous junction
3. biceps brachii, longhead, belly, lower musculotendinous junction
4. brachialis or supinator belly
5. ligaments about carpal lunate bone
6. interosseous belly and tendon of hand
7. intercostal muscle
8. oblique muscles of abdomen
9. psoas, lower musculotendinous junction
10. quadriceps expansion at patella
11. coronary ligament at knee
12. medial collateral ligament in athletes
13. biceps femoris, lower musculotendinous junction
14. musculotendinous junction of anterior tibial
15. posterior or peroneal tibial
16. posterior tibiotalar ligament
17. tendo Achilles in athletes
18. anterior fascia of ankle joint
19. interosseous belly of foot

For deep cross-fiber friction massage to be effective, the exact lesion site must be massaged and the friction must be at right angles to the fibers. It must be of sufficient depth and range to reach and separate the fibers. This author's experience using cross-fiber massage supports Cyriax's claims: healing is rapid and appropriate.

## Trigger Point Massage

Many myofascial pain syndromes can be attributed to trigger points, especially in the lower back, neck, and shoulder, although referred trigger point pain is possible anywhere in the body. J. Travel initiated the research in trigger points and their treatment through procaine injection (Travel [22]; Weeks and Travel [23]). J. Meagher with sports massage [8] and B. Prudden with pain erasure [24] have popularized this work for the athlete and general public by substituting sustained pressure, compression, massage, and cross-fiber

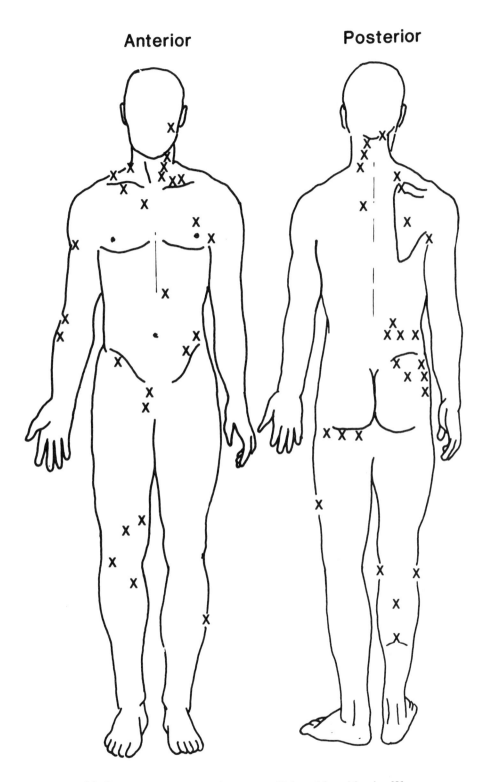

**21–3**    The most common trigger areas. (Adapted from Meagher [8]; Prudden [23]; and Bonica [25]).

massage on the points in place of injection. These massage techniques achieve comparable therapeutic results.

A trigger point is a small localized area of deep tenderness within a muscle. It is hypersensitive, with a lowered pain threshold (Bonica [25]; Travel [22]). Stimulation of the trigger point with mechanical pressure will elicit referred pain in the same remote area in different individuals. Thus, referred pain patterns are predictable and can be mapped and become easily recognized (Travel [22]).

This author's experience leads to the supposition that trigger points are primary or secondary causes of all myofascial pain. A trigger point mechanism may be suspected to be the primary cause of pain when there are no abnormal neurologic findings and when the pain distribution is neither segmental nor follows the peripheral nerve distribution (Bonica [25]). Even when neurologic findings are abnormal, trigger points may be a secondary cause and result in pain that outlasts the original pathology.

Many precipitating causes of trigger points are a part of everyday training for serious competitive and recreational athletes (Travel [22]; Weeks and Travel [23]; Bonica [25]). These include sudden trauma to muscle, tendon, ligament, and bone; unusual or excessive exercise; chilling; immobilization; and acute emotional stress. General fatigue, nutritional deficiencies, nervous tension, and chronic muscle strain produced by repetitive movements or poor posture predispose to precipitating causes of trigger points. To this list might be added muscular stiffness or lack of flexibility, and imbalances between antagonistic muscles.

An active trigger point may elicit enough pain to cause satellite trigger points to appear. Any intense pain can cause new trigger points. Once established, these points can be immediately activated and/or lie dormant to be reactivated only when any of the above factors are present. This has important implications for injury prevention (Meagher and Boughton [8]. If an athlete is kept free of trigger points through massage, the chances of injury can be decreased.

Trigger points usually arise in areas of greatest biomechanical stress. The extremes of repetition inherent in athletic activities (1600 steps per mile) or the one-sided nature of many athletic activities, such as racquetball, subject the athlete's body to greater than normal mechanical stresses. The nature of the sport, and the athlete's physical structure within that sport, define the most common injuries and likewise the most common trigger areas for each sport (see Fig. 21-3) (Meagher and Boughton [8]; Prudden [24]).

## Overuse Injury

Athletic injury not attributable to accident is usually thought to result from overuse. The correlation of overuse with high intensity, such as high mileage in the runner, is a misunderstanding of the term. Overuse is essentially too much, too soon, when the body structures have not adapted to the stresses placed on them. Like massage, appropriate training is both a science and an art, which includes learning to individually recognize the fine line between appropriate stress and adequate time for adaptation, which builds an athlete's body, and excess stress with inadequate adaptation time, which breaks down tissue. Thus, overuse is not a cause of injury solely in athletes training at a high intensity. A study by Pagliano and Jackson [26] indicated that it was the low mileage runner who

**Table 21–2**   Weekly Distance of Injured Runners

| Weekly Distance | % of Injured Runners |
| --- | --- |
| 0–20 miles | 48% |
| 20–40 miles | 32% |
| 40–60 miles | 13% |
| 60–80 miles | 5% |
| 80 + miles | 2% |

most frequently sought injury evaluation and treatment (see Table 21-2). This may be because less experienced runners lack understanding of training principles and body awareness. Massage enhances body awareness by "tuning-in" the person to each part of his or her body. Those who are unaccustomed to massage usually comment that areas of soreness and tension exist that they were unaware of. Massage can aid in overuse injury prevention by making the person recognize problem areas and helping to alleviate them before they become serious.

# Massage and the Healthy Athlete

Massage for the healthy athlete prevents injury and improves function.

## Muscle Soreness

Muscle soreness is a part of all athletic life. It arises when activity level is increased or activity is begun after an inactive lifestyle, when greater than usual effort is expended, or when activities utilize muscle groups in unaccustomed ways. Three theories exist concerning the cause of muscle soreness (Abraham [27]), and each probably plays a greater or lesser role depending on the situation. First is the spasm, metabolic waste theory, which holds that repeated strenuous activity overworks certain muscles, causing accumulation of metabolic wastes such as lactic acid that, in turn, affect muscle fiber osmotic pressure, water retention, and pressure. The wastes irritate nerve endings resulting in pain, muscle contraction, and ischemia.

The second theory, the torn tissue hypothesis, suggests that untrained muscles worked for prolonged periods are especially susceptible to minute tears. Likewise, when metabolic wastes accumulate, muscle strength decreases and continued activity results in small tears in muscle fibers.

The third and most recent theory concerns connective tissue irritation, especially noted with eccentric, negative work, and associated with an increased inflammatory response in muscle components.

Massage can positively affect each of the above processes by increasing circulation, lymph flow, and relaxing muscles. It has been shown that massage is more effective than rest in removing the metabolic wastes produced by exercise (Muller et al. [15]). Massage is especially effective if administered shortly after the strenuous effort, although it decreases soreness at all stages. Athletes have noted that given an equal effort, recovery was greatly enhanced by massage.

## Training Level

Training is based on repeated stressing of the system through specific overload, alternating with recovery and adaptation periods. Adaptation, and thus training, increase in a manner proportionate to the stress applied until maximum stress tolerance is reached, at which point the system begins to break down, causing stress or overuse injuries, fatigue, and decreased performance. Thus, establishing an optimum training program means continually reestablishing a delicate balance.

Massage can help an athlete become aware of and maintain balances between optimum training and overtraining. Massage decreases muscle soreness, and enables muscles to recover from work more rapidly and to perform more work or train at a higher level (Muller et al. [15]). Massage also identifies areas of tension and trigger points and relieves these, making the athlete more flexible, able to perform more easily, and less prone to injury (Meagher and Boughton [8]). Top-class European athletes will not train without regular massage, and attribute the level of training they can handle to the use of massage (Nordqvist [1]).

## Performance Improvement

Experiments concerning the effects of massage on performance have been contradictory. In one study, massage was shown to improve performance of both men and women in swimming 50 m, running 100 m, and riding the bicycle ergometer (Karpovich and Hale [28]). Other studies cited by Karpovich and Hale [28], however, found no effect on performance with massage; these were single experimental situations with standardized massage procedures. The effect of massage on performance, however, is cumulative and should be a regular part of athletic training individually designed for each athlete. With the use of cross-fiber massage and compression on trigger points, it has been said that one may improve performance, endurance, and athletic "lifetime" (Meagher and Boughton [8]).

Muscles work in antagonistic pairs: one pair must relax while the other contracts. Excess tension requires more work from the contracting muscle to overcome the resistance of its antagonist, resulting in loss of power, performance, and coordination (Meagher and Boughton [8]). The body is maintained at a tension level that affects ease of performance. Massage through muscle relaxation and relief of trigger points can reduce this tension and resistance (Nordschow and Bierman [14]).

# Injury Prevention

Prevention of injury is hard to document. Massage may help prevent injury by maintaining muscles in the best state of relaxation, flexibility, and nutrition, and by rapid removal of metabolic wastes. It may furthermore help by finding and alleviating problem areas before they become serious. Finally, it can help reduce chronic or repeated injury by aiding in appropriate healing, as discussed previously.

# References

1. Nordqvist, H. 1979. Massage: A training must. Track and Field News 32(5):50–51.
2. Hansen, T. I., Kristensen, J. H. 1973. Effect of massage, shortwave diathermy and ultrasound on the $^{133}$Xe disappearance rate from muscle and subcutaneous tissue in the human calf. Scand J Rehab Med 5:179–182.
3. Hovind, H., Nielsen, S. L. 1973. The influence of massage on circulation in muscles. Ugeskr Laeger 135(39):2090–2092.
4. Wolfson, H. 1931. Studies on the effect of physical therapeutic procedures on function and structure. JAMA 96:2019–2021.
5. Wakim, K. G., Martin, G. M., Krusen, F. H. 1955. Influence of centripetal rhythmic compression on localized edema of extremities. Arch Phys Med 36:98–103.
6. Bell, A. J. 1964. Massage and the physiotherapist. Physiotherapy 50:406–408.
7. Scull, C. W. 1945. Massage-physiologic basis. Arch Phys Med 26:159–167.
8. Meagher, J., Boughton, P. 1980. Sportsmassage. Dolphin Books, Doubleday and Co., New York.
9. Severini, V., Venerando, A. 1967. Physiological effects of massage on the cardiovascular system. Europa Medicophysica 3:165–183.
10. Wakim, K. G. 1980. Physiologic effects of massage. In: Rogoff, J. B., (ed): Manipulations, Traction and Massage, 2nd Ed. Williams & Wilkins Co., Baltimore.
11. Wood, E. 1974. Beard's Massage: Principles and Techniques. W. B. Saunders Co., Philadelphia.
12. Schneider, E. C., Havens, L. C. 1915. Changes in the blood after muscular activity and during training. Am J Phys 36:239–259.
13. Ladd, M. P., Kottke, F. J., Blanchard, R. S. 1952. Studies on the effect of massage on the flow of lymph from the foreleg of a dog. Arch Phys Med 33:604–612.
14. Nordschow, M., Bierman, W. 1962. Influence of manual massage on muscle relaxation: Effect on trunk flexion. J Am Phys Ther Assoc. 42:10:653–657.
15. Müller, E. A. et al. 1966. The effect of massage on the efficiency of muscles. Int Z Angew Physiol 22:240–257.
16. Licht, S. 1960. Massage, anipulation and Traction. Physical Medicine Library, Vol. 5. Williams & Wilkins Co., Baltimore.
17. Cuthbertson, D. P. 1933. Effect of massage on metabolism: a survey. Glasgow Med J (7th Ed) 2:200–213.
18. Jacobs, M. 1960. Massage for the relief of pain: Anatomical and physiological considerations. Phys Ther Rev 40:2:93–98.
19. Cyriax, J. 1977. Textbook of Orthopoedic Medicine, Vol. 2). Treatment by Manipulation, Massage, and Injection. Ballière Tindall, London.
20. Cyriax, J. 1980. Clinical applications of massage. In: Rogoff, J. B., (ed.): Manipulations, Traction and Massage, 2nd Ed. Rehab Med Lib, Williams & Wilkins Co., Baltimore, pp 152–169.

21. Cyriax, J. 1977. Deep massage. Physiotherapy 63:2:60–61.
22. Travel, J. 1955. Referred pain from skeletal muscle. N Y State J Med 55(2):331–340.
23. Weeks, V. D., Travel, J. 1955. Postural vertigo due to trigger areas in the sterno-cleido-mastoid muscle. J Pediatr 47:315–327.
24. Prudden, B. 1980. Pain erasure. Ballantine Books, New York.
25. Bonica, J. J. 1959. The management of myofascial pain syndromes. Phys Ther Rev 39:6:389–395.
26. Pagliano, J., Jackson, D. 1980. The ultimate study of running injuries. Runner's World 42–50.
27. Abraham, W. M. 1979. Exercise-induced muscle soreness. Phys Sportsmed 7:10:57–60.
28. Karpovich, P. V., Hale, C. J. 1956. Effect of warming-up upon physical performance. JAMA 162:12:1117–1119.

# Chapter 22

# Stretching and Sports[1]

## by Bob Anderson

Few people stretch correctly. Stretching is generally thought of as a form of exercise, and is therefore subject to negative "exercise" jargon such as "the more it hurts, the better it is," or "no gain without pain." Only injuries and pain result from such a stretching philosophy, however.

Correct stretching is not exercise involving rhythmic extensions and contractions of muscles as in walking, running, swimming, hiking, and so on. It involves holding a comfortable stretched position for various lengths of time. There should be no bouncing or bobbing up or down or other movement. When stretching correctly, one is almost as still as a statue.

# The Tendency to Overstretch

Most people stretch with the intention of becoming more "flexible." They therefore stretch as far as possible and, in so doing, constantly overstretch. This tightens the very muscles that they intend to stretch and causes microscopic tears of involved tissues and scar formation. As scars are nonelastic, muscle elasticity is therefore reduced, contributing to muscle pain. Muscle fibers replaced with nonelastic, dense scar tissue interfere with normal blood flow and disturb afferent nerve input, thereby leaving the intact muscle fibers and surrounding connective tissues vulnerable to further injury—a vicious cycle

[1]Illustrations (by Jean E. Anderson) and text of exercises contained in this chapter are excerpted, with permission, from various *Stretching Charts,* © 1979-82 by Bob and Jean Anderson (Stretching Inc., P.O. Box 767, Palmer Lake, CO 80133) and the book *Stretching,* © 1980 by Bob Anderson (Shelter Publications, distributed by Random House, Inc.). No part may be reproduced in any form without prior written approval of both the author and the publisher.

that is repeated each time overstretching occurs. Specifically, overstretching activates the stretch reflex, a monosynaptic reflex response that causes contraction of the muscle(s) that were intended to be stretched. Thus, when a person stretches too far, he or she defeats the purpose of the stretch. It bears repeating: *All overstretching is useless and injurious*.

# Stretching Correctly

When one stretches correctly, on the other hand, the stretch reflex is not activated and muscle tissues are not harmed. Proper stretching elongates the muscles slowly to a point where *mild* tension is felt. For an easy stretch, the elongated position is held 10-30 secs, during which time the subject should not experience discomfort. The longer the easy stretch is held, the less it is felt. If the stretched feeling grows in intensity as the position is maintained, one is overstretching and should ease off into a more comfortable position. The easy stretch is important because it reduces muscle tension, maintains flexibility, and reduces or prevents soreness. The easy stretch does not activate the stretch reflex mechanism and should precede more vigorous stretching to increase flexibility.

After the easy stretch, a fraction of an inch more stretch may be added until a mild increase in tension is felt. This is the *developmental stretch,* which is held for 10-30 secs and should not be painful or increase in intensity. Increasing tension or pain indicates overstretching and stretch reflex activation. If this occurs, ease off slightly into a more comfortable position. If done correctly, the developmental stretch safely increases flexibility, reduces tension, and increases circulation to the stretched muscles.

This basic method of stretching can be learned regardless of age or flexibility. It is based on the ''feel'' method, which should be followed each time a person stretches. It allows one to adjust to daily fluctuations in muscle tension that affect flexibility.

Many people lose muscle elasticity, which adversely affects normal resting muscle length. This happens when the body assumes rigid, fixed positions, such as during sitting or standing for long periods of time and often resulting in muscle pain and excess tension. ''Creeping rigor mortis,'' a slow, but continuous loss of flexibility over the years, describes this condition.

With the gradual loss in flexibility, our muscles become tighter, and we are less able to accomplish things we once did with ease. It has been said that we start losing flexibility by age 8. If this is true, then stretching should be taught in elementary school.

# Preventive Stretching

Stretching is important in preventing muscular injuries, but unless a person has been injured, the motivation for stretching often does not exist. Enthusiasm for stretching usually comes after an injury and is maintained thereafter in an attempt to ward off further injury.

Preventive stretching combines the following:

1. Proper stretch and adequate warm up
2. Regular strength activity
3. Aerobic conditioning through running, swimming, cycling, rope skipping, etc.
4. Proper rest (rest when you are tired)
5. Avoid over-training (understand the law of diminishing returns)
6. Gradual increase in intensity and duration of exercise
7. Plenty of liquid throughout each day (preferably cool, refreshing water)
8. Maintenance of proper body weight
9. Joyful attitude toward physical activity

Stretching after exercise is very important. Slight injuries can be detected during stretching by tightness or soreness of one muscle or another.

Ideally, stretching should be used in conjunction with weight training. Gently stretch the muscles to be used beforehand. Then load them and repeat the stretch. This gives better strength without loss of flexibility. The stretches should be held comfortably; there is absolutely no reason for straining.

This chapter describes 26 basic stretches; regular practice of 8 to 10 stretches, however, is enough to maintain flexibility. Since, as was stated, flexibility diminishes with age, maintaining one's current flexibility is the first goal of proper stretching.

The importance of not overstretching and of relaxing the muscles not being stretched cannot be over emphasized. Learning by doing is the best method: you learn to stretch by stretching.

# Hamstring and Quadriceps Stretches

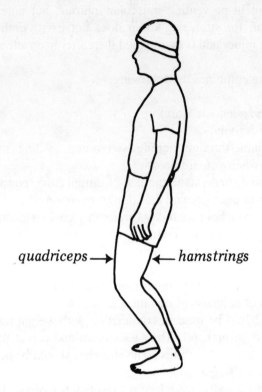

quadriceps →        ← hamstrings

Begin in this bent-knee position. This position contracts the quadriceps and relaxes the hamstrings. Hold for 30 sec. The primary function of the quadriceps is to straighten the leg. The basic function of the hamstrings is to bend the knee. Because these muscles have opposing actions, tightening the quadriceps will relax the hamstrings.

Now, as you hold this bent-knee position, feel the difference between the front of the thigh and the back of the thigh. The quadriceps should feel hard and tight while the hamstrings should feel soft and relaxed.

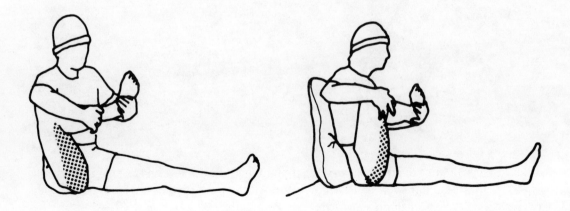

To stretch the upper hamstrings and hip (bottom of page 384), hold on to the outside of your ankle with one hand, with your other hand and forearm around your bent knee. Gently pull the leg *as one unit* toward your chest until you feel an easy stretch in the back of the upper leg. You may want to do this stretch while you rest your back against something for support. Hold for 30 sec. Make sure the leg is pulled as one unit so that no stress is felt in the knee.

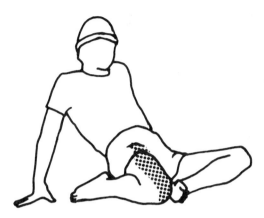

Sit with your right leg bent, with your right heel just to the outside of your right hip. The left leg is bent and the sole of your left foot is next to the inside of your upper right leg. (Try not to let your right foot flare out to the side in this position.) Now slowly lean straight back until you feel an easy stretch in your right quadriceps. Use hands for balance and support. Hold an easy stretch for 30 sec. Do not hold any stretches that are painful to the knee.

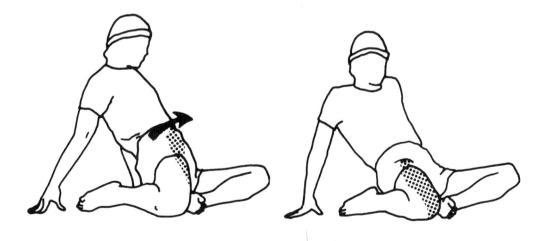

After stretching your quadriceps, practice tightening the buttocks on the side of the bent leg as you turn the hip over. This will help stretch the front of your hip and give a better overall stretch to upper thigh area. After contracting the buttocks muscles for 5–8 sec, let the buttocks relax. Then continue to stretch quad for another 15 sec.

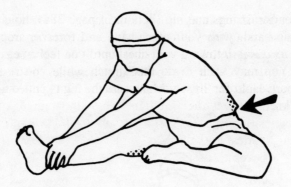

Next, straighten your right leg. The sole of your left foot will be resting next to the inside of your straightened leg. Lean slightly forward *from the hips* and stretch the hamstrings of your right leg. Find an easy stretch and relax. If you cannot touch your toes comfortably, use a towel to help you stretch. Hold for 50 sec. Do not lock your knee. Your right quadriceps should be soft and relaxed during the stretch. Keep your right foot upright with the ankle and toes relaxed.

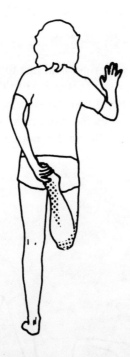

Opposite hand to opposite foot—quadriceps and knee stretch. Grab top of right foot (from inside of foot) with left hand and gently pull, heel moving toward buttocks. The knee bends at a natural angle in this position and creates a good stretch in knee and quad. Especially good if you have had trouble or feel pain stretching in the hurdle stretch position leaning back, or when pulling the right heel to buttock with the right (same) hand. Pulling opposite hand to opposite foot does not create any adverse angles in the knee and is especially good in knee rehabilitation and with problem knees. Hold for 30 sec. Do both legs.

Hamstring pain after injury may last a long time. This can be due to *constant overstretching*, thus stressing the weakened area. An injured area can be stretched, but only *very, very gently*. Overstretching will simply prolong the injury.

The correct way to stretch an injured muscle is to stretch to the point where a slight stretch is felt first, then ease off slowly until no stretch is felt. This position should be held for 20–30 sec or longer. It is very helpful to use ice on the injured area while stretching.

If you can't find a position that does not give pain, the muscle should not be stretched. Prolonged hamstring injuries are helped by proper stretching, but forced overstretching can cause the injury to become chronic.

# Groin and Hip Stretches

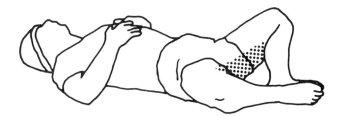

Relax with your knees bent and the soles of your feet together. This comfortable position will stretch your groin. Hold this for 60 sec.

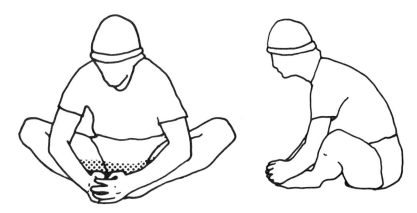

Put the soles of your feet together with your heels a comfortable distance from your groin. Now, put your hands around your feet and slowly pull yourself forward until you feel an easy stretch in the groin. Make your movement forward by bending from the hips and not from the shoulders. If possible, keep your elbows on the outside of your lower legs for greater stability during the stretch. Hold a comfortable stretch for 30–40 sec.

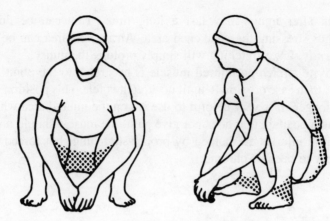

With your feet shoulder-width apart and pointed out to about a 15° angle, heels on the ground, bend your knees and squat down. If you have trouble staying in this position hold onto something for support. It is a great stretch for your ankles, Achilles tendons, groin, lower back, and hips. Hold stretch for 30 sec. *Be careful if you have had any knee problems. If pain is present, discontinue this stretch.*

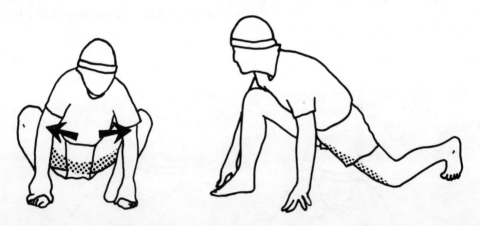

To increase the stretch in the groin, place your elbows on the inside of your upper legs, gently push outward with both elbows as you bend slightly forward from your hips. Your thumbs should be on the inside of your feet with your fingers along the outside borders of the feet. Hold stretch for 20 sec. Do not overstretch. If you have trouble balancing, elevate your heels slightly.

As in the above right drawing, move your leg forward *until the knee of the forward leg is directly over the ankle.* Your other knee should be resting on the floor. Lower the front of your hip downward until an easy stretch is felt in the front of the hip and possibly in your hamstrings and groin. Do this without changing the position of the knee on the floor or the forward foot. Hold the stretch for 30 sec.

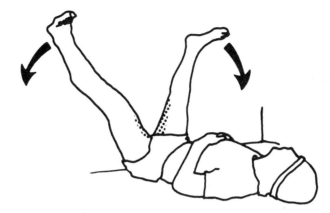

With your heels resting on the wall, slowly separate your legs until you feel an easy stretch in your groin. Be relaxed as you hold the stretch for 50–60 sec.

# Neck and Lower Back Stretches

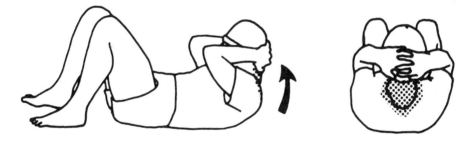

Interlace your fingers behind your head and rest your arms on the mat. Using the power of your arms, *slowly* bring your head, neck, and shoulders forward until you feel a slight stretch. Hold an easy stretch for 5 sec. Repeat three times. Do not overstretch.

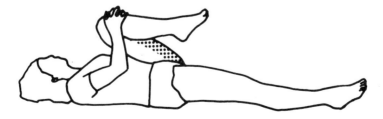

Next, straighten both legs and relax, then pull your left leg toward your chest. For this stretch keep the back of your head on the mat, if possible, but don't strain. Hold an easy stretch for 30 sec. Repeat, pulling your right leg toward your chest.

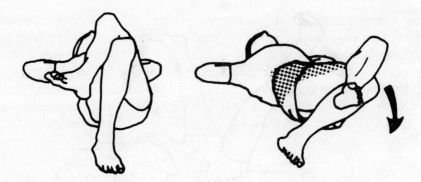

From a bent-knee position, interlace your fingers behind your head and lift the leg over the right leg. From here, use your left leg to pull your right leg toward the floor until you feel a stretch along the side of your hip and lower back. Stretch and relax. Keep the upper back, shoulders, and elbows flat on the floor. The idea is not to touch the floor with your right knee, but to stretch within *your* limits. Hold for 30 sec. Repeat stretch for other side.

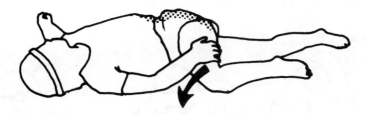

Next, straighten your right leg, and with your right hand pull your bent leg up and over your other leg as shown in the drawing above. Make sure that both of your shoulders and your head are on the floor. Turn your head to look toward your left. Now with your other hand on your thigh (resting just above the knee), control the stretch in your lower back and buttock muscles by pulling your upper leg down toward the floor. Repeat the stretch to your other side. Hold stretch for 30 sec, each side.

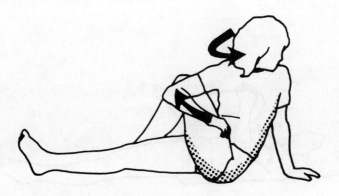

Sit with your right leg straight. Bend your left leg, cross your left foot over and rest it to the outside of your right knee. Then bend your right elbow and rest it on the outside of your upper left thigh, just above the knee. During the stretch use the elbow to keep this leg stationary with controlled pressure to the inside. Now, with your left hand resting behind you, slowly turn your head to look over your left shoulder, and at the same time rotate your upper body toward your left hand and arm. As you turn your upper body, think of turning your hips in the same direction (though your hips will not move because your right elbow is keeping the left leg stationary). This should give you a stretch in your lower back and side of hip. Hold for 15 sec. Do both sides. Do not hold your breath; breathe easily.

# Calf, Achilles, and Iliotibial Band Stretches

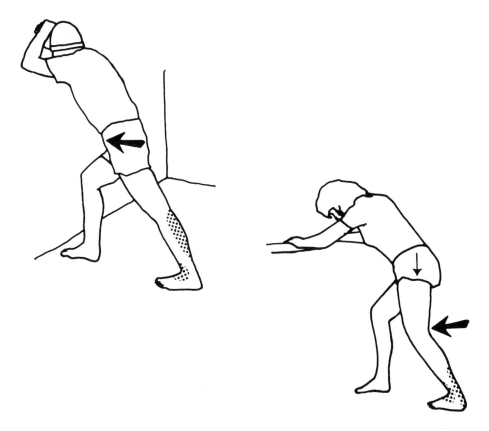

To stretch your calf, stand a little away from a solid support and lean on it with your forearms, your head resting on your hands. Bend one leg and place your foot on the ground in front of you, leaving the other leg straight, behind you. Slowly move your hips forward until you feel a stretch in the calf of your straight leg. Be sure to keep the heel of the foot of the straight leg on the ground and *your toes pointed straight ahead*. Hold an easy stretch for 30 sec. Do not bounce. Stretch both legs.

Now, to stretch the soleus and Achilles tendon, slightly bend the back knee, keeping the foot flat. This gives you a much lower stretch, which is also good for maintaining or regaining ankle flexibility. 15 sec, each leg. This area needs only a *slight feeling of stretch*.

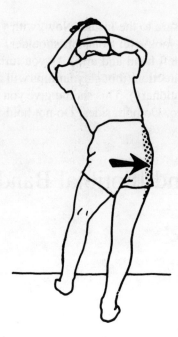

To stretch the outside of the hips and upper leg, start from the same position as in the calf stretch. Stretch the right side of your hip by slightly turning your right hip to the inside. Project the side of your hip to the side as you lean your shoulders very slightly in the opposite direction of your hips. Hold an even stretch for 25 sec. Do both sides. Keep foot of back leg pointed straight ahead with heel flat on ground.

# Arm and Shoulder Stretches

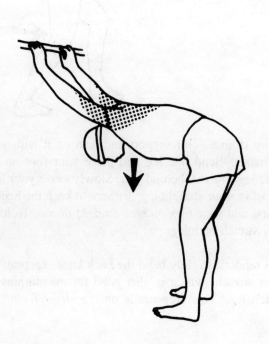

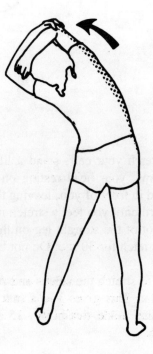

A stretch for the arms, shoulders, and back. Hold onto something that is about shoulder height. With your hands shoulder-width apart on this support, relax, keeping your arms straight and your chest moving downward, and *your feet remaining directly under your hips*. Keep your knees slightly bent (1 inch). Hold this stretch 30 sec. This is a good stretch to do anywhere, at anytime.

With arms overhead, hold the elbow of one arm with the hand of the other arm. Keeping knees slightly bent (1 inch), gently pull your elbow behind your head as you bend from your hips to the side. Hold an easy stretch for 10 sec. Do both sides. Keeping your knees slightly bent will give you better balance.

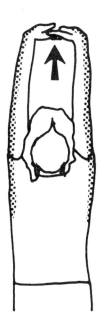 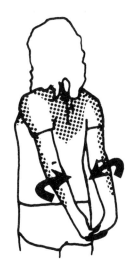

In a standing or sitting position, interlace your fingers above your head. Now, with your palms facing upward, push your arms slightly back and up. Feel the stretch in arms, shoulders, and upper back. Hold stretch for 15 sec. Do not hold your breath. This stretch is good to do anywhere, anytime. Excellent for slumping shoulders.

The next stretch is done with your fingers interlaced behind your back. Slowly turn your elbows inward while straightening your arms. An excellent stretch for shoulders and arms. This is good to do when you find yourself slumping forward from your shoulders. This stretch can be done at any time. Hold for 5-15 sec. Do twice.

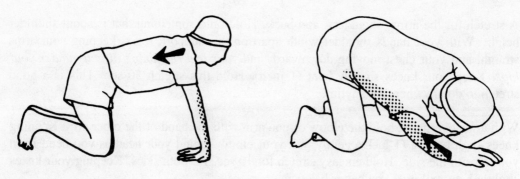

From the position illustrated on the left above, with your palms flat and fingers pointed back toward your knees, slowly lean backwards to stretch the forearms and wrists. Be sure to keep your palms flat. Hold a comfortable stretch for 20-25 sec. *Do not overstretch.* Stretch for a good feeling. Enjoy stretching.

With legs bent under you, reach forward with one arm and grab the end of the mat, carpet, or anything you can hold onto. If you cannot grab onto something, just pull back with your arm straight while pressing down slightly with your hand. Do likewise pulling on end of mat. Hold stretch for 20 sec. Stretch each side. Do not strain. You should feel the stretch in your shoulders, arms, sides, upper back, or even in your lower back.

# Chapter 23

# Biomechanics of the Foot and Lower Extremity

## by Robert M. Parks

## Introduction

The clinical application of lower extremity biomechanics has received increased attention in recent years, partly because of computer availability, refinements in photography, and the search for ways to improve athletic performance. The axiom, structure dictates function, is now more clearly appreciated by sports physicians. Normal structure often results in superior performance, and abnormal body mechanics frequently correlate with poor performance and athletic injuries. The coach, trainer, and medical clinician who understand the musculoskeletal system in motion will be more effective in their respective roles.

## History

Investigation of lower-extremity biomechanics arose from the need to treat post-World War II amputees more effectively. Thorough understanding of joint motion and function was necessary in order to build better limb prostheses. Researchers at the University of California established normal values for ranges of motion in the major joints of the foot and ankle. Podiatric physicians (Root et al. [1-3]; Sgarlato [4, 5]) confirmed these findings clinically and have found them to be of value in treating common foot and leg disorders. Practitioners can now distinguish normal from abnormal function and can determine the degree of deviation from normal by basic measurements. Many developmental osseous and soft-tissue disorders of the foot and leg benefit by biomechanical evaluation and treatment.

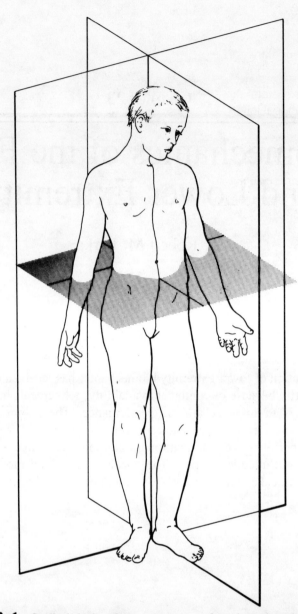

**23–1** Cardinal body planes—transverse, frontal, and sagittal. (From Sgarlato, T.E. 1971. A Compendium of Podiatric Biomechanics. College of Podiatric Medicine Corp., San Francisco. Reprinted with permission.)

# Biomechanics in Sports and Medicine

The ability to categorize extremity types through quantitative biomechanical assessment is invaluable in sports research and clinical medicine. The researcher can roughly predict an athlete's maximum potential and can more effectively help him or her overcome problems. Sports medicine practitioners can now uncover the athlete's "weak link" during the

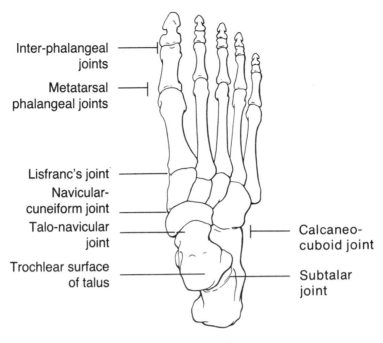

Inter-phalangeal joints

Metatarsal phalangeal joints

Lisfranc's joint

Navicular-cuneiform joint

Talo-navicular joint

Trochlear surface of talus

Calcaneo-cuboid joint

Subtalar joint

**23–2**   Dorsal view of foot.

stress of athletic participation. The cause of injury is identified and corrected rather than the practitioner's providing treatment based on symptoms. Prediction of future injury is also possible through biomechanical analysis. Preventive medicine can then be practiced by altering variables of training, environment, exercise, and equipment.

The study of lower extremity biomechanics is not a concrete science, and accepted principles should be evaluated critically. The intent of this chapter is to help the reader understand mechanics of the lower extremity and foot.

# Anatomic Considerations

The bony anatomy of the foot is complex, and each part allows many movements (Fig. 23–1). From proximal to distal, bones of the foot can be categorized as the greater tarsus, lesser tarsals, metatarsals, and phalanges (Figs. 23–2, 23–3). The greater tarsus includes the talus and calcaneus; the lesser tarsals are the navicular, cuboid, and the first, second, and third cuneiforms. There are five metatarsals. Each digit has three phalanges, proximal, intermediate, and distal, except for the hallux, which has two. The metatarsals and phalanges are long bones; the tarsal and lesser tarsal bones are not long bones and, in contrast, have multifaceted articulations supported by interconnecting ligaments.

The talus is one of three bones of the ankle joint. Its superior articulating surface forms an arc, which permits flexion and extension of the ankle. Its medial and lateral borders form angles of approximately 90° to its superior surface and articulate with the tibial and fibular malleoli, respectively. This architecture does not permit transverse and frontal

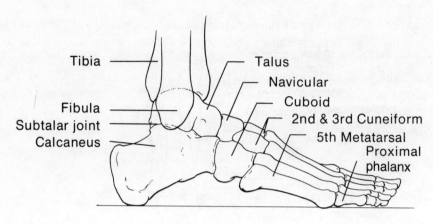

**23–3** Lateral view of foot.

plane motion within the ankle joint. Transverse plane movement of the talus at the subtalar joint is transmitted directly into transverse plane leg rotation. The bony architecture of the ankle joint and weight bearing prevent ankle inversion and eversion. Medial and lateral collateral ligaments function only when a subluxatory force is present and, therefore, do not provide frontal plane stability. The inferior surface of the talus articulates with the calcaneus to form the subtalar joint. This joint consists of three facets, the surfaces of which lie near the transverse plane of the body. When the subtalar joint moves, all facets glide simultaneously. This motion, although derived from a common axis, lies oblique to the three cardinal planes of the body and is termed triplane. The two movements of the subtalar joint are supination (turning-in of the foot) and pronation (out-turning of the foot) and will be discussed in more detail later.

The calcaneus articulates with the talus on its superior surface; the plantar aspect is the surface of the heel that strikes the ground. The distal part of the calcaneus articulates with the cuboid bone to form the calcaneocuboid joint. The articulating surface of the cuboid is somewhat egg-shaped and lies on the frontal plane of the body with greatest dimensions running in a dorsoplantar direction. The calcaneocuboid joint forms the apex of the lateral arch of the foot and functions in unison with the talonavicular joint. The two joints combined form the midtarsal joint, which moves around two separate axes. The longitudinal axis of the midtarsal joint, although providing triplane motion, functions maximally in the frontal plane. The oblique axis of the midtarsal joint, also triplane, allows for a predominance of sagittal plane motion.

The distal aspect of the talus articulates with the navicular (boat-shaped) bone. This joint is similar to the calcaneocuboid joint and, as previously mentioned, the two together comprise the midtarsal joint.

The three cuneiform (wedge-shaped) bones lie adjacent to one another from medial to lateral and articulate proximally with the navicular bone. The external cuneiform articulates laterally with the cuboid bone. In a normal foot, the shape and close proximity of the bones of the lesser tarsal joints permit only minimal movement. In cases of altered foot mechanics, increased sagittal plane motion may occur. The distal surfaces of the medial, middle, and external cuneiforms and the cuboid articulate with the five metatarsals to form the Lisfranc's joint. Motion at this location results in sagittal plane movement of the metatarsals. The second, third, and fourth metatarsals function around a common axis, while the first and fifth metatarsals function independently. Ground reactive forces tend to dorsiflex and invert the first metatarsal. The fifth metatarsal responds to plantar pressure by dorsiflexing and everting. The metatarsal heads articulate with the proximal phalangeal bases to form the five metatarsal-phalangeal joints. These joints are condyloid in nature, permitting primarily sagittal plane motion (flexion, extension) with lesser degrees of transverse and frontal plane motion. The interphalangeal joints are hinge-like, permitting only sagittal plane motion (flexion, extension).

# Physical Principles of Joint Function

To understand the mechanics of weight-bearing joints, one must appreciate basic physical principles that govern their function. Body movement abides by the Newtonian laws of motion and modern physics. Weight-bearing joints of the body have a dual function: They allow movement and provide support and stability. Stability is necessary for upright posture and locomotion. It is generally accepted that more mobile joints are also more unstable. Lack of stability arises from intrinsic or extrinsic forces. What, then, allows a weight-bearing joint to be both mobile and stable simultaneously?

First consider the angle that joint surfaces form in respect to the ground. In the knee, for example, forces acting when the extremity strikes the ground are the result of body mass multiplied by body acceleration (force = mass × acceleration). This force is equalized at heel contact by an equal and opposite force of ground resistance, termed *ground-reactive force,* which enters the knee perpendicular to the joint surfaces and compresses them together. This *joint compressional force,* applicable only during weight bearing, maintains joint congruity by bone-on-bone compression.

When joint alignment is oblique to ground-reactive forces, the resulting stress may produce joint subluxation. This is successfully resisted when body function is normal. A force producing joint instability is termed *joint rotational force.* Factors other than joint compression help maintain joint stability. These include articular surface configuration and the axis on which it functions. A joint surface with a deep socket or curves and irregularities has greater ability to resist rotational forces. Abnormal ranges of joint motion result in a jamming effect on the opposing joint surfaces. This locking mechanism can be overcome only if rotational forces exceed joint compressional forces.

The axis of joint motion not only indicates its direction of movement but also the direction of force from which the joint can maintain stability. Joint motion occurs at 90° to a joint axis (examine the mechanics of a door and note that movement occurs 90° to the supporting hinge) (Fig. 23–4). Forces directed obliquely to a joint must increase as the angle of applied force decreases from 90°. No force parallel to an axis can produce motion.

Soft tissue, as well as bone, help maintain joint stability. Tendons crossing joints serve a dual function in providing both motion and stability. A tendon's ability to resist rotational forces and provide motion depends upon the lever arm length and direction in relation to a joint axis. A tendon with a long lever arm coursing perpendicular to a joint axis provides maximum stability. Ligaments do not stabilize joints moving within their normal range. When a normal range of motion is exceeded, ligaments become taut and help resist subluxation and possible dislocation.

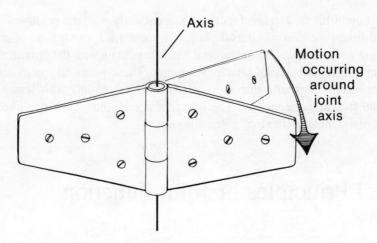

**23–4**   Axis of motion around hinge.

## The Gait Cycle

Upright locomotion in humans results from functional integration of many body segments. Walking requires corresponding movement from the head, arms, torso, and lower extremities. The apparent fluidity of forward progression is actually the result of movement in all body planes simultaneously. Muscles accelerate, decelerate and stabilize at the same time. It is only through this mechanical complexity that human beings can propel and maneuver with such great precision.

Observation of gait is the clinician's way of assessing segmental body locomotion. A full gait cycle is the period beginning with heel contact of one foot and ending with heel contact of the same foot. This includes the entire interval of foot support (stance phase of gait) and also the period when the extremity is swinging forward in preparation for heel strike (swing phase of gait). The gait cycle is further divided by percentages, so that muscle function and joint motion can be assessed in relation to a specific time within the gait cycle.

## The Swing Phase of Gait

The swing phase of gait begins immediately after toe-off and ends with heel contact of the same foot. This phase of gait carries the extremity from one step to the next and is also referred to as the stride. The hip and knee joint flex during this period, allowing for ground clearance of the swinging limb. The ankle and subtalar joints dorsiflex and pronate, respectively, to assure forefoot and digital ground clearance. The stride length in walking or running is influenced by the degree of hip flexion, speed of progression, and limb length. When a person walks, body weight transfers from limb to limb with a corresponding shift in the center of gravity. In running, a double-float phase or period occurs, during which both limbs are off the ground. When heel contact ensues, the runner's center of gravity must be balanced above one limb to prevent falling toward the

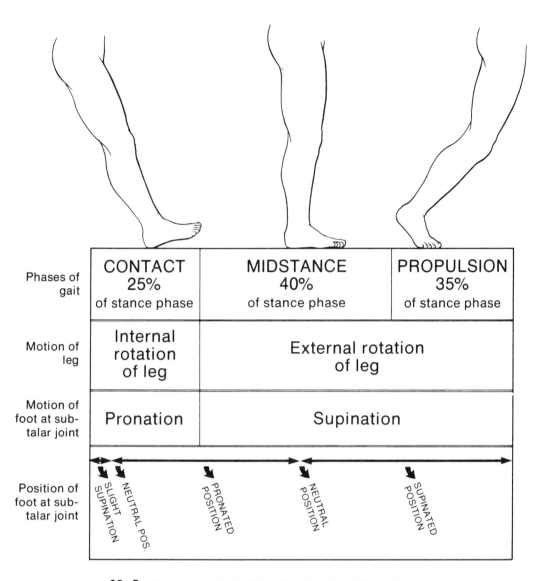

**23–5**   Stance phase of gait. (From Sgarlato, T.E. 1971. A Compendium of Podiatric Biomechanics. College of Podiatric Medicine Corp., San Francisco. Reprinted with permission.)

nonweight-bearing side. The center of gravity for the runner is nearly, therefore, a straight line of progression, and shifts forward (anterior) according to speed of progression.

As a runner attains greater speeds, the upper extremity swings forward with hip flexion. Acceleration of swing phase requires increasing hip flexion for adequate extremity ground clearance. Just prior to heel contact, the forward-progressing limb extends to approximately 175° at the knee joint, and the foot supinates in preparation for body support.

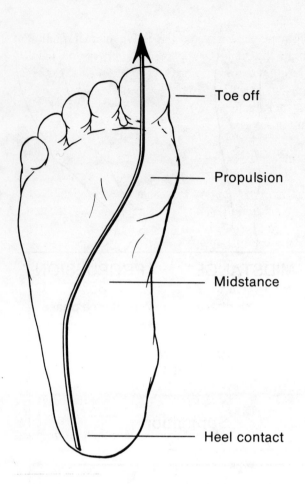

— Toe off

— Propulsion

**23–6** Force curve: Weight-bearing forces as they occur from heel contact to toe-off.

— Midstance

— Heel contact

## The Stance Phase of Gait

The stance phase of gait is subdivided into contact, midstance, and propulsive phases (Fig. 23–5). The three phases are analyzed sequentially below.

**The Contact Phase of Gait**   The contact phase of gait, which comprises 25% of the stance phase, begins with heel contact and lasts until the forefoot meets the ground. Two important functions of the foot during this period are to dissipate shock resulting from heel strike and to adapt to variations in terrain.

The lower extremity absorbs heel-contact shock by slight knee flexion, ankle plantar flexion, and subtalar joint pronation. The unweighting effect of these movements dissipates shock. Vertical ground-reactive forces during walking do not approach the force of body weight until the midstance phase of gait. During the contact phase of gait, the foot functions much like a universal joint, to accommodate for variations in ground terrain. This is achieved through subtalar joint pronation, which is associated with calcaneal eversion, plantar flexion, and adduction of the talus.

As indicated previously, adduction of the talus cannot occur without simultaneous internal rotation of the leg. The tibia and fibula, therefore, rotate internally throughout the contact phase of the gait. Internal rotation of the leg is transmitted to the femur and hip joint since the knee does not permit transverse plane motion. Excessive internal rotation of the limb can be assessed by examining the transverse plane rotation of the patella. Normally, the patella rotates inward during the contact phase of gait to the same degree that it externally rotates during propulsion. If inward rotation is favored over external rotation, the cause is likely to be excessive subtalar joint pronation, if it may be assumed that there are no abnormalities at the hip or knee.

**The Midstance Phase of Gait**    The midstance phase of gait normally comprises 40% of the stance phase and begins with cessation of contact and ends with heel-off. At the beginning of midstance, the weight-bearing limb begins to externally rotate and the foot to supinate. In contrast to the foot's function as a mobile adapter during the contact phase, at midstance the foot must now be ready for full weight bearing, so propulsion muscles can function around stable bony segments. Stress-related injuries of the foot and leg occur when muscles are required to stabilize an otherwise unstable foot and also function as prime movers.

Supination of the foot is initiated by external rotation of the hip. Again, the closed-chain effect of transverse plane rotation is transmitted distally into the foot, producing external rotation and dorsiflexion of the talus. The calcaneus inverts simultaneously with rearfoot supination. Muscular contraction also plays an important role in foot supination. All posterior leg muscles with a supinating action at the subtalar joint, particularly the gastrosoleus group and the tibialis posterior, assist in foot supination. This reversal of motion can be visualized by external rotation of the patella and inversion of the heel.

The foot actively supinates from its pronated position, achieving joint neutrality half-way through the midstance phase of gait. It must be noted that the terms *supination* and *pronation* refer to motion, and *supinated* and *pronated* refer to position. With the "rearfoot" in a functionally stable position, the ball of the foot accepts greater amounts of body weight. For maximum stability, body weight rests on a triangle of support, the heel posteriorly and the first and fifth metatarsals distally. Weight transference continues from heel to "forefoot" as the tibia moves anteriorly over the foot and the posterior leg muscles continue to fire.

**Propulsive Phase of Gait**    The propulsive phase comprises the last 35% of the stance phase of gait. This begins at the instant of heel elevation and terminates with toe-off.

Efficient foot propulsion depends upon osseous stability and normal muscular function. Most of the foot's propulsive stability is due to the extremities' preparation during midstance. Dynamic balance and stability is, therefore, necessary during contact and, particularly, during midstance for normal propulsion to occur.

Subtalar joint supination continues throughout the propulsive phase of gait. Although the subtalar joint no longer directly contacts the ground by means of the calcaneus, its position continues to account for distal stability. The midtarsal and lesser tarsal joints are subjected to the greatest load during propulsion. As the foot plantarflexes at the ankle for forward acceleration, weight transmitted through the forefoot clearly exceeds body weight. Osseous restraint and stability are, therefore, essential to prevent subluxation of the lesser tarsal joints.

During the propulsive phase of gait, weight is transferred from the lateral metatarsals medially (Fig. 23–6). This medial shift in weight is necessary for the foot to obtain its most efficient propulsive lever, the first metatarsal phalangeal joint. The metatarsal

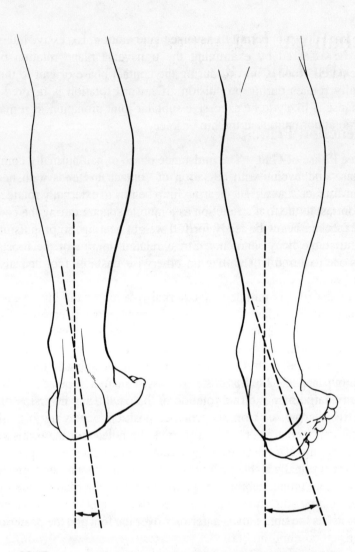

**23–7**   Nonweight-bearing subtalar joint, total range of movement. (From Root, M.L. et al. 1977. Normal and Abnormal Function of the Foot. Clinical Biomechanics Corp., Los Angeles. Reprinted with permission.)

parabola (length pattern) and the peroneal muscles are responsible for this weight shift. The peroneus longus muscle stabilizes the first metatarsal until the final moments of toe-off. Efficient propulsion from the hallux, as stabilized by the first metatarsal, is then possible. Most extrinsic muscles attaching to the mid- or rearfoot that coordinate foot position during contact and midstance cease to function midway through the propulsive phase of gait. The majority of extrinsic and intrinsic muscles that have digital insertions function until toe-off. The completion of stance phase propulsion initiates swing phase of the same limb and weight bearing of the opposite limb.

# Biomechanical Determinants of Foot and Leg Stability

## "Chain-Reaction Principle"

Early investigators believed that ligamentous and muscular tension were largely responsible for maintenance of a normal arch and efficient foot function. Today, we understand that the precise function of each segment of the lower extremity and foot determines efficiency of motion. Root et al [3] state: "No bone can be stabilized at a joint if the bones proximal to it are unstable." This phenomenon of joint mechanics relates to the absolute dependence of one foot segment's stability on another segment's function, a principle this author refers to as the "chain-reaction principle."

**Subtalar Joint Function**    The largest and most proximal joint in the foot is the subtalar joint. This joint is sometimes called the "universal joint" of the foot, since it allows the plantar aspect of the foot to accommodate for variations in terrain. The motion in this joint, termed triplane, is oblique to all body planes. The collective triplane motions are called supination (turning in of the rearfoot) and pronation (turning out of the rearfoot) (Fig. 23–7). Subtalar joint motion can be assessed by measuring frontal plane excursion of the heel bone in relation to the distal leg. Although the total range of motion of the subtalar joint is approximately 30°–40° (measured on the frontal plane), the normal range used during gait is only about one-fourth of this. The subtalar joint range of motion must be maintained within this narrow range to assure maximum foot efficiency. This joint must unlock itself by pronating during the contact phase of gait and then quickly begin supinating prior to heel-off so the foot may become a solid foundation from which to propel. The posterior aspect of the heel should remain nearly vertical during stance and ambulation. Structural abnormalities, such as tibial vara, genu valgum, or frontal plane deformities of the forefoot and rearfoot that require subtalar joint compensation, excessively pronate or supinate this joint.

**Midtarsal Joint Function**    The midtarsal joint is important in allowing independent movement of the forefoot and the rearfoot in all three body planes. Motion available at the midtarsal joint is derived from two independent axes. The oblique axis allows the forefoot to dorsiflex and plantarflex on the rearfoot. (This motion is actually triplanar, but the greatest movement occurs in the sagittal plane.) The longitudinal axis allows the forefoot to invert and evert in relation to the rearfoot. Longitudinal axis motion is also triplanar, but its greatest movement is in the frontal plane.

The articular surfaces of the midtarsal joint, like almost all other lesser tarsal joints, are at near right angles to ground reactive forces. The midtarsal joint depends mainly on muscular and ligamentous tension to withstand rotation forces, unlike the subtalar and ankle joints, where compressional forces are great. Chronic subluxations, therefore, frequently occur in the lesser tarsal joint as a result of ineffective bone and soft-tissue support.

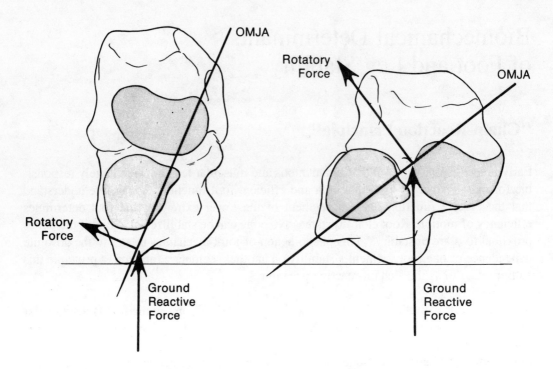

**23–8**   Change of position of subtalar joint affecting stability of midtarsal joint. OMBJ, oblique midtarsal joint axis. (From Root, M.L. et al. 1977. Normal and Abnormal Function of the Foot. Clinical Biomechanics Corp., Los Angeles. Reprinted with permission.)

Like the subtalar joint, the midtarsal joint locks and unlocks, depending on the phase of gait and compensatory requirements. The midtarsal joint must be mobile during initial ground contact and become rigid or locked prior to heel-off. If the oblique axis is mobile at midstance, the midtarsal joint or instep sags with body weight. This presents clinically as a low instep or an abducted forefoot in relation to the rearfoot.

Midtarsal joint stability depends on the position of the subtalar joint. When the subtalar joint is neutral or supinated, the talonavicular joint is superior to the calcaneocuboid joint. (These two joints make up the midtarsal joint [Fig. 23–8].) If the subtalar joint pronates, the two joints are almost side by side. In the first instance, the oblique midtarsal joint axis is almost parallel to ground reactive forces. Weight bearing is thereby met with osseous resistance. In the second case, ground reactive force during gait is sufficient to dorsiflex the forefoot on the rearfoot. This results in skeletal imbalance and hypermobility.

It is then clear that the positions of the talus and calcaneous are determined by the subtalar joint, and their relationship determines the longitudinal and oblique axes of the midtarsal joint, which in turn determine the midtarsal joint's stability. Midtarsal joint stability therefore depends upon subtalar joint stability.

A second means of attaining osseous stability of the midtarsal joint is based upon differences in joint congruity existent with varying positions of the talonavicular and the calcaneocuboid articulations (Elftman [6]) (Fig. 23–9). The articulating surfaces of both

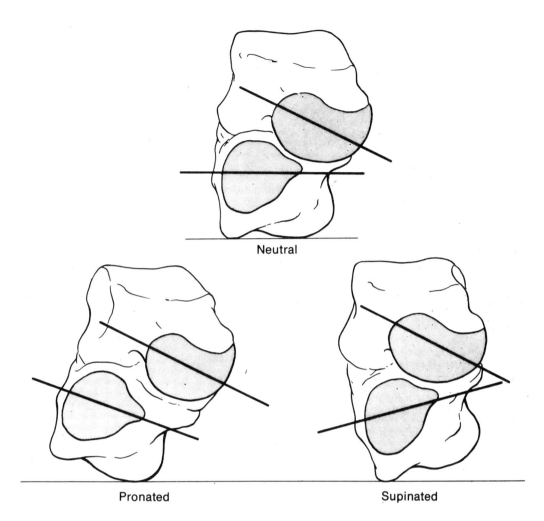

Neutral

Pronated                    Supinated

**23-9**   Axial locking of midtarsal joint. (From Root, M.L. et al. 1977. Normal and Abnormal Function of the Foot. Clinical Biomechanics Corp., Los Angeles. Reprinted with permission.)

joints are egg-shaped. When the subtalar joint is neutral or supinated, the long axes of the joint surfaces are oblique to each other. Weight bearing results in stability based on joint incongruity. If the subtalar joint pronates, the long axes of the joints become more parallel, creating a common axis for movement. Motion and the tendency for joint instability is, therefore, increased.

**Lesser Tarsal Joint Function**   The lesser tarsal bones are wedge- or cube-shaped. Their articulating surfaces are subjected to large rotational forces during weight bearing, which must be resisted by both osseous and soft-tissue structures. The lack of motion between the lesser tarsal bones allows them to function as a unit, and their position is determined by the subtalar and midtarsal joints. Protection against subluxation in the lesser tarsal region depends on the multifaceted nature of the articular surfaces and the strength with which the joints are held together by muscles and ligaments.

A second osseous locking mechanism is responsible for lesser tarsal joint stability as well as for metatarsal-tarsal joint (Lisfranc's joint) stability. This is derived from the midtarsal joint's position. When the midtarsal joint is neutral or supinated, the lesser tarsal region becomes dorsally convex from medial to lateral. The bones move closer together and ground-reactive forces are resisted. If the midtarsal joint pronates, the lesser tarsal bones are more parallel to the ground, joint compressional forces are reduced, and ground-reactive forces result in saggital plane hypermobility of the forefoot.

The ligaments of the lesser tarsus, normal muscular function, and bony restraints provide local stability. Muscular support is from the medial pull of the tibialis posterior and the lateral pull of the peroneus longus and brevis; retrograde stability is assisted by intrinsic foot muscles.

**Metatarsal Function** The greatest motion of the metatarsals occurs on the sagittal plane, with lesser movement occurring on the transverse plane. Stability of the second, third, and fourth metatarsals is derived from osseous resistance and normal muscular function. Proximal bony stability is necessary for metatarsal stability with each muscle contraction.

The first metatarsal functions independently of other metatarsal bones. It is the largest of the metatarsals and carries approximately twice the weight of the lesser metatarsals. The first metatarsal and first cuneiform normally move as a unit called the first ray. First ray motion is triplanar, although the largest movement is in the sagittal plane (dorsiflexion, plantarflexion). During the propulsive phase of gait, weight is transferred from the lateral metatarsals medially. The first metatarsal must be stable when weight is borne on the first metatarsal phalangeal joint; otherwise the foot pronates as the medial aspect of the foot collapses.

First metatarsal stability depends upon the function of the peroneus longus muscle (Fig. 23–10). The peroneus longus enters the foot laterally, goes below the cuboid on the plantar surface of the foot, making a near right-angle turn to insert medially at the base of the first metatarsal and cuneiform. The stability of the cuboid allows the peroneus longus to function like a pulley to increase its effective force from medial to lateral. The peroneus longus abducts the foot and plantar-flexes the first ray, and the position of the rearfoot (subtalar joint) determines which function predominates. Stability of the first ray depends on the ability of the peroneus longus to plantar-flex the first ray (not its ability to abduct). When the subtalar joint pronates, the medial arch of the foot approaches the supporting surface. As the first metatarsal and cuneiform descend, the peroneus longus approaches the transverse plane. Muscular contraction under these circumstances results in transverse plane motion or abduction of the foot. Supination of the subtalar joint allows the base of the first metatarsal and cuneiform to rise above the cuboid. Contraction of the peroneus longus pulls downward on the first ray to plantar-flex and stabilize the first metatarsal. It is, therefore, necessary that the subtalar joint cease contact phase pronation and reverse into a neutral or supinated position prior to midstance and foot propulsion. Only under these circumstances is the medial column of the foot prepared for weight bearing and toe-off.

The fifth metatarsal functions around an independent axis much like the first metatarsal. As the fifth metatarsal dorsiflexes, it simultaneously everts and abducts; as it plantar-

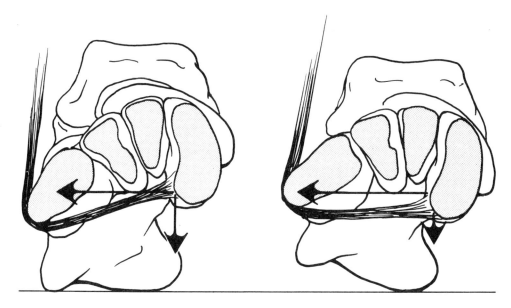

Neutral           Pronated

**23–10** Changes of peroneus longus force vectors at insertion into first ray. (From Root, M.L. et al. 1977. Normal and Abnormal Function of the Foot. Clinical Biomechanics Corp., Los Angeles. Reprinted with permission.)

flexes, it inverts and adducts. The fifth metatarsal articulates proximally with the fourth metatarsal base and cuboid. This bony segment, like other bones of the lesser tarsus and forefoot, depends on subtalar joint position for stability. The fifth metatarsal is the first bone of the forefoot to make ground contact during gait. Stability of the fifth metatarsal depends largely upon subtalar joint position, which, in turn, determines midtarsal joint stability and the degree of frontal plane rotation of the cuboid. As the midtarsal joint pronates around its oblique and longitudinal axis, the cuboid abducts, dorsiflexes, and everts. This author believes that the change in position of the cuboid flattens the transverse metatarsal arch and causes the fourth metatarsal to descend in relation to the fifth. The osseous restraint between the fourth and fifth metatarsals diminishes, allowing greater freedom of movement of the fifth ray. Midtarsal joint pronation permits hypermobility at the calcaneocuboid joint and is another means for sagittal plane compensation of the lateral forefoot. Joint resistance and stability of the fifth metatarsal is attained in converse fashion as the subtalar joint supinates. Soft tissue assists fifth metatarsal stability in a way similar to that mentioned for the second, third, or fourth metatarsals.

# Conclusion

The foot is the foundation of body support. Its two major functions are to provide stability and to aid in body propulsion. The subtalar joint of the rearfoot determines the way in which forces are transmitted through the foot and lower extremity. Subtalar joint function is responsible for frontal plane stability of the ankle and mechanical efficiency of the knee and hip, as determined by transverse plane position. Sagittal plane positioning of the pelvis and its effect on the lumbosacral angle are also influenced by subtalar joint position. In the foot, subtalar joint alignment directly or indirectly determines tarsal and lesser tarsal stability as well as efficiency of muscle function. Osseous instability resulting in biomechanical imbalances is the major cause of injuries to the endurance athlete. Clinicians must be aware of the important role improper body mechanics play in injury processes and learn to alter mechanical imbalances whenever necessary.

# References

1. Root, M.L., Weed, H.H., Sgarlato, T.E., Bluth, D. 1966. Axis of motion of the subtalar joint. J Am Podiatry Assoc 56b(4):149–155.
2. Root, M.L., Orien, W.P., Weed, J.W., Hughes, R.J. 1971. Biomechanical Examination of the Foot. Clinical Biomechanics Corp., Los Angeles.
3. Root, M.L., Orien, W.P., Weed, J.H. 1977. Normal and Abnormal Function of the Foot. Clinical Biomechanics Corp., Los Angeles.
4. Sgarlato, T.E. 1965. The angle of gait. J Am Podiatry Assoc 55(9):645–650.
5. Sgarlato, T.E. 1971. A Compendium of Podiatric Biomechanics. College of Podiatric Medicine Corp., San Francisco.
6. Elftman, H. 1960. Transverse tarsal joint and its control. Clin Orthop 16:41–44.

# Chapter 24

# Biomechanics and Sports Injury Treatment

## by Robert M. Parks

The sports physician must differentiate between injury cause and effect. The success of treating the effects of overuse injury, such as pain and swelling, may be dramatic, but is ultimately short-lived. Successful overuse injury treatment may require altering the participant's body mechanics and style of movement, in addition to weight and flexibility training, changes in equipment or shoes and modifications of training technique.

This chapter deals with treatment of sports injury based on biomechanical principles discussed in Chapter 23.

The clinical application of biomechanics in treating sports injuries does not require a full understanding of anatomy or the concepts presented in Chapter 23. Coaches, trainers, and athletes themselves can administer successful biomechanical treatment. Unfortunately, the recent marketing of biomechanical paraphernalia, such as runner's shoe wedges and instant orthotic devices, and the overuse of rigid orthotic appliances may have distorted the value of biomechanics as applied to sports injury. The effective "sports biomechanist" appreciates the indications and limits of biomechanics and can integrate this treatment into a multifaceted therapeutic program.

The following discussion of common overuse injuries provides examples of how biomechanics may be important in sports injuries and their prevention. Treatment modalities presented are biomechanically oriented only and are not intended to be complete.

## The Subluxed Cuboid

Lateral instep or lateral arch pain occurs frequently in running sports and may also be associated with inversion-type ankle sprains, a condition often misdiagnosed and mistreated. Pain from this syndrome may be located on the dorsal aspect of the calcaneocubiod joint, the lateral surface of the cuboid, or around the fifth metatarsal-cuboid joint. This syndrome most commonly occurs during long runs on asphalt or concrete surfaces or in runners with poorly maintained shoes. Quick movement sports may also precipitate "cuboid" pain if the heel twists (inverts or everts) in relation to the forefoot.

The "cuboid syndrome" is caused by ligamentous or capsular sprain of the above-mentioned joints from bony instability. Any acute or chronic joint movement beyond the normal range places excessive strain on soft-tissue supporting structures in the area. The "cuboid syndrome," also called "subluxed cuboid," refers to a positional change between the cuboid and calcaneus, and an important method of treatment involves manipulation. The cuboid and the attaching fifth metatarsal bone dorsiflexes, abducts and everts in relation to the calcaneus when subjected to abnormal weight bearing forces. The manipulative technique for correction, therefore, involves quick plantar flexion and inversion of the forefoot on the heel. An audible click occurs when the manipulation is successful, and the patient experiences sudden pain relief. Other investigators believe the pathology of the "cuboid syndrome" involves slippage of the peroneus longus tendon from its groove under the cuboid, and the click during manipulation occurs when the tendon moves into place. Whether the pathology of the "cuboid syndrome" results from joint subluxation and subsequent inflammation or abnormal tendon position, the abnormal foot mechanics are often the same and the above treatment is usually successful.

The lateral column of the foot, or lateral arch, comprised of the calcaneus, cuboid, and fifth metatarsal, normally forms a concave arch laterally. This is high in the high-arched foot (pes cavus) and low in the flat or pronated foot. It is not clear why the lateral column often becomes progressively higher in severe pes cavus, but the cause of breakdown and associated pain within the lateral column is well-accepted.

Stability of the calcaneocuboid joint (the outer half of the midtarsal joint) is determined by factors described in Chapter 23, the most important being heel position as dictated by subtalar joint position. If the foot is pronated during gait, calcaneocuboid joint stability is lost, allowing the lateral column to dorsiflex, evert, and abduct on the rearfoot. If the fourth and fifth metatarsals are unstable, similar movement occurs and the result is strain of the capsules and ligaments on the top of these joints. The cause of the "cuboid syndrome" is inherent biomechanical weakness of the foot. If the foot is highly unstable, normal walking may bring about symptoms. If the foot is more stable, worn shoes, severe jarring of the lateral column from running on hard surfaces, or trauma may instigate pain.

Pain of the "cuboid syndrome" is dull and deep and interferes with running and sometimes walking, but little pain is felt during nonweight bearing, unless swelling is present. A crippling type of pain often occurs when the patient arises from bed; such pain usually dissipates with ambulation. Pain becomes progressively worse with persistence of running.

On physical examination, palpation produces pain directly below the extensor digitorum brevis muscle belly on the dorsolateral aspect of the foot and more distally along the lateral column. This should not be mistaken for pain arising from the sinus tarsi or from a previous ankle sprain with injury to the anterior talofibular ligament. Pain occasionally spreads distally as far as the fifth toe. Joint movement through a full range is pain-free, and weight-bearing is necessary to bring about symptoms. Fractures should be ruled out radiographically. The subluxation of the cuboid is usually not apparent on X-rays. One should attempt to alleviate symptoms and then assess the mechanical causes. Runners should train to tolerance on soft surfaces and apply ice as necessary. Running shoes with superior heel counter-stability and good shock absorption are important. For runners with this problem, the author recommends Adidas, Tiger, and Etonic training shoe models. A ⅛- to ¼-inch heel lift in both shoes that artificially heightens the lateral column and reduces plantar fascia and Achilles tendon stress may be surprisingly effective. A tight Achilles tendon can strongly pronate the foot, so this should be stretched daily. Manipulation by trained personnel is worth trying. The patient should massage the painful site daily, and foot strapping may be used to stabilize the rearfoot and plantar fascia. If these measures relieve early symptoms, it is of diagnostic significance. If progress does not occur, other means to enhance foot stability may be required. A varus wedge or over-the-counter arch supports help control subtalar joint pronation and heel position. Some clinicians find that a silver dollar-sized ⅜-inch pad under the lateral arch reduces discomfort. If the latter modalities are employed, the heel lifts should be removed. When the therapeutic response continues to be less than optimal, and nonbiomechanical causes have been ruled out, functional orthotic devices made from neutral foot casts should prove successful. Rigid foot orthotics worn during sport and nonsport activities will establish dynamic foot stability that is often difficult to obtain by other means.

# Heel Spur Syndrome and Plantar Fasciitis

Heel and plantar fascial injuries are common complaints of runners. The high rate of injury is related to their important weight-bearing roles. The heel sustains the largest and most direct impact at heel contact, and the plantar fascia aids in maintaining the foot's arch during stance. Since running sports increase the foot's load three to five times that of walking, it is no wonder that injuries develop. Heel spur syndromes occur at the medial plantar tubercle of the calcaneus, where the plantar fascia originates; this is located at the distal plantar aspect of the heel medial to the center. The cause of heel spur syndrome has been attributed to tension or pull of the plantar fascia on the calcaneus. The continual pull causes the periosteum to become inflamed (periostitis), and subsequent calcification produces the radiologically evident heel spur. A bony spur does not have to be present to produce pain or the heel spur syndrome.

The same strain or pulling force within the fascia that causes the heel spur syndrome produces plantar fasciitis. Patients often describe fasciitis-type pain just previous to the onset of heel pain. Plantar fasciitis pain is usually in the center of the medial longitudinal arch but can occur in any area of the fascia. The mechanism of injury to both the heel and plantar fascia appears similar. In the author's practice, heel pain is more prevalent than fascial pain. Some athletes may associate plantar fasciitis pain with fallen arches or arch fatigue and not seek medical advice for the problem. Excessive foot pronation during gait predisposes to symptoms of fasciitis or heel spur. This foot type has a normal arch during nonweight bearing, but flattens out when the subject stands or walks. Excessive mobility and movement of the pronated foot appears to be more significant than the static arch height in producing symptoms. The congenital flat foot with little or no arch when the subject is sitting or standing is less likely to develop heel and arch symptoms.

The mechanics of foot pronation that precipitate plantar fasciitis begin at the subtalar joint. Subtalar joint pronation unlocks the midtarsal joint, causing the arch to sag and the foot to elongate. Elongation of the foot stretches the plantar fascia at the center of the arch or at its origin on the heel, this stretching eventually produces inflammation and pain. Examination for plantar fasciitis and heel spur syndrome shows tenderness to palpation in the arch or on the undersurface of the heel. Clinical signs of inflammation are generally not seen with either problem. Visible or palpable swelling may indicate acute injury.

Treatment for plantar fasciitis and heel spur syndrome is similar, since they have a common cause. If attention is sought soon after onset of symptoms, simple measures are likely to alleviate the complaint. If the condition is long-standing, however, quick recovery is less likely. Initial care should be directed at reducing inflammation in the acute stage.

Tape strapping of the foot to support the plantar fascia, if applied correctly, reduces symptoms immediately. A ¼-inch to ⅜-inch shock-absorbing heel lift in both shoes reduces plantar fascia tension and dissipates heel contact shock. The author prefers rubberized cork with a Spenco® top cover or ¼-inch Sorbathane®, and has not found that heel cups or heel pads with central cutouts reduce heel or arch pain. Street shoes with rigid shanks and firm heel counters should be worn during daily activities. If sports activities are allowed, cardboard-lasted shoes with good heel counter-control are preferred. Achilles stretches therapeutically stretch the plantar fascia and should be performed twice daily. If heel lifts are ineffective, attempts should be made to control foot pronation, using the same criteria for foot supports as for the cuboid syndrome. When abnormal foot mechanics are present in conjunction with chronic fasciitis or heel spur syndrome, the use of functional foot orthotics is mandatory. In the author's practice, the use of orthotic devices for chronic fasciitis is nearly 95% effective, and in heel spur syndrome, almost 85% effective.

# Achilles Tendonitis

The Achilles tendon and calf muscle provide foot plantar flexion and propulsion, and are frequently injured. Runners are especially prone to Achilles tendonitis, since their sport is unidirectional, requiring continuous propulsion from the calf and hamstring muscles. Muscular imbalance from inflexible calf muscles is the major cause of overuse Achilles injuries. Daily stretching of the calves and hamstrings is imperative to avoid injury. Calf and hamstring flexibility testing can identify athletes who are prone to Achilles injury. Subjects with tight Achilles tendons, whether acquired or congenital, tend to have an early heel-off or bouncy gait. When these people are injured, they should have heel lifts for their shoes to reduce the tension within the tendon.

Abnormal foot pronation may also precipitate Achilles tendonitis. The Achilles attachment on the heel tolerates an unlimited range of sagittal plane motion (caused by contraction of the tendon and its antagonist) and the small amount of frontal plane motion that normally occurs with foot pronation and supination. If the heel everts past normal ranges, however, it pulls on the tendon in two planes instead of one and the result is often injury.

The treatment for Achilles tendonitis should begin with calf muscle-stretching exercises. Achilles contractures may be divided into hereditary and acquired categories. This can be done by testing ankle dorsiflexion with the knee both extended and flexed. Hereditary deformities are usually associated with lack of dorsiflexion in both knee positions, and result from long-standing contractures of both the soleus and gastrocnemius muscles. Hereditary Achilles contractures respond poorly to stretching exercises, although they should be recommended. These athletes may perform more efficiently with heel lifts, whether or not they are injured. Clinicians should recommend icing and other physical therapy modalities as indicated. Shoes with good shock absorption and heel counter-control to lessen the shock of heel contact are recommended, and abnormal foot pronation should be controlled with appropriate wedging, arch supports and functional orthotic devices as necessary.

# Shin Splints

Historically, any athlete with pain between the knee and ankle was thought to have shin splints. The cause of shin splints was unknown and treatment was usually unsuccessful; many running careers were interrupted or terminated because of this problem. Today, sports physicians can classify leg injuries anatomically, and often are able to treat them successfully without interruption of training.

Each muscle compartment in the leg is separated by thick fascia and serves a specific locomotive function. If muscle balance is not maintained by proper training, one compartment may overpower another, resulting in overstress and injury. Shin splints may occur in either the anterior or posterior compartment. Either type results from pulling of the involved muscle away from its tibial origin. Anterior shin splints, an injury seen most often in beginning runners, affects the front of the leg on the outer side of the tibia. Posterior shin splints, the more common of the two injuries, occurs along the back and inside border of the tibia and affects more seasoned athletes.

The injured muscle responsible for posterior shin splints is the tibialis posterior. It originates on the medial side of the tibia and becomes tendon above the inside ankle bone (medial malleolus); it then makes a right angle turn around the medial longitudinal arch. The tibialis posterior muscle supports the arch and supinates the foot. Abnormal biomechanics leading to injury occur if the foot pronates excessively during gait. This motion places undue strain on the muscle tendon near its insertion. As the strain continues the pull is transmitted to the ankle bone (functioning as a pulley) and into the muscle belly where it pulls at its origin, the tibia. The tibial periosteum becomes inflamed from chronic tension and posterior shin splint pain ensues. Posterior shin splints also occur if the posterior compartment muscles are not stretched regularly. These muscles become progressively tighter and inflexible. Fast running on hard surfaces or poor footwear are, therefore, more likely to cause injury when the tightened muscles are strained. Posterior shin splint pain occurs along the lower mid-portion of the tibia, starting 3–4 inches above the medial malleolus. When the leg is straightened horizontally and the belly of the calf hangs freely, palpation along the tibia produces exquisite pain. Swelling may also be found. The swelling will be dispersed and soft if the injury is acute or subacute. If the nodules are firm, the injury is long-standing. There are no other clinical findings. Tibial stress fractures must not be mistaken for shin splints. They usually occur in the lower or upper one-third of the tibia and are associated with circumferential bone swelling.

Early treatment for posterior shin splints should include ice massage. A good method for application is freezing water in a styrofoam cup. The top inch of the cup is then peeled away and the denuded ice is used to massage along the length of painful bone. Ten to 15 min of ice massage twice daily, and especially after sports activity, is recommended. Athletes should stretch the posterior leg compartment (calf stretch), which includes the tibialis posterior muscle, three times per day. Foot dorsiflexion exercises strengthen the anterior compartment muscles and maintain equilibrium between compartments.

Foot structure of athletes with posterior shin splints should be evaluated and structural deformities that result in abnormal pronation should be supported. Varus wedges lessen the stress on the tibialis posterior muscle at heel contact, and a Morton's pad under the first metatarsal controls pronation during the propulsive phase of gait. Appropriate taping to support the arch may reduce the pronatory stretch on the effected muscle. If the severity of the structural abnormality of the foot and its relationship to injury is not clear, the above treatment may be used for diagnostic purposes. If foot support improves symptoms, the mechanical etiology is verified. Heel lifts can reduce the stress within the posterior compartment that occurs during walking or running. If heel lifts and arch supports or varus wedges are used together, heel lifts of lesser height should be placed under the heel of the supports or on top of the heel wedges. Running shoes should have superior heel counter stability. If biomechanical therapy fails and functional foot control is needed, rigid orthotic devices are the next step. These offer a favorable prognosis in selected patients.

Anterior shin splints result from overuse of the tibialis anterior muscle. This muscle originates from the upper lateral tibia, crosses the front of the ankle and attaches to the medial side of the foot. The function of the tibialis anterior muscle is to dorsiflex the foot at the ankle joint. During gait, the tibialis anterior muscle raises the foot during swing phase to allow toe clearance, and at heel contact, slowly lowers the forefoot to the ground preventing foot-slap.

In most cases, the cause of anterior shin splints is strictly from overuse and is not due to biomechanical abnormalities. Sports such as running produce muscle fatigue, and the tired muscle can no longer protect itself from injury. Tight calf muscles may contribute to anterior shin splint injury. The calves' antagonistic function adversely affects the tibialis anterior function and its ability to dorsiflex the foot. When more muscular effort is needed to resist the opposing pull of the calf muscle, the anterior leg muscles fatigue prematurely and injury results. Pain from anterior shin splints is felt along the mid-portion of the lateral tibia, and nodule formation may be present, as in posterior shin splints.

Pain and stiffness within the entire anterior compartment, but not necessarily along the bone, is a separate entity called "anterior compartment syndrome." The cause of this injury is the same as shin splints, although the pain results from muscle swelling in response to exercise instead of pulling of muscle from bone.

Treatment for anterior shin splints includes icing, stretching, and strengthening similar to that used for posterior shin splints. The anterior leg muscles should be stretched with forced plantar flexion of the foot. Running, speed, and stride length should be reduced and training should be on natural surfaces. Running shoes should be those that provide good midfoot shock absorption.

# Knee Injuries

Athletic knee injuries occur frequently, due to its principal role in providing body support and locomotion. Each knee must individually support and dissipate ascending forces from heel strike that may reach three to five times body weight. Local anatomic variation and faulty body posture most frequently contribute to injury. Knee injuries are usually traumatic or overuse in nature. Acute traumatic injuries will not be discussed.

Overuse knee injuries may involve the medial, anterior, lateral, and less often, the posterior aspects of the knee. Soft-tissue structures that cross the knee to lend support or provide motion may be injured, with the exception of the collateral ligaments that require a subluxatory force for damage to result. Knee ligament injury suggests the presence of a severe torque, trauma, or preexisting injury as the primary etiology. The biomechanical treatment of overuse knee injuries may be based on the location of pain. However, it is preferable to define the structure involved.

## Medial Knee Injuries

Medial knee injuries may involve the tendons making up the pes anserinus, which include the sartorius, semitendinosus, and gracilis. Repetitive valgus and rotatory stress from abnormal foot pronation and flat feet generally cause tendonitis and pain in these structures. Foot deformities resulting in abnormal foot pronation always result in simultaneous internal knee rotation (see Chapter 23). Excessive internal knee rotation during gait imposes a valgus torque that pulls on the medial knee tendons with each foot strike and often results in injury. The knee that has a structural valgus may sustain a similar injury. This knee type directs the body's center of mass to the inside of the feet, causing compensatory foot pronation that, in turn, rotates the knee. It is important to recognize and treat the primary deformity causing abnormal knee function. Athletes must be evaluated during weight bearing, nonweight bearing, standing still, and in motion.

Medial knee pain presents with pain to palpation at the insertion of the pes anserinus onto the medial tibial condyle and may also be present at the medial joint margin. Injuries to the medial collateral ligament, medial joint capsule, and medial meniscus must be ruled out. If palpatory pain is exquisite, bursal inflammation may be involved. Bursitis in areas of tendon insertion is an occasional finding with most types of overuse injuries. Knee bursitis must be differentiated from other soft-tissue injuries.

Range of motion testing of the knee is usually pain-free with medial knee pain. Forced adduction of the leg against resistance may produce pain in these patients. Pes anserinus tendonitis, in both acute and subacute stages, is cared for by icing and stretching. Biomechanical therapy should reduce rotational or valgus torque in the knee. Shoes with good tortional stability and heel counter-control are best. Varus heel wedges in running shoes relieve pain. Morton's pads under the forefoot control pronation during the propulsive phase of gait. If symptoms persist and foot pronation is significant, arch supports or functional orthotic devices should be tried.

# Anterior Knee Pain

Injuries resulting in anterior knee pain may involve the quadriceps and its retinacula, the patella, or patellar tendon. Since these structures function as a unit, injuries to them may be classified as extensor mechanism disorders. The patella enhances the power of the quadriceps by increasing the distance of the tendon from the knee's axis of motion, creating a greater lever arm and more efficiency in extending the knee. The V-shaped articulation between the patella and the femoral condyle prevents subluxation and controls patellar tracking within its groove. The quadriceps muscle extends the knee from a flexed position during the swing phase of gait and supports the knee in an extended position during heel contact. The four individual muscles that make up the quadriceps attach into the patella by retinacular fibers, and the patella attaches to the tibial tuberosity via the patellar tendon.

The quadriceps mechanism, particularly the patellofemoral joint, is highly susceptible to injury at heel contact. Ground-reactive forces tend to buckle the knee and must be adequately countered by the extensor mechanism. The quadriceps contracts firmly, driving the patella against the femur resulting in strong compressional forces between the two bones. If patellar tracking is altered by anatomic variants or by faulty extremity mechanics, injuries are apt to occur.

The most common athletic injury to the anterior knee is patellofemoral syndrome, characterized by pain and swelling within the patellofemoral joint. Bone or cartilaginous changes are not visible on arthroscopy or X-rays in the early stage of injury. As this injury progresses, erosion develops on the undersurface of the patella resulting in chondromalacia patellae. Treatment is more effective during the early stages of injury. Related injuries may affect the extensor retinaculum or patellar tendon. These injuries result from similar causes and respond to similar therapy. Pain within the quadriceps muscle may occur in those participating in ballistic sports and should be treated as a muscular injury. Tibial tuberosity pain in adolescents, consistent with Osgood-Schlatter disease, should be differentiated from overuse injury and treated accordingly. Pain within the patellofemoral joint may be due to structural deformities of the knee such as patella alta, patella baja, or an abnormally high Q angle. All of these deformities adversely affect patellar tracking within the femoral condylar grooves. Structural deformities either extrinsic or intrinsic to the foot, resulting in abnormal foot pronation, may contribute to patellofemoral disorders. Internal rotation of the knee initiated by foot pronation shifts the patella laterally in the femoral groove and may produce articular irritation. Knee alignment and Q angle should be examined during weight bearing and nonweight bearing, since functional disorders from biomechanical causes are not evident during nonweight bearing.

Patellofemoral pain should be evaluated with the athlete supine. The ankle is grasped and the knee is taken through a full range of motion, while lightly compressing the patella with the opposite hand, checking for crepitation throughout the range of motion. Next, the patella is compressed firmly with the knee in 160° of extension. The patient is asked to contract the quadriceps and the examiner feels for crepitation or pain. The examiner should palpate around the patella carefully, checking for discomfort. With the aid of appropriate testing to rule out the presence of other knee pathology, and a thorough history, the diagnosis of a patellofemoral disorder should be established.

Treatment includes reduction of sports activities to tolerance. Isometric strength-building exercises for the quadriceps should begin at once, with emphasis on the vastus medialis. Hamstring stretching is helpful in reestablishing muscular equilibrium between the posterior and anterior thigh muscles. The knee joint should be evaluated radiographically and appropriate measures instituted. The patella should be examined during static stance and throughout gait for internal positioning caused by excessive foot pronation. If abnormal pronation is present, proper shoes, varus wedges, and orthotic therapy is indicated.

## Lateral Knee Injuries

Overuse injuries to the lateral knee commonly affect the iliotibial band, popliteus tendon, or long head of the biceps femoris. Injuries near the insertion of the iliotibial band appear to be most common in runners. The popliteus tendon is near the iliotibial band on the lateral femoral condyle, so differentiation of injuries of these two structures may be difficult. Fortunately, treatment for popliteus tendonitis and iliotibial band syndrome are similar. Tendonitis of the biceps femoris at the head of the fibula, although located laterally, is best discussed with posterior knee complaints.

Mechanical stresses adversely affecting the lateral knee may result from structural deformities such as rigid pes cavus (high arched feet), rearfoot varus, and tibial varum (inverted positioning of the heel or leg, respectively). The shock of weight bearing in these conditions is directed laterally at the knee joint. Deformities of this nature apply a frontal plane traction of the lateral leg on the femur and result in repetitive stress to all lateral soft-tissue structures. Many of these deformities appear as bowed legs and, if viewed from behind the lower leg and heel, appear to be grossly inverted in relation to the floor. Gait analysis shows jarring at the knee and quadriceps and an abrupt heel contact. When the above-mentioned deformities are flexible and allow the foot to compensate with pronation, an internal rotatory torque is applied to the knee joint. The transverse plane torque resulting from excessive pronation of the foot twists the knee-supporting structures and promotes injury with each step. Twisting, pulling, and poor shock dissipation are, therefore, three components of injury that must be considered when treating lateral knee pain.

## Iliotibial Band Syndrome

The iliotibial band is a fascial structure that helps to stabilize the hip, thigh, and knee during heel contact. It originates proximally from the iliac crest where it is called fascia lata. The iliotibial band then descends along the lateral thigh to become tendon-like just above the knee where it attaches on the anterolateral tibia called Gerdes tubercle. The iliotibial band is easily seen by having the athlete extend the involved extremity. Injury occurs most often over the lateral femoral epicondyle, a bony prominence that contacts the iliotibial band during knee flexion and extension, and may produce inflammation around the band. To palpate this structure, the patient is asked to flex the knee joint approximately 20° and the examiner then compresses the epicondyle. In this position, the iliotibial band lies directly over the epicondyle and is usually painful. Palpation may also induce pain at its tibial insertion. Prolonged running aggravates pain in either of these two areas. Iliotibial band pain may radiate proximally, and fascia lata pain, particularly in females, may radiate distally. If pain is worse proximally, one should think of leg length discrepancy. Iliotibial band syndrome of the knee should be distinguished from pain within the lateral collateral ligament and other conditions involving internal knee derangement.

Iliotibial band syndrome responds well to icing. Specific stretches for the lateral thigh and hip, and strengthening exercises for thigh abductors are recommended. Running should be reduced to tolerance, and speed and stride length should be decreased. Athletes with rigid, high-arched feet should purchase running shoes with good heel and midsole shock absorption, and those who pronate excessively should use wedges and Morton's pads. Resistant cases may require functional orthotic devices.

## Posterior Knee Injuries

Injuries of the posterior aspect of the knee largely result from ballistic sports and sprinting. Muscle strains and tears are the most frequent injuries to the hamstrings. Tendonitis at the knee is common in distance runners and is nearly always related to poor flexibility. Therapeutic measures for these injuries include ice massage and stretching. Fast running and sprinting should be restricted. Biomechanical faults are rarely implicated in hamstring injuries.

# Chapter 25

# Physical Therapy in Maintenance of Athletic Performance

## by William J. O'Brien

The weekend athlete, the serious runner, and the professional athlete all have one thing in common: the biomechanical and physiologic characteristics of their bodies. In the resting state, the body displays certain biomechanical and physiological adaptations. Exercise by definition is a perturbation of the resting state, accompanied by its own physiologic and biomechanical adaptations to that perturbation.

## Stretching and Warmup

Since exercise is a form of stress, one must prepare the body for it. This requires a gradual warmup of 5 to 10 min that includes stretching of muscles to be exercised. Joint movement allows stretching of soft tissues—joint capsules, ligaments, and muscle, and spreads synovial fluid over the cartilage for lubrication to maintain it as a shock absorber during impact. Stretching muscles and tendons facilitates blood flow into the area, which "warms up" the peripheral nerves for better impulse conduction. The muscle spindles and joint receptors provide feedback information on muscle length and movement to the spinal cord and are "biased" to expect the changes in length and tension that accompany exercise.

The type of exercise dictates the style of warmup and stretching. A jogger or runner will place great demands on his hamstrings for deceleration. Therefore, emphasis must be placed on stretching the hamstrings.

Physical differences among individuals are expressed by the person's stance, gait, and sleeping posture. A person's unique posture predetermines the muscle groups that will be tight. If one sits most of the day, one will have tight hip flexors and hamstrings; special attention should, therefore, be given to stretching those muscles. Flexibility requires a stretching program based on knowledge of biomechanics and anatomy. No universal formula can be uniformly applied to all body types for all exercises.

After exercise, the body must cool off and return to its resting state gradually. Adequate cardiac output depends upon venous filling of the heart. During exercise, extremity muscular contraction and abdominal and thoracic movements facilitate venous return mechanically. When exercise stops, mechanical compression ceases abruptly while peripheral vasodilatation persists. Therefore, the venous return and, hence, cardiac output may fall to dangerously low levels. This usually causes ''dizziness'' and the person lies down which increases venous return and the ''dizziness'' clears. For similar reasons, one should not take a hot shower immediately after exercise.

Training specificity is well documented (Morehouse and Miller [1]); a sprinter trains by sprinting and a swimmer by swimming. An athlete's physical prowess is, however, determined by his or her vascular, biochemical, and muscular makeup, which is genetically determined. By training, optimum performance based on genetic potential can be achieved (Al-Amound et al. [2]; Peckham et al. [3]; Pette et al. [4]; Riley and Allin [5]; Salmons [6]; Salmons and Henriksson [7]). Most individuals have muscles that are heterogenous in fiber type, but are capable of adaptations in response to training (Salmons and Henriksson [7]).

# Training and Muscle Fiber Adaptations

A specific training program can be designed to stress and cause adaptation of the appropriate muscle fiber type. Rapid, large increases in tension require maximum effort for short time periods. This favors Type II—fast-twitch muscle fibers. An intense effort is needed to activate these fibers, a process that can be explained by Henneman's spinal neuron recruitment theory (Henneman et al. [8]). According to that theory, big motor units are innervated by large anterior horn cells that require a large excitatory input before they fire. These large motor units contain many muscle fibers that can rapidly increase tension with maximum effort. Because the smaller, slower motor units are already active, explosive anaerobic exercise stresses the fast-twitch motor units and are appropriate for weight lifting, sprinting, or similar activities.

Regular exercise increases oxidative enzymes and skeletal muscle mass. The former is evidenced histologically by increased numbers of mitochondria and greater capillary density, changes that facilitate oxygen delivery. Increased muscle fiber diameter that depends on the type of exercise program also occurs. Heavy resistance anaerobic exercises result in the greatest hypertrophy (Salmons and Henriksson [7]). Weight lifting is not only anaerobic exercise, but can also be a useful aerobic program.

# Application of Modalities

The physical therapist is often called upon to treat athletic injuries with heat or cold application or special exercises. During the acute phase of injury, cold is the modality of choice, since it slows local metabolic activity, decreases inflammation, and minimizes vasodilatation (Grant [9]; Gucker [10]). Reduced venous dilatation limits edema since the capillary bed hydrostatic pressure is influenced by venous pressure. Swelling can hide bony and ligamentous injuries; therefore, it is important to minimize it, using cold early. Cold also slows peripheral nerve conduction and decreases pain. A basic rule for modality application is that the area to which it is applied should have normal sensation and the patient should be capable of communicating his or her sensations to the person applying the modality.

Generalized soreness after exercise often improves with heat (Gucker [10]). Whirlpool therapy is relaxing and comfortable, but the high temperature can cause significant peripheral vasodilation that may interfere with adequate cardiac filling and hence cardiac output. A person going into the whirlpool must have recovered fully from exercise, e.g., have resting respiratory and heart rates.

Heat facilitates edema formation in dependent extremities and may make examination of an injured joint or bone difficult, but during healing, the vasodilatory effects of heat are beneficial. In chronic, noninflammatory athletic injury, heat is often used to increase local circulation (Gucker [10]) and tissue healing. Local heating modalities include whirlpool, hot packs, short-wave diathermy, microwave, or ultrasound (Grant [9]; Gucker [10]; Griffin and Karselis [11]; McCluskey et al. [12]).

On occasion, an injured extremity must be immobilized prior to moving the patient (McCluskey et al. [12]; Malone et al. [13]). This can be achieved by using prefabricated or air splints or even rolled magazines. Immobilization is important in fractures to prevent pain and vascular tears by boney fragments or nerve injury from compression or laceration. The injured extremity should be immobilized without compromising blood supply and should be kept elevated until examined by a physician. If a physician is not immediately available, the immobilized extremity can be cooled with ice packs. One should remember to inspect periodically.

Physical therapy of athletic injuries requires understanding of the principles stated earlier: cold application, inflammation and the associated pain and edema. It should not be used after the acute stage of injury. A good rule of thumb is if the injured part is warm, red, or swollen, elevate and cool. Once the injured area has passed through the acute warm, red, and swollen stage, circulation can be improved by warming (Gucker [10]).

Injuries are cooled by ice and water applied in plastic bags held in place with an elastic bandage. Elevation decreases pain, edema, and inflammation. The injured area should be examined periodically to prevent additional damage by the modality itself, and ice should be removed if the area becomes completely anesthetic. It should warm up until sensation returns. Generally, ice packs are applied for 15 to 20 min. Other means of applying cold include chemical cold generation packs, or fluoromethane spray.

Heat applications can be provided by a variety of modalities, from hot towels to pulsed short-wave diathermy. The depth of penetration ranges from superficial infrared and hot packs, to microwave, short-wave, pulsed-short-wave diathermies, and ultrasound, which provides the greatest depth of penetration (Griffin and Karselis [11]). The modality

**Table 25-1**   Heat Modalities

| Modality | Contraindications |
|---|---|
| Infrared<br>Hot Packs | Do not administer over "artificial hair" wigs<br>Diabetes or peripheral vascular disease<br>Areas of abnormal sensation |
| Microwave Diathermy<br>(2450 Megacycles [Mc]) | Areas of abnormal sensation<br>Diabetes or peripheral vascular disease<br>Metastatic disease<br>Obesity |
| Short Wave Diathermies<br>(13.56 and 27.12 Mc) | Areas of abnormal sensation<br>Diabetes or peripheral vascular disease<br>Metastatic disease<br>Metal in or on field |
| Ultrasound<br>(1 Mc) | Growth plates in bones of children<br>Do not administer directly over bone<br>Do not apply over stellate ganglion<br>Diabetes or peripheral vascular disease |

selected for heat application should be based on the area to be treated and patient comfort. Contraindications for various modalities are shown in Table 25-1.

The most common sports injuries referred to physical therapists involve the ankle, knee, elbow, and foot, and occasionally, the shoulder and back.

# Ankle Injuries

Ankle injuries are often seen first by orthopaedists or emergency room physicians. Physical therapy of ankle sprains depends upon the grade of the sprain. The basic management includes ice and elevation initially, followed by a graded exercise program. Grade I sprains should be taped to limit subtalar motion, inversion, and eversion. The patient should be taught a partial weight-bearing gait with the aid of crutches, and the ankle should be elevated and iced, when the patient is not walking, for 3 to 5 days (McCluskey et al. [12]; Connolly [14]; Starkey [15]).

Grade II sprains should be taped, iced, elevated, and the patient mobilized with a partial weight-bearing gait and crutches (McCluskey et al. [12]; Connolly [14]; Starkey [15]).

Grade III sprains require cold, compression, elevation, and massage and, occasionally, surgical repair of ruptured ligaments. The patient is often fitted with a below-knee, short-leg cast. Partial weight-bearing ambulation with crutches is permitted (McCluskey et al. [12]; Connolly [14]; Starkey [15]).

Nonoperated cases are treated with ankle exercises alternating with elevation and icing. The exercises for eversion, inversion, dorsiflexion, and extension are at first isometric and progress to full resistive exercises as the patient's condition improves. Commercial exercise devices are available to strengthen the muscles that move the ankle joint. An inner tube can be cut to shape to be used throughout the day. The uninjured foot anchors one end of the rubber loop and the injured foot inserted into the other end pushes, pulls, inverts, or everts against the resistance of the rubber.

Complete rehabilitation of a severe ankle sprain can take 4 to 8 months and requires motivation of the patient to achieve full range of motion (McCluskey et al. [12]; Connolly [14]; Starkey [15]). Rehabilitation consists of an ankle range-of-motion exercise against resistance followed by elevation and icing if post-exercise swelling occurs (McCluskey et al. [12]; Connolly [14]; Starkey [15]).

Isokinetic testing on a Cybex® machine allows comparison of work performance of the muscles of the injured ankle with those of the uninjured side and objectively measures progress before permitting the patient to return to athletics.

# Knee Injuries

Knee injuries are common in contact sports like football. However, significant knee damage can also occur in dancers and runners, is often accompanied by pain and swelling, and accounts for many referrals to physical therapists (Davies et al. [16]).

The biomechanical complexity of the knee joint leads to significant problems when the joint is unstable (Derscheid and Malone [17]; McLeod and Hunter [18]).

The basic management of acute knee injuries includes elevation, icing, compression, and ambulation with use of crutches and partial weight bearing. After surgical procedures, 6–8 weeks of immobilization with a cylinder cast or cast brace and nonweight-bearing walking with the aid of crutches may be necessary followed by graded institution of a full resistive exercise program. To permit active knee motion is a difficult decision because the longer the joint is immobilized, the more difficult it is to obtain full range of motion.

For knee sprains accompanied by pain and joint effusion, elevation, compression-wrap, and ice for 3 to 5 days or until the knee is no longer warm or swollen are indicated (Connolly [14]; Derscheid and Malone [17]). During this time, patients should perform isometric quadriceps exercises and straight-leg raising throughout the day. Following the acute phase, if significant joint damage has not occurred, active range of motion exercises on a stationary bicycle and/or exercise table may be started. Initially after each bout of exercise, the knee is elevated and iced; later it is elevated and iced only if the exercise causes pain and edema. If active range of motion is tolerated, the patient may then progress on an exercise table, bicycle, or isokinetic exercise device like the Orthotron® or Fitron®. Joint instability may be increased by the use of free weights.

Patients with surgically treated knee injuries should be instructed preoperatively in isometric quadriceps exercises, and these should be done for 5 to 10 min every hour postoperatively (Connolly [14]).

Patients should then be taught partial or nonweight-bearing ambulation with crutches depending on operative procedure. The postoperative knee can also be elevated and iced. Gentle active range of motion exercises are in order about 10 days postoperatively, depending on the surgical procedure. Active knee exercises followed by icing, if necessary, may then progress to full resistive exercises with the above-mentioned equipment. Maximum exercise with minimum pain and edema is a measure of progress. Knee function can be evaluated objectively by Cybex® testing and comparison with the contralateral healthy side. The power output ratio of the quadriceps to the hamstrings is an important guide for return to active sports. When this is favorable and range of motion is full, the patient should again be able to participate successfully in athletic activities.

The reestablishment of quadriceps and hamstring power is often the major goal of rehabilitation. Joint flexibility of both the knee and proximal and distal joints must be maintained by stretching exercises. The hip flexors, abductors, extensors, and adductors are best gently stretched by using positions that isolate these muscles. Special attention should be paid to obtaining a full range of motion at the ankle, and the gastrocnemius group may be stretched by passive foot dorsiflexion; i.e., face a wall and place the palms against the wall, back away with knees and hips straight so that by leaning against the wall, body weight stretches the posterior calf muscles.

# Elbow Injuries

Elbow injuries have escalated with the increase in popularity of racketball, tennis, and golf. Previously, most elbow injuries occurred in baseball players.

The typical elbow injury is from overuse. In baseball pitching, a valgus thrust to the arm results in medial collateral ligament stress and injury (Connolly [14]). A top-spin forehand in tennis places great demand on the forearm extensors to decelerate forearm pronation, and the racket weight stresses wrist extensors as the follow-through tends to flex the wrist.

Acute overuse elbow injuries are treated with elevation, ice, compression, and rest. Active elbow motion may be resumed as the pain, swelling, and heat subside.

Nonoperative management of elbow overuse also includes taping to restrict wrist movement, and support of the medial and lateral collateral ligaments with tape or special elastic bands.

Resistive exercises followed by icing for the first few weeks strengthen the muscles originating from both medial and lateral epicondyles. Specific resistive exercises for the forearm pronators (pronator teres and quadratus) and supinator include use of a hammer or a rotational exercise device. Most elbows nonsurgically treated for overuse improve within 6 to 8 weeks.

# Foot Injuries

Injuries to ligaments and muscles of the feet occur more often today because of the increased popularity of running. A common problem is calcaneus spurs. These bony elongations of the calcaneus resemble a bird's beak, and mark the origin of the long plantar ligament of the foot. They are acutely painful to palpation, and may be treated with phonophoresis of 5%-10% hydrocortisone cream. Ultrasound is less painful, and a good response can be expected after six to eight 10-min treatments. Arch support with padding over the painful area and stretching exercises for the gastrocnemius soleus muscle group are recommended.

# Shoulder Injuries

Common shoulder injuries result from falling on the outstretched arm or from an acute exacerbation of bursitis. Acromial separations can be managed with ice and a figure-eight bandage and/or an arm sling. Ice is applied when the shoulder is swollen and hot. After the acute inflammation subsides, simple active range of motion exercises can be done. Initially, the patient can let the arm hang and gently swing it to and fro ("Codman's" exercises), and then should progress to active shoulder motion using a shoulder wheel, wall ladder or simple overhead pulleys. If the shoulder remains painful after exercise, icing may be necessary. Resistive shoulder exercises using weights, pulleys, or isokinetic apparatus are the next step. Resistance is applied to the internal and external rotators, the shoulder abductors, flexors, and extensors. When the patient performs these exercises without pain, he or she may return to previous activities. Power can be measured with a Cybex® isokinetic testing unit and compared with power output curves of the uninjured side.

# Back Injuries

Most acute back injuries result from occupational activities superimposed upon bad postural habits, and rarely occur in athletes. The lumbosacral fascia and paravertebral muscles shorten with longstanding lordosis and failure to stretch them. In this situation, even a minor twist may cause severe and long-lasting pain.

Application of ice packs or ice massage usually relieves acute muscle spasm, but to correct the long-standing problem, education of the patient is needed. Once the spasm, swelling, and pain resolve, gentle exercises to increase back flexibility are in order. These include classic Williams flexion exercises to stretch paravertebral and hamstring muscles, along with strengthening of abdominal muscles. Obesity aggravates back pain by perpetuating poor posture; proper body weight minimizes the stress placed on the back. Heat modalities such as whirlpool, hot packs, diathermy, and/or ultrasound can be used after the acute phase in conjunction with massage to gently stretch and relax the paravertebral muscles. Combined electric stimulation and ultrasound Medco-sonlator® are often relaxing during recovery.

Paravertebral muscles should be strengthened to support the vertebral column. Situps with knees and hips flexed are good abdominal strengthening exercises and half a twist can be added as the patient progresses. Back extension exercises are as follows: the patient lies across several tightly rolled pillows and extends the upper trunk. Hip extensors can be strengthened by extending one leg at a time with progression to extension of both legs as they get stronger.

# Preventing Injury

The key to prevention of injuries is flexibility and balanced power between opposing muscle groups. If the body is structurally sound, it will work well as long as it is in balance with the forces acting on it. It is that balance that physical therapy endeavors to maintain or restore.

# References

1. Morehouse, L.E., Miller, A.T. 1976. Skill development. In: Physiology of Exercise, 7th Ed. C.V. Mosby Co., St. Louis, pp 287–288.

2. Al-Amound, W.S., Buller, A.J., Pope, R. 1973. Long-term stimulation of cat fast-twitch skeletal muscle. Nature 244:225–227.

3. Peckham, P.H., Mortimer, J.T., Vander Meulen, J.P. 1973. Physiologic and metabolic changes in white muscle of cat following induced exercise. Brain Res 50:424–429.

4. Pette, D., Smith, M.E., Staudte, H.W., Vrbova, G. 1973. Effects of long-term electrical stimulation on some contractile and metabolic characteristics of fast rabbit muscles. Pfleugers Arch 338:257–272.

5. Riley, D.A., Allin, E.F. 1973. The effects of inactivity, programmed stimulation and denervation on the histochemistry of skeletal muscle fibre types. Exp Neurol 40:391–413.

6. Salmons, S. 1967. An implantable muscle stimulator. J Physiol (Lond) 188:13.

7. Salmons, S., Henriksson, J. 1981. The adaptive response of skeletal muscle to increased use. Muscle Nerve 4:94.

8. Henneman, E., Somjen, G., Carpenter, D.O. 1965. Functional significance of cell size in spinal motoneurons. J Neurophysiol 28:560–580.

9. Grant, A.E. 1964. Cold: Massage with ice (cryokinetics). Arch Phys Med 45:233–238.

10. Gucker, T. 1965. Heat: The use of heat and cold in orthopaedics. In: Licht, S. (ed): Therapeutic Heat and Cold. Elizabeth Licht, New Haven, pp 398–406.

11. Griffin, J.E., Karselis, T.C. 1982. The infra red energies; ultraviolet light; ultrasound energy. In: Physical Agents for Physical Therapists, 2nd Ed. Charles C Thomas, Springfield, Ill., pp 177–309.

12. McCluskey, G.M., Blackburn, T.A., Jr., Lewis, T.A. 1976. A treatment for ankle sprains. Am J Sports Med 4:158–161.

13. Malone, T.R., Blackburn, T.A., Wallace, L.A. 1980. Knee rehabilitation. Phys Ther 60(12):1602–1609.

14. Connolly, J.F. 1981. Mechanisms of Injuries: The Management of Fractures and Dislocations. W.B. Saunders Co., Philadelphia, pp 1802–1808.

15. Starkey, J.A. 1976. Treatment of ankle injuries by simultaneous use of intermittent compression and ice packs. Am J Sports Med 4:142–144.

16. Davies, G.J., Wallace, LA., Malone, T.R. 1980. Mechanisms of selected knee injuries. Phys Ther 60(12):1590–1595.

17. Derscheid, G.L., Malone, T.R. 1980. Knee disorders. Phys Ther 60(12):1582–1589.

18. McLeod, W.D., Hunter, S. 1980. Biomechanical analysis of the knee: Primary functions as elucidated by anatomy. Phys Ther 60(12):1561–1565.

# Chapter 26

# Equipment for Sports

## by Art Gardenswartz

Improvements in equipment have kept pace with changes in recreation. With increased leisure time, people are devoting more energy to hobbies, sports, and other pleasures. Athletic equipment has changed radically in the last 10 years, reflecting the boom in sports in our society, and in particular, the boom in specialty sports. Participants have demanded and been granted dramatic improvements in equipment.

## The Changing Sports Scene

During the 1970s, one of the fastest growing consumer demands in the United States was for recreational equipment, clothing, and services. Between 1970 and 1980, recreational expenditures in this country increased from 41 billion dollars to 106.4 billion dollars, or a 260% jump. During this period the percentage of total personal income expended for recreational purposes increased to a high of 6.8% in 1975 (Fig. 26–1). Since then, the percentage has fluctuated between 6.4% and 6.8%. This leveling-off is likely the result of inflation and the need for individuals to spend a greater part of their income on necessities. That Americans have placed greater value on outdoor recreation is indicated in Table 26–1 which shows that recreational expenditures are climbing when discretional spending growth is near zero, as was the case in 1961, 1970, and 1974. Many consumers have become accustomed to a particular level of physical activity and are reluctant to reduce it even in the face of income decline or increased living costs.

In 1965, all tennis rackets were wood. Today, there are at least five different types of rackets: wood, graphite, fiberglass, composite, and metal (aluminum and steel). There are internally and externally strung rackets. Tennis in the United States has grown from less than 5 million participants in the mid-1960s to 25 million in the late 1970s.

The increasing number of individuals involved in participant, as opposed to spectator, sports has been a significant factor in the improvement of equipment in many sports. Prior to 1970, athletic participation was limited to junior high, high school, and college

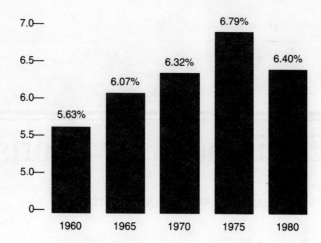

**26–1** Recreation as a percentage of total personal consumption expenditures, 1960–1980. (From Oshman's Sporting Goods. 1981. Oshman's Sporting Goods 1981 Annual Report and 10-Year History. Houston. Reprinted with permission.)

populations, with relatively few active participants over the age of 25. At that time, most Americans were content to watch younger people compete. Now, there are almost monthly increases in active participants in racquetball, running, tennis, cross-country skiing, slow pitch softball, soccer, and hiking. Little or no growth has occurred in sports that require less activity, such as golf, hunting, fishing, or organized football, and yet improved technology has altered performance and safety in these sports also (Monthly Sports Census [1]).

The most dramatic increase in participation has been the running/jogging boom throughout the world. For example, there were about 100,000 runners in 1968 in the U.S.A., but by 1979 the number had increased to 27 million (Cooper [2]).

Running has changed from a conditioning activity for another sport to a sport in its own right. The 270-fold growth in running appealed to business interests in our society, and shoe companies became interested in developing products for consumers who engaged in running. As a consequence, running shoes have improved dramatically in the last several years. In 1968, two large European manufacturers of athletic shoes were in competition with each other. American manufacturers made a tremendous effort and today new American companies are more important in supplying the American market.

Every sport has its own shoe type—basketball, tennis, racquetball, football, baseball, soccer, wrestling, hiking, golf, etc.—but shoes are 90% of the required equipment for runners and are of two types, training and racing. The main purposes of the running shoe are comfort, protection from injury, and cushioning. There is no simple answer to the question, "What is the best running shoe?" A number of variables should be considered: weight of the shoe, speed of the runner, toe or heel impact, running style, and degree of pronation. These variables determine whether one does best with shoes of greater shock absorbency or more flex. A jogger (a person whose pace is 8.5–11 min/mi) strikes heel first; for him, the heel shock absorbence of his shoe is more important than flex or forefoot shock absorbence. With increasing running speeds (6–7 min/mi), heel shock absorbence is less important and forefoot cushion and flex are more important. A heavier person

**Table 26–1**    Recreation Expenditures and Discretionary Spending in the U.S., 1961–1981.*†

| Year | Discretionary Spending ($ Billions) | % Change Previous Year | Recreation Expenditures ($ Billions) | % Change Previous Year | Recreation Expenditures as % of Discretionary Income |
|------|------|------|------|------|------|
| 1981 | $705.1 (E) | 6.14% | $122.4 (E) | 15.0% | 17.36% |
| 1980 | 664.3 | 2.94 | 106.4 | 7.4 | 16.02 |
| 1979 | 645.6 | 23.34 | 99.1 | 8.7 | 15.35 |
| 1978 | 523.3 | 18.21 | 91.2 | 12.3 | 17.43 |
| 1977 | 442.7 | 8.71 | 81.2 | 11.2 | 18.34 |
| 1976 | 407.2 | 20.44 | 73.0 | 9.8 | 17.93 |
| 1975 | 338.1 | 5.39 | 66.5 | 9.1 | 19.67 |
| 1974 | 320.8 | 1.90 | 60.9 | 10.3 | 18.98 |
| 1973 | 314.8 | 12.22 | 55.2 | 12.4 | 17.53 |
| 1972 | 280.5 | 11.57 | 49.1 | 12.4 | 17.50 |
| 1971 | 251.4 | 8.22 | 43.7 | 12.3 | 17.38 |
| 1970 | 232.3 | − .01 | 41.0 | 7.5 | 17.65 |
| 1966 | 190.4 | 8.55 | 28.9 | 9.9 | 15.18 |
| 1961 | 129.9 | − .05 | 19.5 | 6.6 | 15.01 |

†Source: *A Guide to Consumer Markets,* 1980/1981. Conference Board Report and July issues of the *Survey of Current Business.* (E) = estimate.
*From Oshman's Sporting Goods. 1981. Oshman's Sporting Goods 1981 Annual Report and 10-Year History. Reprinted with permission.

needs more heel cushion than one who weighs less. Other qualities to consider are heel control and flexibility.

The best way to select a running shoe is to look at independent test results of heel cushioning, forefoot cushioning, and stability, in conjunction with biomechanical knowledge of one's own lower limbs.

America leads in recreational product manufacture. We have a great deal of leisure time, and consider recreation a necessity, not a luxury. We are "health conscious." An example of how the world market is oriented toward the American customer is seen in suppliers of equipment and clothing for skiing. The world population of skiers is approximately 50 million; 10 million of those are in the United States. Ski shops in Europe give little floor space to equipment, but are mostly concerned with fashion. Montebelluno, in Italy, makes 75% of the world's ski boots. Italian ski boot companies market for the American consumer even though their biggest sales are elsewhere. American consumers have become more sophisticated, spend more money, and, because the equipment is of great importance to them, are more conscious of its value. If a product sells successfully in America, the rest of the world will follow in purchasing that particular product.

The sociologic importance of athletic participation has influenced pricing practices both in the U.S. and abroad. In established sports, it is no longer acceptable, for example, to use cheap equipment even though it might be just as serviceable. Counterculture trends, however, particularly among runners, are apparent, and a big toe showing through the top of a worn running shoe may be the mark of a tough long-distance runner.

# Technological Improvements

Technologic improvements have changed equipment dramatically. In addition to new materials, new design and the computer have made their marks.

Regarding materials, graphite is a carbon-based material more responsive, stronger, and lighter in weight than fiberglass that is being used increasingly in sports equipment manufacture. Fishing rods made of graphite are significantly changing fly fishing, where timing is important. Graphite is also used in water- and snow skis. Graphite ski poles are stronger and lighter and are now standard in cross-country ski racing. As a further example of improvements in materials, fiberglass bowling balls are replacing the rubber and plastic balls.

Wind resistance is a drawback in timed competitions. Improvements reducing wind resistance include the use of skin-tight Lycra suits in downhill and cross-country ski suits, speedskating, running, and bicycling. Swimming trunks and caps of Lycra decrease water resistance in swimming competition. These new garments are, however, three times more expensive than conventional attire, and last only half as long. Bike components and frames are also made specially to decrease wind resistance.

In other clothing for sports, Gortex, a waterproof, yet breathable material, has proven excellent for outdoor clothing for camping and backpacking, tents, sleeping bags, warm-up suits for bikers, and protective suits for runners in bad-weather conditions.

In terms of equipment design, tennis racket design has changed from the old 75 square inches to new rackets with well over 115 square inches of hitting surface. Most expert, recreational, and weekend players perform better with the larger racket.

The compound bow in archery, experimental only 4 years ago, has now outdated the usual long bow. This design improvement uses a system of pulleys, cams, and levers that facilitate the draw and allow faster and more powerful release of the arrow.

Integrated boots and bindings for downhill skiing are an innovation that has made skiing safer by providing more stability and edge control. Integrated bindings designed for cross-country ski racing are more flexible and weigh less.

The aluminum baseball bat is now produced with a crooked handle that allows the bat to be in front of the wrist when contact is made with the ball, thus improving the delivery of power.

Design changes in golf equipment have occurred rapidly and include tapered and fluted golf shafts, low profile graphite or aluminum irons, and dimpled golf balls.

Not surprisingly, computers are making inroads in sports manufacturing. For example, computers help in the design and manufacture of some skis that are made with a foam injection system. The computer is used to vary the density of the foam, which changes the flex of the ski to best fit its length. Computers are also used in sole design for running shoes, therefore samples no longer need be handmade.

# Aspects of Consumer Buying

Most American sports participants tend to over-equip themselves, thereby creating a huge market for sports commodities. This tendency gives manufacturers incentive to improve the quality and also fashion aspects of their products.

Serious athletes will go to almost any extreme to improve their sport even slightly. For example, a golfer may spend double the amount of money for golf balls to get three to five yards more per stroke. Or a cyclist will spend $300 to $500 to obtain a bike that is two to three pounds lighter.

Since recreational equipment is often used in a social setting, a particular brand of golf balls, tennis racket, or running shoes may be purchased, more to increase one's self-esteem than perhaps performance.

These aspects of consumer buying encourage manufacturers to make more sophisticated equipment and to market to sophisticated needs. As business and budgets improve, manufacturers, in turn, are engaging in more research. For example, Nike, Inc. was projected to spend 7 to 10 million dollars on research and development in 1982. Their research has produced several patented items, including Air Sole®, a sealed chamber of air inside running and basketball shoes that improves cushion. Nike, Inc. has also designed running shoes for runners of various weights.

## Sports Popularity Cycles

A definite pattern or cycle exists for a sport, from its infancy to maturation, and the accompanying equipment changes drastically during this time. For example, running, racquetball, and tennis each quadrupled in participants within 5 years. During the initial phase of popularity of a sport, a demand for inexpensive equipment exists. As the sport matures and popular interest subsides, participants become more sophisticated and demand higher-quality merchandise. For example, little demand exists today for cheap jogging shoes, cheap racquetball rackets, or cheap prestrung tennis rackets. In 1981, for instance, the best-selling racquetball racket in the United States was the Electalon 250G that retailed from $90 to $105. This racket is a combination of graphite and fiberglass and offers many advantages over cheaper rackets. When demand for a product is high, manufacturers have incentive to improve it. Wind surfing, on the other hand, is a sport in its infancy; consequently, the bigger market for windsurfing or sailboards is at the lower end of the price structure. Eventually, as the market saturates with entry level equipment, the sport will mature and participants will demand more exotic, high quality, and performance-oriented equipment.

Seldom does a sporting goods product last for more than 2 years before another, more functional and fashionable version appears that replaces it.

As both amateur and professional sports enthusiasts demand more from their equipment, technology and industry respond with increasingly sophisticated and individualized equipment. Innovations in sports equipment respond not only to increasingly higher levels of athletic performance, but also to the consumer's growing awareness of and concern for health and safety.

# References

1. Monthly Sports Census. 1979. The sporting goods dealer December: 11–19.
2. Cooper, K. 1979. Runner's World December: 23–29.
3. Oshman's Sporting Goods 1981 Annual Report and 10-year History.

# Index